Child Health

Care of the Child in Health and Illness

Anne Keene

Stanley Thornes (Publishers) Ltd

First published in 1999 by:
Stanley Thornes (Publishers) Ltd
Ellenborough House
Wellington Street
CHELTENHAM
GL50 1YW
United Kingdom

99 00 01 02 03 / 10 9 8 7 6 5 4 3 2 1

A catalogue record for this book is available from the British Library.

ISBN 0 7487 3651 4

Typeset by Columns Design Ltd, Reading
Printed and bound in Great Britain
by Redwood Books, Trowbridge, Wiltshire

Contents

Biographical note

Anne Keene, MA, comes from a background of nursing, midwifery and Health Visiting. Until 1998 she managed childcare programmes at Basford Hall College. She has now established MTW International, a childcare training and recruitment agency, which aims to recruit high quality childcare workers for families, childcare establishments, out of school clubs and playschemes. The agency also provides a range of traditional and customised training in the childcare field. Services to business include advice and guidance in establishing on-site childcare facilities and assistance in meeting the individual childcare needs of their employees.

She can be contacted at MTW International at:

Rothesay
10 Bromley Road
West Bridgford
Nottinghamshire
NG2 7AP
Tel: 0115 9811 566
email: annekeene @mtwcarers.demon.co.uk
website: www.mtwcarers.demon.co.uk

Acknowledgements

I am indebted to all the childcare students who have, over many years, taught me how to make information accessible to them.

Thanks to Irene Tipping for the use of several photographs of young children at play.

Many thanks to my family – Paul, Ryan, Hayley and Chloe – for their patience and humour during the production of this book. Special thanks to Hayley for the 'Get back to work' screensaver which appeared after two minutes of keyboard inactivity, and kept me 'on task'!

The author and publishers are grateful to the following for permission to reproduce copyright material:

- Dorling Kindersley for permission to reproduce the symptoms charts on pages 138–9, 144–5, 146–7 and 160–1, from Valman, Bernard, *The British Medical Association Children's Symptoms*, Dorling Kindersley, 1997.
- Working Party on Personal Child Health Records for permission to reproduce the *Contents page of a Personal Child Health Record* (page 109)
- Professor Barry McCormick, Children's Hearing Assessment Centre Nottingham, for permission to reproduce the form *Can your baby hear you?* (page 98)
- Nottingham Community Health NHS Trust for permission to reproduce *Be Safe in the Sun* (page 237)
- Royal College of General Practitioners for permission to reproduce the cover of *You and Your GP at Night and Weekends* (1997), published by the Royal College of General Practitioners, London (page 119)
- Her Majesty's Stationery Office for permission to reproduce *The Safety Challenge* (page 5) and *Reduce the Risk of Cot Death* (page 58): Crown copyright is reproduced with the permission of the Controller of Her Majesty's Stationery Office
- UK Growth Standards, © Child Growth Foundation for permission to reproduce the percentile charts (pages 111–13).
- The Health Education Authority for permission to reproduce the leaflets *Enjoy Fruit & Veg* (page 5); *Weaning Your Baby* (page 12); *Sexual Health Matters* (page 13); *Drinking for Two* (page 46); and *Keeping Baby Teeth Healthy* (page 52).

Photo credits
- Great Ormond Street Hospital – Rubella rash, Chickenpox rash (plate 1); Tonsillitis (plate 3).
- St. John's Institute of Dermatology – Chickenpox (plate 1); Urticaria, Impetigo, Eczema, Psoriasis, Tinea pedis (athlete's foot), Tinea capitis (ringworm) (plate 2); Warts, Verrucae (plate 3), Port-wine stain (plate 4).
- John Radcliffe Hospital, Oxford – Scabies (plate 3).
- Science Photo Library – Koplik's spots (plate 1); Jaundice (plate 4).
- Wellcome Trust – Mumps (page 200); Measles, Meningococcal rash (plate 1); Otitis externa, Dental caries, Oral thrush (plate 3); Foreign body in cornea, Mongolian blue spot, Rhinovirus (common cold), Influenza virus (plate 4).

Introduction

This book is presented in three parts covering all aspects of child health.

- **Part One** concentrates on the positive aspects of children's health and how to keep children healthy.
- **Part Two** describes the signs and symptoms of illness and explains how to detect early signs of illness in children, continuing with detailed descriptions of several conditions which may affect children. To enable the book to be used as an easy reference tool a simple format of headings has been used in this part: 'What is . . .?', 'What causes . . . ?', 'How to recognise. . .', 'Immediate action', 'Ongoing care', 'Possible complications', and 'Further information'.
- **Part Three** examines aspects of caring for children with acute and chronic illnesses, and explains the support services that are available for children and families.

The following features, spread throughout the book, have been used to assist readers and users of the text.

- **Good practice** points are made to help students and childcare workers to provide the most appropriate care.
- **Remember** points stress important information that students and professionals should not forget in certain situations.
- **Case studies** help understanding by describing actual scenarios.
- **Activities** encourage students to further their understanding by applying what they have read and learnt to different situations; or to conduct further research.
- **Progress checks** at regular intervals throughout the book contain questions for students to answer. The answers are contained in the previous section.

This approach makes the book a valuable resource for students following childcare programmes. It caters for the child health aspects of a range of courses such as CACHE DNN, CCE, ADCE, NVQ 2 and 3 Early Years and NVQ 2, 3 and 4 Playwork, EDEXCEL (BTEC) National Diploma in Childhood Studies, and GNVQ options covering childcare.

Childcare workers in any establishment will find *Child Health* to be an invaluable reference book. The colour photographs, combined with descriptions of childhood diseases, will assist them in identifying conditions and will also reinforce their own knowledge and skills.

I hope that this text generates further enthusiasm for keeping children healthy and provides some helpful information about the role of childcare staff in this endeavour.

Part 1: The Healthy Child

Part One highlights the importance of keeping children healthy. Child health promotion, including health surveillance and childhood screening, is explained in detail. The role of childcare workers in maintaining and improving the health and well-being of children in their care is also detailed. Childcare workers, together with parents and health professionals, are part of a large team whose aim is to encourage children to flourish and achieve their potential. Knowledge of the services available to children, the screening programme in childhood and the role of health care professionals will enable childcarers to work in partnership with parents and support health professionals. There are many influences on child health and it is important for carers to know how they can affect growth and development. Although carers may not have the power to change some of the negative factors, they can provide a positive influence on the health and well-being of children in their care.

Understanding how diseases are transmitted and how the spread of infection can be minimised will increase awareness in students and professional carers. By providing consistently high standards of care in safe, secure and stimulating environments, children can grow and develop to their full potential.

Chapter 1 Keeping children healthy: the prevention of illness

This chapter includes:
- Health promotion
- Child health surveillance
- Disease prevention
- Health education
- Health education in childcare establishments
- Meeting needs
- A holistic approach to child health

There are references in this chapter to 'Chapter 4, Screening' and 'Chapter 5, Health care professionals' which should also be consulted.

There are many important factors involved in maintaining children's health and keeping them safe from illness. Identifying and meeting the needs of children, both as individuals and in group situations, will promote development and encourage a sense of security and well-being. Childcare workers have a unique professional role, because as they stimulate the whole child they are also meeting the child's physical, social, emotional and health needs. Children cared for in a climate of health awareness are more likely to adopt healthy lifestyles themselves.

This chapter explores the concept of health promotion related to children, including the value of national health promotion campaigns and providing ideas of how to put these policies into practice.

Childcare establishments and individual childcarers can have an impact on the health of the children in their care. By providing routines and activities which increase knowledge and understanding of good health for both adults and children they can heighten awareness and enrich the lives of children.

This includes the necessity for offering accurate information about the risks associated with certain child-rearing practices, and enabling informed decision-making on the part of parents and carers. Parents and childcare workers together provide healthy patterns for life.

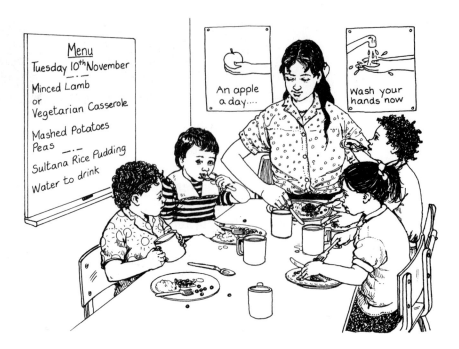

Dinner time in the nursery

Health promotion

Health promotion means encouraging positive and healthy lifestyles by promoting good health practices. It aims to help everyone to understand how to keep fit and healthy by identifying areas of risk and dealing with them appropriately. It is also concerned with the environment and how it can be changed or adapted to improve the general health of the population and the well-being of individuals.

Health promotion is not only the responsibility of statutory authorities but can be assisted by every person who cares for and takes an interest in others, including childcare workers and teachers.

Health promotion aims to:

- change government health policy where necessary
- promote the positive aspects of improving and maintaining health.

Child health promotion

Child health promotion is an umbrella term which includes:

- child health surveillance – a programme of care to monitor children's health and prevent illness
- health education – the education of parents and carers about child health, growth and development
- screening – the examination of apparently healthy children to find those who probably do have a condition from those who probably do not (see Chapter 4).

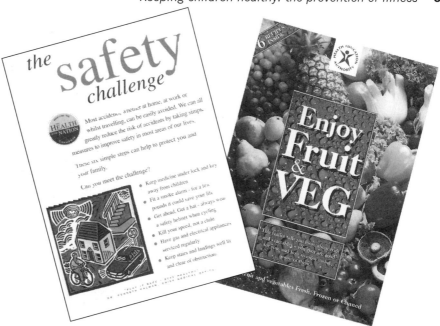

Samples of current health
promotion leaflets

Strategies to improve health in children are performed mainly by
members of the primary health care team, assisted by the school health
service, dentists and other health care professionals (see Chapter 5).
Health visitors are the only health workers who routinely and regularly see
children from 0 to 5 years regardless of their health status (see page 121).

Good Practice

Childcare workers should take every available opportunity to promote
positive health practices. They should:
- respect and value the views of parents and their child-rearing
  practices
- be effective role models for healthy lifestyles
- observe children at regular intervals to monitor their development
- have access to accurate information and/or referral routes for families
  who request health-related advice.

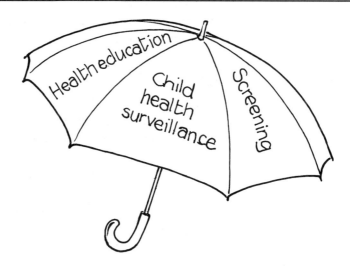

Child health promotion

The primary objective of child health promotion is to enhance child development and growth within the context of promoting the health of the family by:

■ encouraging healthy lifestyles such as breast-feeding if possible, and immunisations in childhood. The prevention of illness and accidents may be achieved by advising carers and families about meeting children's needs such as balanced nutrition and travel safety

■ detecting any deviations from the 'norm', for example babies and children who are not following the expected patterns of development or behaviour, or who are displaying signs of illness. These children can then be referred for specialist investigation and/or treatment where necessary

■ detecting any areas of potential difficulty early and offering appropriate advice or practical assistance. For example, parents in stressful situations may have difficulty in providing consistent and stimulating care for their children. A health visitor may be able to help relieve their situation by helping them to apply for family centre assistance, or a nursery place for their child.

 Progress check

1 What does health promotion aim to do?
2 What is 'child health promotion' an umbrella term for?
3 Who may be involved in health promotion?
4 Describe the three elements of child health promotion.

Child health surveillance

Child health surveillance is more than the surveillance of vision, hearing, development and specific medical problems. It includes the surveillance of growth, illness, behaviour and child abuse as well as health education and immunisation. It is involved with looking at the whole child throughout their childhood and not relying on occasional checks.

Surveillance also concerns promoting development. It is effectively performed by parents, childcare workers and teachers as well as professionals trained in screening.

Developmental surveillance

Developmental surveillance is a continuous process which is not restricted to particular ages. It monitors a child's whole progress including the development of particular skills and milestones. Developmental surveillance means looking at a child as a whole and being aware of all-round development, not only whether they are crawling, walking or talking. This approach accepts that all children are individuals, each developing at their own pace.

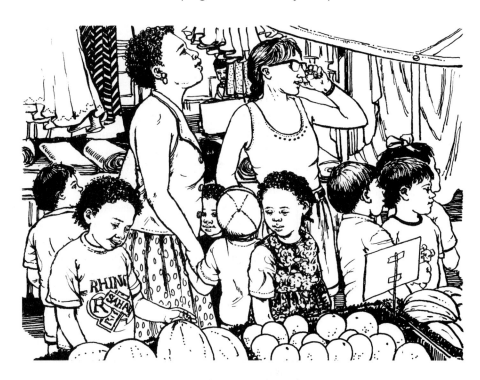

All children are individuals

Principles of child health surveillance

For child health surveillance to be as effective as possible there are several factors which must be incorporated.

Child health surveillance should:

- recognise the importance of parental co-operation. Partnership with parents is vital – they are the experts and know their own child better that anyone else. They are in the best position to recognise problems in health, development and behaviour and should be respected and taken seriously.
- be a positive experience for children and parents
- be based on good communication and teamwork between the health care workers involved with a child or family
- be a learning experience for parents and health care workers which involves the exchange of information
- provide an opportunity for tactful guidance on health care topics and health promotion
- be carried out by observation and talking with parents and carers, with tests and formal assessments to complement the process
- offer flexibility by providing opportunities for extra reviews if necessary, and conducting programmes to suit the requirements of the child and family.

Assessment

The term assessment is often used to describe any sort of check, but it should be used only to describe what happens when a child is being

Remember

Parents are the experts who know their own child better than anyone else. Their views should always be asked for and respected.

assessed to detect what the problem is (when the diagnosis is being made).

A child who fails a screening test or is found through surveillance will be referred to a specialist who will:

■ give a detailed examination with other tests
■ confirm or exclude the presence of a problem
■ recommend or supply treatment, counselling or further referral.

 Progress check

1 What is child health surveillance?
2 What is the difference between health surveillance and assessment?
3 What are the principles of child health surveillance?
4 What is the role of the childcare worker in child health surveillance?

Case study

Kyle is 12 months old and has attended a private day nursery since he was 3 months old. Both his parents work full-time and Kyle is their first child. He is usually contented and smiles and laughs a lot, seeming to benefit from the company of the other babies and the high quality care provided by the nursery staff. He has not attended the child health clinic, or seen the health visitor, since his last immunisation at 4 months of age. Kyle's childcare worker is concerned about his development. He cannot sit unless he is supported by an adult or by several cushions. He is not yet showing any signs of being mobile – he cannot roll, crawl or bottom-shuffle. He does not weight-bear or try to pull himself up to stand on the furniture. The officer-in-charge of the nursery has asked to see the parents to discuss Kyle's progress – she wants to tell them about her concerns and to suggest that Kyle is seen by the health visitor, GP or community paediatrician. He may need to be referred for assessment by a specialist in child development.

1 Kyle appears to be delayed in one area of development. Given the opportunity, what questions would you ask the nursery staff or parents about his all-round development ?
2 What skills do childcare workers need to approach parents when there is a possible problem?
3 What might the assessment of Kyle's development by a specialist result in?
4 How do you think that Kyle's difficulty could have been dealt with earlier?

Disease prevention

Preventing disease has three distinct parts: primary prevention, secondary prevention and tertiary prevention.

Primary prevention

This involves attempts to reduce the number of children being affected by a disease or disorder, by promoting preventative health measures such as:

■ immunisation to reduce the number of children affected by a particular disease
■ safety to reduce the number of accidents
■ balanced diet to reduce the incidence of diet-related disorders such as dental caries or obesity.

Secondary prevention

This includes efforts to detect departures from good health early, so that the effects can be reduced sooner, by:

■ screening (see Chapter 4) to detect any abnormalities so that treatment can be started
■ changing habits that are detrimental to health such as poor diet, or unprotected sunbathing.

Tertiary prevention

This is aimed at reducing the effects of a particular disease or condition and minimising the suffering caused. It includes:

■ efforts to help children and parents to adjust to life changes which result from an impairment or disability
■ helping children to achieve their full potential.

 Progress check

1 What are the three stages of disease prevention?
2 How can a childcare worker contribute towards the prevention of disease?
3 Suggest three ways that a childcare worker could have a positive contribution to disease prevention for each stage i.e. primary prevention, secondary prevention and tertiary prevention.

Good Practice

Childcare workers can provide valuable contributions to all stages of disease prevention. By providing a safe environment and a well-balanced diet for children, they are offering primary prevention. Reporting any deviations from the developmental norm to senior staff and parents and reinforcing the value of good health practices provides secondary prevention. Encouraging children to achieve their individual potential regardless of gender, culture or disability and meeting individual needs, thereby reducing suffering, is tertiary prevention.

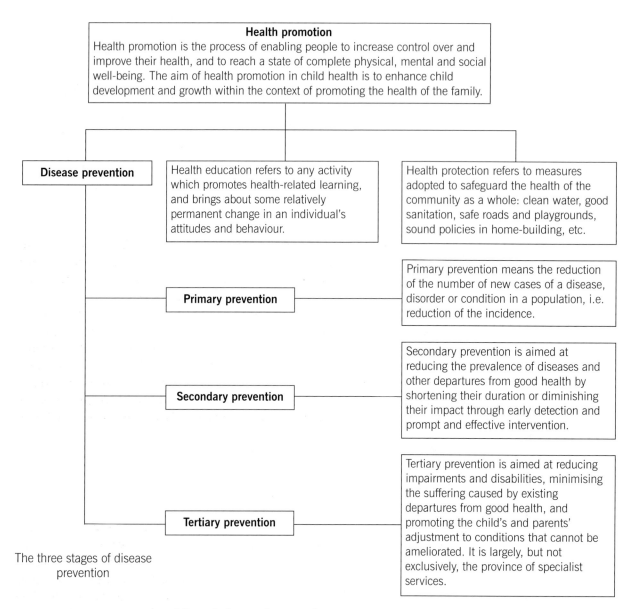

Health promotion
Health promotion is the process of enabling people to increase control over and improve their health, and to reach a state of complete physical, mental and social well-being. The aim of health promotion in child health is to enhance child development and growth within the context of promoting the health of the family.

Disease prevention

Health education refers to any activity which promotes health-related learning, and brings about some relatively permanent change in an individual's attitudes and behaviour.

Health protection refers to measures adopted to safeguard the health of the community as a whole: clean water, good sanitation, safe roads and playgrounds, sound policies in home-building, etc.

Primary prevention

Primary prevention means the reduction of the number of new cases of a disease, disorder or condition in a population, i.e. reduction of the incidence.

Secondary prevention

Secondary prevention is aimed at reducing the prevalence of diseases and other departures from good health by shortening their duration or diminishing their impact through early detection and prompt and effective intervention.

Tertiary prevention

Tertiary prevention is aimed at reducing impairments and disabilities, minimising the suffering caused by existing departures from good health, and promoting the child's and parents' adjustment to conditions that cannot be ameliorated. It is largely, but not exclusively, the province of specialist services.

The three stages of disease prevention

Health education

Defining health

Health is a difficult word to define because it means different things to different people. Some may consider themselves to be 'healthy' because they do not smoke, others because they have not been ill recently. Being healthy involves more than our physical condition and may include being fit, not being ill and living to a very old age.

The World Health Organisation in 1947 defined health as: 'A state of complete physical, mental and social well-being and not merely the absence of disease or infirmity.'

This definition recognises that there are three aspects of health – our physical, social and mental states – which will all affect overall health.

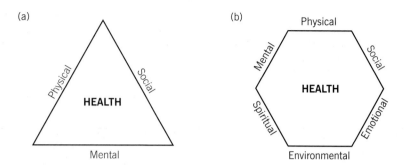

(a) The health triangle and (b) the health hexagon

However, this definition has been criticised for being too idealistic, because it makes a healthy status out of reach of a large proportion of the world's population. Poverty or disability may affect health, but their presence need not imply that poor health is inevitable.

The World Health Organisation also states that: 'The enjoyment of the highest attainable standard of health is one of the fundamental rights of every human being without distinction of race, religion, political belief, economic or social condition . . .' This may seem to be more reasonable – especially when applied to children whose health is dependent upon competent and caring adults. One of the main issues in health is the person's capacity to make their own choices. These choices may be based on:

■ the traditions of the cultural group
■ the family
■ self-awareness
■ knowledge.

Adults make choices for themselves and also on behalf of their children, for instance when to wean and which foods to offer babies, whether to immunise, or what car and road safety is provided. Most adult/child interaction and involvement can directly or indirectly affect the health and welfare of the child concerned. The choices made by childcarers should be made with full knowledge of the implications. The Health Education Authority and health professionals seek to inform the population about health issues so that they can make their own informed choice.

Current health concerns

Despite the original expectation that the cost of treatment would gradually reduce with the improved health of the population after the introduction of the National Health Service in 1948, costs have rocketed. Lifestyles have changed and become less active, living standards have improved for most people but high morbidity (illness) and mortality (death) rates still exist. Although people are living longer they are suffering from chronic illness. The following diseases are responsible for most of the deaths in the adult population:

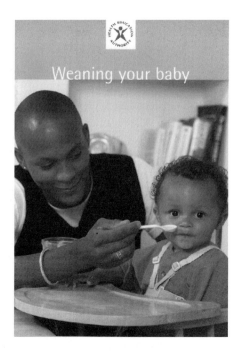

The Health Education
Authority publishes leaflets
about child health issues

- cancer
- heart disease
- strokes.

Although there may be an inherited tendency to any of these diseases, healthier lifestyles could help to prevent their occurrence.

Positive steps encouraged by health professionals and the Health Education Authority to reduce mortality rates include:

- stopping smoking
- exercising regularly to strengthen the heart and reduce stress
- eating a high-fibre and low-fat diet to maintain optimum weight, encourage bowel health and reduce the risk of heart disease.

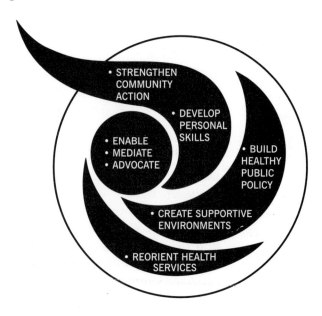

Symbol of the World Health
Organization Charter, which
emphasises aspects of
health education

Aims of health education

The main objective of health education is to improve the general health of the population and to enable people to take responsibility for their own and their children's health. The aims are:

- to change behaviour and/or attitude
- to provide knowledge and raise awareness
- to empower people to choose their own lifestyle and be aware of the implications of their choices
- to promote the interests of a particular group
- to meet local and/or national targets in health, e.g. promoting self-examination of the breasts to detect breast cancer.

Health education campaigns

There have been many health education campaigns in recent years to make the public aware of issues such as:

- the reduction of disease, e.g. by immunising children
- increasing healthy living practices, e.g. balanced, healthy diets, exercising regularly
- the risks of potentially harmful practices, e.g. smoking, sunbathing
- personal safety.

Each campaign has to consider its 'target group' – that is the part of the population who will benefit most from the information provided – and address the information to them using appropriate language, presentation, emphasis and content.

Language

The language used is important. Adolescents, for example, will respond more positively to words and phrases they use themselves and understand. Literature should also be available for people whose first language is not English.

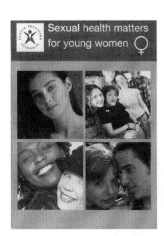

Sexual health matters for young women ♀

This health education leaflet on sexual health targets a young adult audience

Presentation

Presentation in the form of pictures, photographs, diagrams and/or cartoons will be suitable for different groups of the population. Some campaigns may shock, others may need to gently encourage.

Emphasis

The information given will emphasise the most important aspects of the campaign, for example anti-smoking campaigns will emphasise the need to give up.

Content

This should be accessible and interesting. Providing too much or too little information may make the target group 'switch off' and not absorb any new knowledge.

Activities

1 Plan a health education campaign in your college or workplace, with the co-operation of tutors and/or workplace supervisors. Follow the planning schedule and evaluate how effective you have been. The stages in planning an effective health education campaign must be worked through logically.

Planning a health education campaign

Planning stage	Examples
1 Deciding which health issue to promote	Immunisation to prevent disease Dental care Accident prevention
2 Identifying your target group	Parents in the day nursery Children at Key Stage 1
3 Aims and objectives	Aim: to raise awareness of the dangers of baby walkers Objective: 1) to prepare a display about accidents caused by baby walkers 2) to distribute information about mobility in children under 1 year to parents (Be specific with objectives – the achievement of them will help to evaluate the success of the campaign)
4 Method of presentation	Video Display Workshop Demonstration
5 Resources and equipment	Will depend on how much space is available, the cost of the equipment, whether it is accessible by the target audience
6 Planning the presentation	Working out precisely how the information will be delivered
Implementation and review	**Process**
1 Implementation of the campaign	Relax, don't panic and try to enjoy the presentation experience! Try and gauge how effective the programme is as it progresses
2 Evaluation	Try using an evaluation form so that the target group can report back about their perceptions of the campaign. Activities like this are always a learning experience – whether you judge them to have been successful in achieving the aims and objectives, or not.

2 You are a member of the target group for a current or recent national health education campaign. It could be about drug awareness, breast screening, drinking and driving, or any topical issue. Find all the evidence you can about the campaign e.g. cuttings of press articles and advertisements,

TV programmes and TV advertisements, leaflets, etc. Evaluate how effective this campaign has been:

■ to you personally
■ to your peers.

For example, was the information directed at the target group? Was it informative and useful, or was it patronising? Has it resulted in a change of attitude or behaviour? Has it heightened awareness of the particular issue?

If your answers conclude that the campaign has been ineffective in any of these areas, decide how the health education message could have been given more effectively.

 Progress check

1 Write a description of what good health means to you.
2 What may influence individual people's health choices?
3 Why is it important for adults to know about health issues that may affect children?
4 What do 'morbidity' and 'mortality' mean?
5 What positive steps to reduce mortality have been encouraged by the Health Education Authority?
6 What are the aims of health education?
7 Why is consideration of the 'target' group so important?
8 What are the stages of planning a health education campaign?

Case study

Jane is a newly qualified nursery nurse working in a mainstream nursery unit for 3 to 5 year olds. During her EDEXCEL training she completed an in-depth assignment about children's accidents and has continued to be very interested in the subject. In the two terms she has been at the nursery, seven children have attended the accident and emergency department at the local hospital and two children have been admitted to hospital as the result of accidents in the home. Several other children have been involved in accidental mishaps at home which have not required hospital treatment. The nursery team have decided to try to reduce the incidence of such accidents. The nursery teacher is aware of Jane's interest and asks her to co-ordinate a health promotion campaign to raise awareness about accidents in the home.

1 Who are the target groups for Jane's campaign?
2 What sort of strategies can she use to increase awareness of the potential risks to children and how they can be avoided?
3 How can she measure how effective her campaign has been?

Health education in childcare establishments

There are many different ways for childcare workers to encourage healthy lifestyles for children and to raise awareness of health issues.

Health education for children should:

■ be relevant to the child and linked to their knowledge and experiences
■ contain simple and clear messages which are constantly reinforced
■ explain the reasons for rules
■ contain 'real' examples.

Guidelines for health education in childcare settings

Childcare workers have a responsibility to the children in their care to both keep them healthy and prepare them for a healthy life. The following suggestions will help to ensure good practice in health education in childcare and education establishments, and should underpin good practice.

1 A structured health education programme should be in place which includes:

 ■ a variety of up-to-date resources – models, pictures or collections that will initiate discussion
 ■ practical activities which enable children to see, feel and handle objects
 ■ a range of teaching and learning methods to include information-giving, the development of skills and exploring attitudes and values (see suggestions for health related activities below)
 ■ activities which can be completed in 15 to 20 minutes for 5- to 7-year-olds at Key Stage 1.

2 Health issues should be dealt with as they arise. Gentle reminders about health and hygiene will reinforce healthy life skills.

3 Every opportunity should be taken to increase children's self-esteem. Selecting activities which are within a child's capabilities will promote a sense of achievement. Children who feel good about themselves are more likely to develop independence and form positive relationships which will improve their health status.

4 Supportive policies should be in place to deal with bullying, safety issues, and so on. Clear rules which are adhered to will not only reduce the number of accidents and promote safety, but will also increase feelings of security.

5 Reward systems for positive behaviour, such as reinforcing acceptable behaviour with lots of attention and praise discourages unacceptable or negative behaviour and promotes a climate for learning.

6 An equal opportunities policy should be in place. Meeting the individual needs of all children and promoting positive images and role models should be evident in both the care and the curriculum provided by any childcare establishment.

7 Childcare workers must accept responsibility as role models. Children

are born imitators and should be witness to positive actions and behaviour in relation to health.

8 The physical environment should be safe and stimulating. Safety reduces the incidence of accidents and increases awareness of dangerous situations, such as road safety or meeting strangers.

9 Meals and snacks should offer healthy choices that promote eating fresh foods containing protein and vitamins and reducing fat and sugar intake.

10 A smoking policy should be in place. Childcare establishments should be designated no-smoking areas. Children who see their carers smoke are more likely to believe that smoking is acceptable and go on to smoke when older.

11 Parents/carers should be actively encouraged to take part in the life of the establishment. Discussion and promotion of positive health practices can take place on an informal basis, via parents' groups, children's activities, and so on.

12 Health professionals and other agency involvement should be encouraged and welcomed. Speakers from the health service and related agencies can provide information and promote positive health, for example the school nurse, health visitor, midwife or dietician.

13 Children can make links with community groups and local services by visiting establishments which welcome children's participation and help; and by organising and/or participating in fund-raising activities for voluntary organisations based locally or nationally, for example a particular local cause or the NSPCC.

> **Remember**
>
> Childcare workers have a responsibility to the children in their care to both keep them healthy and to prepare them for a healthy life.

Activities

1 Relate the guidelines for health education to what happens in your workplace. Are all these practices in place? Think about any areas that could be improved and how this could be achieved.

2 Prepare a topic or curriculum plan with an area of health as the primary focus. It could be 'Looking after ourselves', 'People who help us', 'Diet', 'Dental Care', 'Exercise', etc.

Be specific about the learning outcomes for the children and be especially careful to relate the plan to the age group of children you are working with. Encourage parents/carers to participate. Link your plan to the Desirable Outcomes for children aged 3 to 5 and National Curriculum at Key Stage 1 for children from 5 to 7 years.

Health-related activities

There are numerous activities which can be offered to children to raise their awareness and promote good health. They must be appropriate for the developmental stage of the child concerned so that they are accessible and offer achievable goals, but they should also be interesting, exciting and stimulating. Health information can be offered in many ways.

■ Structured and imaginative play in an area set up as a hospital, dentist's surgery, greengrocer's shop or café will promote role-play, decision making, familiarity with procedures and understanding.

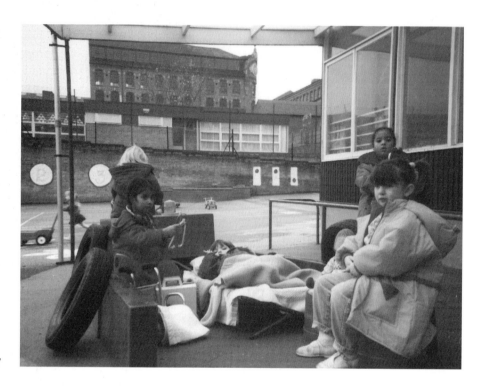

Hospital play at the nursery

■ Visits from people who help us such as the health visitor, school nurse, road crossing patrol or dietician add interest.
■ Visits to places of interest, such as farms, can increase awareness of meeting needs, caring and how things grow.
■ Daily routines such as hygiene routines and safety issues can be reinforced by consistent procedures.
■ Sorting activities with models, pictures and so on, can raise awareness about things that are good or bad for health, or safe and unsafe places.
■ Children's literature, including cassettes, pictures, books and stories, is available which emphasises health topics in an accessible way. Choosing songs and rhymes which reinforce these messages will increase the impact.
■ Drama and using music and movement helps to practise expressing emotions, facial expressions and physical activity.
■ Pictures and photographs and other relevant visual aids can be used to promote discussion about any topic
■ Puppets can be used to convey any health message in an interesting and visual way.

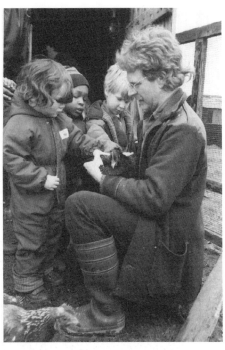

Visiting farms offers an experiential learning experience

■ Games such as board games created with an aspect of health in mind will also encourage co-operation and reinforce important issues.

■ Demonstrations of washing hands efficiently, brushing teeth, brushing hair, and crossing the road safely are useful.

■ Drawing and writing will encourage children to display their understanding visually.

■ Displays and interest tables based around children's work on a health education topic will include all the benefits of general display being child-centred, accessible and educational.

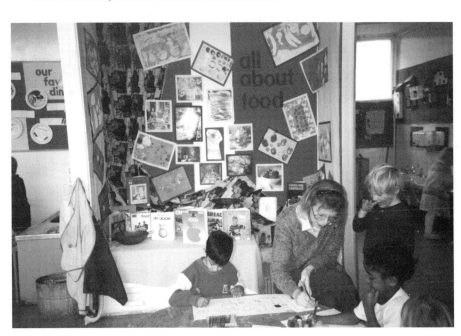

Health education is reinforced by using displays of children's work

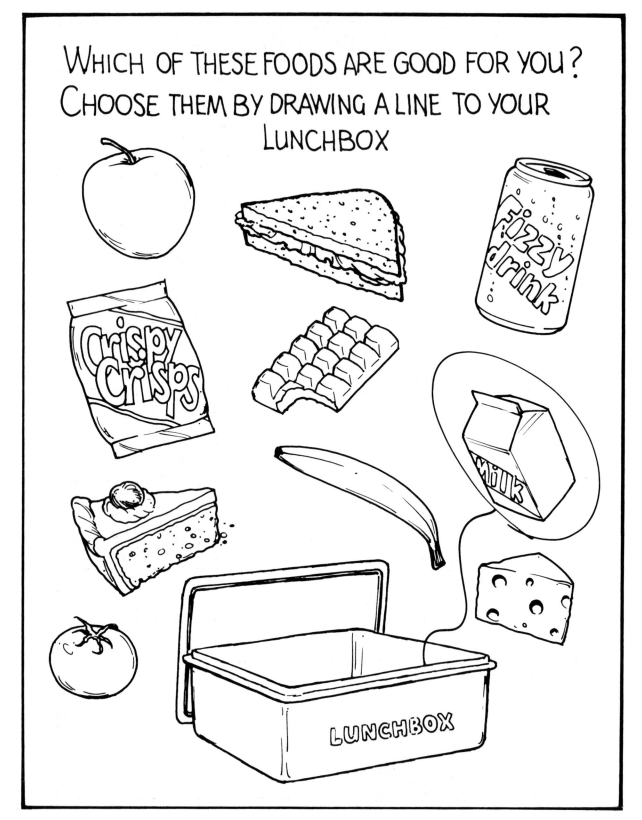

Sorting activities can be used to raise children's awareness of dental health

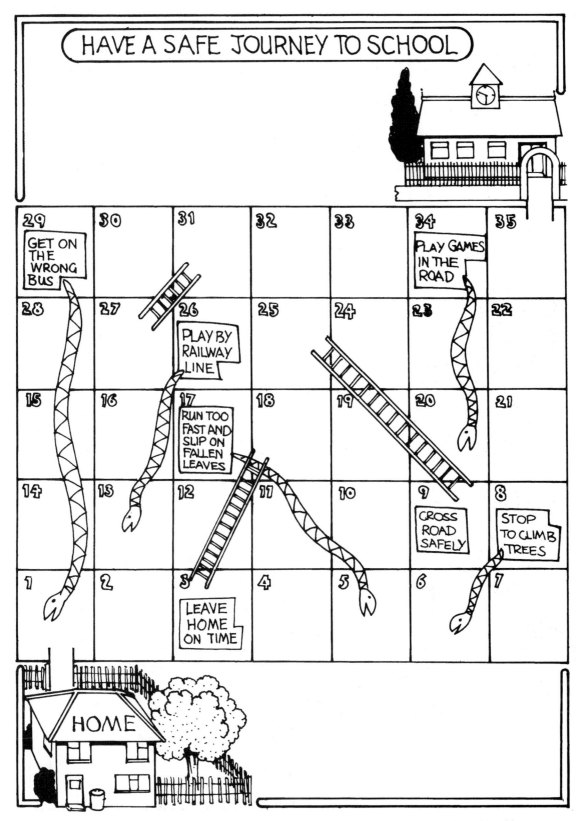

Classroom board games can be used to teach children about keeping safe and healthy

WHAT I EAT

	MONDAY	TUESDAY	WEDNESDAY	THURSDAY	FRIDAY
Breakfast					
Breaktime					
Lunch					
Breaktime					
Tea					
Snacks					

Children can be encouraged to keep a food diary

✅ **Progress check**

1 List ten methods that childcare workers can use to encourage healthy lifestyles for children.
2 What factors should childcare workers consider when planning health related activities for children?
3 Which health related activities do you consider are most appropriate for children aged 1 to 4 years?
4 Which health related activities do you consider are most appropriate for children aged 4 to 7 years?

Meeting needs

The needs of children are well documented and can be categorised as physical needs, social and emotional needs and healthy lifestyles.

Physical needs

Physical needs include:

- food – a nutritionally balanced diet and water
- warmth – clothing suitable for both the season and developmental stage of the child
- shelter – comfortable, dry and clean housing
- fresh air and sunlight – regular access to safe outdoor play and ventilation in the home and childcare establishment
- exercise – the opportunity to play energetically and pursue sporting activities
- rest and sleep – the provision of restful activities and an environment conducive to sleep when tired
- physical comfort – cuddles and hugs are also emotionally rewarding
- safety and protective care – the removal of hazards from the environment: including the home, travelling, and places of care and education
- access to medical care – regular health surveillance and emergency care if required
- prevention of infection – a hygienic environment and provision of immunisation.

Social and emotional needs

Social and emotional needs include:

- love and continuity of care from trusted adults
- security – consistency of care and established routines
- stimulation – for all areas of development comprising a mixture of familiar and new experiences and encouragement for children to progress at their own pace

- independence and responsibility when appropriate – from feeding themselves and going to the toilet unassisted to looking after a pet of their own
- training in life skills acceptable to the social and cultural group e.g. toilet training, mealtime behaviour, and forming and maintaining relationships
- praise and recognition of their achievements, great or small
- discipline and respect – having clear boundaries for what is acceptable and unacceptable behaviour.

Maslow's hierarchy of needs places needs in an order of priority. This can be illustrated as a triangle with the basic needs at the bottom working up to a pinnacle of complete well-being, through the various levels of need.

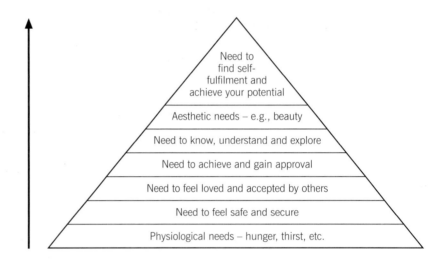

Maslow's hierarchy of need

Maslow's idea is that each level must be satisfied before children can progress to the next stage, for example physiological needs (food, water etc.) are essential for survival. If these needs are not met they become a priority and energies are devoted to satisfying them, preventing any higher level needs from being met. There is some overlap between the stages but, in general, if the low level needs are met the child is able to progress to the pinnacle of the triangle and operate at its peak, when all needs are satisfied.

If this is so, children will only achieve self-fulfilment and achieve their potential if they have been cared for physically, and positively encouraged to progress in a suitable environment.

Healthy lifestyles

For children to grow and develop healthily, needs must be met.

Babies and young children need a safe yet stimulating environment if they are to grow and develop to their full potential. They need space and encouragement to develop a new skill, and the opportunity to practise and perfect their technique. A positive atmosphere in which adults praise children's efforts and recognise their achievements will encourage trust and progress. This is why all childcare workers need a thorough knowledge of child development. With this information they can provide the correct environment for the child to progress at their own individual pace.

To stimulate development, carers need to provide:

- space
- opportunity
- freedom to learn from experience
- reassurance
- praise
- access to some equipment.

When caring for disabled children it is vital to remember that every child is a unique individual with specific needs, which will depend on their own abilities and capacity for independence. Remember that disabled children are children first. Each achievement should be encouraged and praised so that they develop a high self-esteem. Adapting the environment to suit their individual needs will help their progress.

Providing a safe environment

Children are the responsibility of the adults who are caring for them. It is of prime importance to keep the child safe and in doing so, prevent accidents. Most accidents that occur to children could be prevented with care and thought.

Fresh air

All children need regular exposure to fresh air and preferably an opportunity to play outside. If conditions are not suitable for outdoor play, the play area should be well ventilated to provide fresh air and to prevent a build up of carbon dioxide.

The benefits of fresh air are:

- it contains oxygen – breathing in oxygen gives energy and stimulates exercise
- it contains fewer germs than air indoors; germs are killed by the ultra-violet rays in sunshine
- exposure to sunlight causes the skin to produce vitamin D.

Exercise

Exercise is a necessary and natural part of life for everyone. It is especially important for young children who need to develop and perfect physical skills. All physical exercise strengthens muscles, and encouraging exercise from an early age will lay the foundations for a life-long healthy exercise habit.

Rest and sleep

Rest is necessary after physical exercise, and children will know when to stop their vigorous activity as they begin to feel tired.

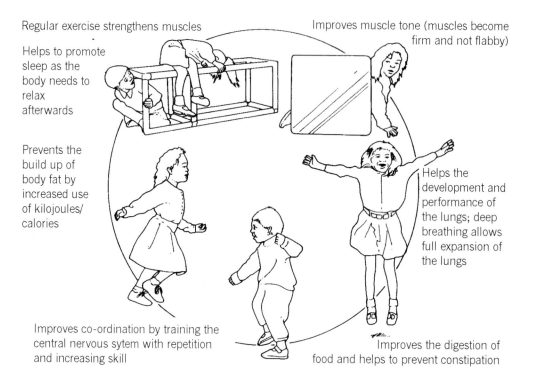

Regular exercise strengthens muscles

Improves muscle tone (muscles become firm and not flabby)

Helps to promote sleep as the body needs to relax afterwards

Prevents the build up of body fat by increased use of kilojoules/calories

Helps the development and performance of the lungs; deep breathing allows full expansion of the lungs

Improves co-ordination by training the central nervous sytem with repetition and increasing skill

Improves the digestion of food and helps to prevent constipation

The physical exercise cycle

The benefits of rest are:
- to allow tissues to recover
- to allow the heart rate to fall
- to allow oxygen to be replaced
- to allow body temperature to drop
- to allow the central nervous system to relax
- to take in food if required
- to prevent muscles from aching and becoming stiff after heavy exercise.

Children should exercise regularly to promote their strength, suppleness and stamina, but they must be allowed to rest. This may be relaxation, sleep or just a change of occupation. One of the values of relaxing, or of quiet areas in nursery and school, is in providing children with the opportunity to rest and recharge their batteries. Children need not be challenged all the time; it is beneficial to sometimes give them toys or activities that are relatively easy to complete.

Activity

Compile a list of resources and activities which enable children to have quiet, restful periods and/or sleep.

1 Consider which are most appropriate for children aged 0 to 1 year, 1 to 4 years and 4 to 7 years.
2 Suggest suitable childcare environments for these activities and/or resources e.g. child-minders, nannies, private day nurseries, state nurseries and infant classes.
3 Explain how children may be encouraged to participate e.g. routines.

Sleep

Everyone needs sleep but has different requirements. The sleep needs of children will depend on their age and stage of development, the amount of exercise taken and their own personal needs.

Sleep is a special kind of rest which allows the body to rest and recuperate physically and mentally.

Babies and children need varying amounts of sleep. Some children wake often at night even after settling late. There is little that can be done apart from following a sensible routine. This will involve:

- patience
- not stimulating the child, remaining quiet, calm, and not encouraging interaction
- remaining upstairs (do not take the child to where there is any activity)
- encouraging daily exercise
- trying to reduce stress or worries
- being prepared to use the carer's bed, as this may resolve waking in the night.

Social and cultural expectations of children may include letting them stay up later at night. As long as the child is given the opportunity for an adequate amount of sleep it should not create a difficulty.

For successful settling to bed at night it is important to have a regular routine. The same process each night helps the child to feel secure and comfortable and so aids sleep. Using a familiar routine and giving reassurance that carers are nearby may encourage children who are unwilling to go to bed to settle more willingly.

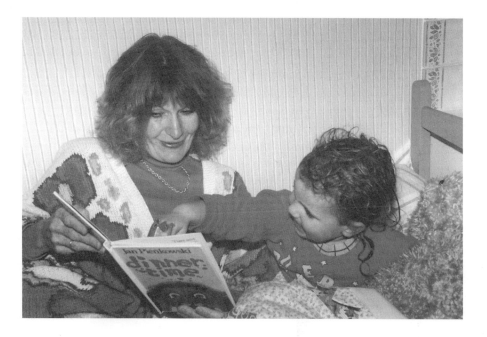

Bedtime routines help children to settle

Good Practice

It is important to work in partnership with parents/carers and to meet the child's individual rest and sleep needs. Children need opportunities for rest and sleep in all childcare settings.

Look at the routines in your establishment. Do they meet the needs of ALL the children ?

Do they incorporate flexibility?

Plan suitable areas and activities to enable children to take advantage of quiet times when they need to rest.

Toilet training

There are many different theories of when and how to train babies and children in the use of potty and toilet.

A child will only become reliably clean and dry by the age of 2 to 3 years, at whatever age the potty is introduced. There does not seem to be any point in rushing this skill. It is much more easily achieved if it is left until the child is 2 years at least, unless they show an interest earlier.

Children usually become dry at night of their own accord. Accidents are common and should be treated with understanding and not displeasure. There is no need for concern about occasional accidents unless the child is upset. Seeing a sympathetic doctor or health visitor should help.

Hygiene: care of the hair, skin and teeth

All children need adult help and supervision in their personal hygiene requirements. Good standards of hygiene in childhood are important for the following reasons:

- they help to prevent disease
- they increase self-esteem and social acceptance
- they prepare children for life by teaching them how to care for themselves.

Because the skin has so many important functions and because it is the first part of the body to come into contact with the environment, it must be cared for adequately. This does not mean obsessive cleaning of the skin: too much cleaning can be as harmful as too little because it may make the skin dry and sore and also wash away the sebum which protects it.

- Wash the face and hands in the morning and before meals.
- Wash hands after going to the toilet and after messy play.
- Keep the nails short by cutting them straight across. This will prevent dirt collecting under them.
- A daily bath or shower is necessary with young children who play outside and become dirty, hot and sweaty. Dry them thoroughly, especially between the toes and in the skin creases, to prevent soreness and cracking.

Remember

Carers should listen to parental wishes and liaise with them about toilet training issues.

Remember

Childcare workers should seek parental permission before cutting a child's nails.

The benefits of good hygiene are:

- infection is prevented (it can spread from child to child from dirty hands and nails)
- health is maintained
- good habits give a pattern for life
- it allows the skin to perform its functions
- treats skin problems, for example eczema or sweat rash. Itchy, sore skin can prevent sleep and make the child irritable and restless. This may affect all-round development
- clear, glowing skin and shiny hair which are a sign of good health
- the child looks attractive and feels well, and develops a positive self-image
- washing is a tonic; children feel healthy as a result.

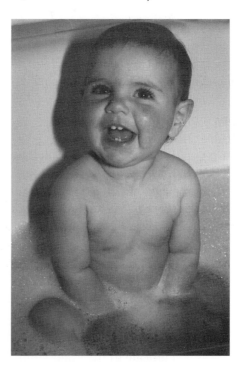

Bath time is fun!

Encouraging independence in hygiene

There are several ways in which carers can encourage a child to develop independence in personal hygiene:

- provide positive role models
- establish caring routines that encourage cleanliness from early babyhood
- make hygiene fun: use toys, cups and containers, and sinkers and floaters in the bath
- provide the child with their own flannel, toothbrush, hairbrush, etc. that they have chosen themselves
- allow the child to wash themselves and participate at bath time. Let them brush their hair with a soft brush and comb with rounded teeth

- provide a step so that they can reach the basin to wash and clean teeth
- make haircuts fun too: some barbers and hairdressers specialise in cutting children's hair.

Teeth

Teeth may appear at any time during the first two years of life. It is usually expected that they will begin to erupt during the first year but this is not necessarily so. The first 20 teeth are called the 'milk teeth' and they will usually be complete by the age of 3 years. From 5 to 6 years these teeth begin to fall out as the adult teeth come through. There are 32 permanent teeth, and the care they are given in childhood will help them to last a lifetime.

Care of the teeth

Provide a soft toothbrush for a baby to use and become familiar with. Teach older children how to clean their teeth. A dental hygienist will be able to offer professional assistance – the dentist will arrange this. Ensure that cleaning the teeth becomes a habit: in the morning after breakfast and after the last drink or snack before bed. Cleaning the teeth after meals should be encouraged, but this may not always be possible.

Diet

Encourage healthy teeth and prevent decay by providing a healthy diet that is high in calcium and vitamins and low in sugar. Avoid giving sweet drinks to babies and children, especially in a bottle or soother: this coats the gums and teeth in sugar and encourages the formation of acid which dissolves the enamel on the teeth. Sugar can penetrate the gum and cause decay before the teeth come through. This is common in babies and children who are frequently offered sweet drinks.

If you do need to feed a child between meals, provide food that needs to be chewed and improves the health of the gums and teeth, like apples, carrots and bread.

Fluoride

Fluoride in the water supply has been proven to strengthen the enamel on the teeth, and so prevent decay. In areas where the fluoride content is low, drops can be given daily in drinks. Fluoride toothpaste also helps to prevent decay.

The dentist

Visit the dentist regularly. A baby who attends with an adult, and then has her own appointments, will feel more confident about the procedure. Prepare children for their dental appointments by explaining what will happen and participating in role play. *Never* pass on any adult feelings of terror, fear or anxiety about the dentist.

Clothing and footwear

Toddlers and children work hard at their play, and this will mean that they get dirty. Although they are often washed for their health and comfort they

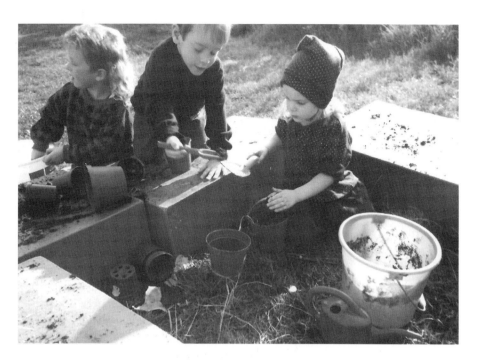

Children will inevitably get dirty as they play

will soon be dirty again. The attraction of a muddy puddle, digging soil and exploring the sandpit will see to that! This is all natural and should be encouraged. Children should not be pressurised into keeping clean, or the spontaneity and excitement of play will be lost.

Clothing

Clothing must be comfortable and loose enough for easy movement but fitted well enough to prevent loose material from catching and hindering movements. It should be able to be easily washed; children *do* get dirty. This should be expected and not disapproved of.

Footwear

The bones of the feet develop from cartilage, and are very soft and vulnerable to deformity if they are pushed into badly fitting shoes or socks. Shoes should not be worn unless it is absolutely necessary, and not indoors. Shoes are not necessary until a child will be walking outside, when they protect the feet and preserve warmth.

Feet grow two to three sizes each year until the age of 4. The primary carer is responsible for making sure that footwear fits correctly. This should be done by regularly checking the growth of the feet. They must be checked every 3 months by an expert trained in children's shoe fitting. Both the length and width are important.

Shoes should:
- protect the feet
- have no rough areas to rub or chafe the feet
- have room for growth
- have an adjustable fastener, for example a buckle or Velcro
- be flexible and allow free movement

- fit around the heel
- support the foot and prevent it from sliding forwards.

Socks must be of a size to correspond to the size of the shoe. Stretch socks should be avoided.

Children reared in a climate of health awareness are more likely to develop a life-long habit of good health. Parents and childcare workers can together establish patterns for life.

 Progress check

1 What are children's physical needs?
2 What are their social/emotional needs?
3 Describe Maslow's theory of needs.
4 Describe the value of rest and sleep.
5 Describe any traditions or family circumstances which may promote varying attitudes to sleeping patterns for young children.
6 How can adults encourage independence to enable children to take responsibility for their own hygiene?
7 How can dental hygiene be encouraged ?
8 What special care should be taken to promote healthy growth of the feet?

Activity

Plan a daily hygiene routine which will meet the needs of a child aged 1 to 4 years. Include all aspects of care related to the child's needs and development:
- encouraging independence
- sleeping requirements
- opportunity for rest and exercise
- stimulation
- safety factors
- awareness of the needs of the family.

How can a childcare worker ensure that all the physical needs are provided for in the early years of childhood ?

A holistic approach to child health

The holistic approach to child health means meeting the needs of the **whole child** and not concentrating on one part at a time. For example when a child attends a clinic for a routine hearing test, enquiries and observations should be made about the health and development of the child in all other areas, not only whether or not they can hear sounds. It also relates to the care provided by parents and carers, who not only supply the physical requirements to maintain a healthy life, but also the social and emotional benefits of consistency of care in a safe and stimulating environment.

A holistic approach implies that childcarers recognise that a child's health is dependent on many factors, all of which are inter-related. For instance, poor housing in damp conditions may result in frequent illness. See Chapter 2 for factors affecting health. The main factors which influence health are related to:

■ personal health status
■ environmental factors.

A holistic approach also involves accepting the value and potential benefits of varied child-rearing practices, including acknowledging the use and value of complementary medicines and treatments.

Complementary medicines and treatments

Complementary medicine does not simply treat symptoms of illness, but provides a holistic approach i.e. cares for the whole child or person. Physical, emotional, mental and spiritual factors are all taken into account to provide individual therapy and treatment. Complementary health care can be effective as part of a programme of health promotion.

Complementary medicine is not an alternative to traditional medicine, nor a replacement, as the two should work together in harmony.

Homeopathy

Homeopathy was established in the late 1700s and early 1800s by Dr Samuel Hahnemann who acknowledged the role of nature as a healer. There continues to be some controversy about the use of homeopathy, but it is important to remember that this is not simply an alternative to traditional medicine. It is a natural complement to modern medicine which treats the individual as a whole, not simply treating the signs and symptoms of a disease. It is based on using natural substances to treat a wide range of conditions.

The three principles of homeopathy are:

■ a substance which causes symptoms in a healthy person can be used to treat those symptoms in an ill person
■ homeopathy treats the whole person and not just the illness
■ diluting homeopathic medicines increases their curative powers and avoids unwanted side-effects.

Some doctors offer homeopathic remedies for minor ailments within their National Health Service practice. Qualified homeopaths can be consulted – the Society of Homeopaths publishes a register of qualified and experienced homeopaths who have agreed to abide by the society's code of ethics.

It is possible to buy homeopathic medicines in most pharmacies without a prescription – they are safe if the instructions on the pack are followed carefully.

It is important to remember not to rely on homeopathy if symptoms persist or are severe. Children can become seriously ill very quickly and a doctor should be consulted without delay.

> ### Remember
> - Read the label and follow the directions on the pack.
> - Do not give a child food or drinks or contact with toothpaste for half an hour before or after taking a homeopathic medicine.
> - Keep all medicines out of the reach of children in a locked medicine cabinet.
> - If symptoms persist or are severe consult a doctor without delay.

Some examples of homeopathic remedies

Tea-tree oil
Tea-tree oil and eucalyptus oil are effective in dealing with head lice (see page 240).

Chamomilla
This is useful for sleeplessness in crying, angry and restless children especially when teething or suffering from colic. It is a useful remedy for teething babies.

Arnica
Arnica is helpful for all injuries which may lead to bruising.

Cantharis
Cantharis aids the healing of burns and scalds. It helps to relieve the burning sensation after an insect sting; and helps the discomfort of sunburn.

> ### Remember
> Childcare workers should never administer complementary medicines or treatments to a child without parental permission.

Aromatherapy

Aromatherapy involves using natural oils from flowers, fruits and other parts of plants to improve physical and mental well-being. In common with other complementary treatments, aromatherapy aims to treat the 'whole person' by recognising physical and emotional symptoms. It can be used to deal with a wide range of common problems and is safe to use with children of all ages if the instructions are followed carefully.

Many plants contain valuable essential oils each with their own special characteristics and healing properties – they can refresh, relax, soothe or stimulate the body and mind. These oils work in two ways:
- smell – picked up by the sensory cells in the nose
- absorption – through the skin and into the bloodstream in very small quantities.

Pure essential oils are the basis for all aromatherapy treatments and they can be used in baths or as an inhalant.

Essential oils should be selected according to their general effect and traditional uses. Charts are available from chemists and pharmacies which contain details of the 'fragrance families' and the properties of all the oils in those families. It is possible to blend two or three essential oils together.

> ### Remember
> Never apply essential oil directly onto the skin. It should always be diluted first in a 'carrier oil', such as sweet almond or jojoba oil.
> Sometimes both the effects of smell and absorption work together, for example during a massage.

Some examples of essential oils

Pine

Pine helps to ease the symptoms of colds by refreshing the nasal passages. It is used as an antiseptic for cuts and abrasions.

Frankincense

Used to comfort cracked skin, frankincense assists in the healing of minor wounds.

Tea tree

Tea tree is used as an antiseptic to ease cold sores, warts, minor burns, spots and insect bites. It is used to prevent infestations by head lice and it also eases the symptoms of colds, coughs and flu.

Lavender

Lavender comforts the symptoms of headaches. It comforts and eases painful joints and sprains. It helps to soothe minor burns and helps in the repair of scar tissue.

Reflexology

Reflexology is a deep foot massage which stimulates nerve endings (reflexes) in the foot and hopes to return the body to a state of equilibrium or balance – good health depends upon all parts the body working in co-operation with each other.

By massaging the reflexes it is possible to treat the different areas of the body. Reflexology can be used to treat ill health and to maintain good health by preventing illness and to provide deep relaxation.

Osteopathy

Paediatric osteopathy works with the natural movement of the body's water content. The qualified osteopath exerts very light pressure and painlessly pushes tissues, ligaments, muscles, bones and joints back into their correct positions. This helps to untrap nerves and it frees muscle spasms, drains mucus membranes and helps the digestive, circulatory, and lymphatic systems to work efficiently.

Children who may be helped with this treatment are those with glue ear, asthma, epilepsy, learning difficulties, behavioural problems, developmental disorders, headaches, allergies and sleep problems.

Other complementary therapies

Other complementary therapies include:

■ relaxation
■ massage
■ Chinese traditional medicine
■ acupuncture.

In some areas of the country complementary health groups for parents offer a range of complementary therapies aimed at promoting health by reducing stress. This positive experience will enrich children's lives too – parents who have an increased awareness and ability to manage their health and stress, will be more receptive to their children and better able to provide for their needs.

Case study

After his parents separated six months ago Joseph, aged 3 years, lived with his mother Barbara and older sister Caroline in the family home. He had been prone to nightmares and disturbed sleep since his father moved out, sometimes waking seven and eight times a night. The disturbed nights were more severe when he had been for his fortnightly weekend visit with his father and his new girlfriend. Barbara tried everything she could think of to reduce Joseph's anxieties; she explained that mummy and daddy could not live together any more but they still loved him very much and would always be there for him. When he woke up in the night, Barbara took him into her bed to settle him back to sleep. The GP and health visitor tried to help the family to resolve their difficulties with suggestions for helping Joseph, but the nightmares continued. A friend suggested trying her homeopathist who could offer a holistic approach to Joseph's health. Barbara was dubious about complementary therapy but thought it must be worth a try. At the first consultation the homeopathist prescribed an individual blend of natural substances to relieve Joseph's distress and help him to sleep. That night Joseph woke twice, and over the next week he began to sleep through the night. Barbara was impressed and decided to see the therapist herself and take Caroline too.

1 Why do you think this homeopathic treatment worked?
2 What other forms of complementary therapy may help Joseph?

✔ Progress check

1 What does a 'holistic' approach to child health mean?
2 What is homeopathy?
3 What are the three principles of homeopathy?
4 What is aromatherapy?
5 Which two ways do essential oils work?
6 What is paediatric osteopathy?
7 Which conditions can paediatric osteopathy help?

Key terms

You need to know what these words and phrases mean. Go back through the chapter and find out.

aromatherapy	osteopathy
assessment	physical needs
complementary medicines	primary prevention
developmental surveillance	reflexology
health education	screening
health promotion	secondary prevention
holistic	social and emotional needs
homeopathy	surveillance
Maslow's hierarchy of needs	tertiary prevention

Chapter 2 *Factors affecting child health*

This chapter includes:

- Pre-conceptual factors
- Pregnancy – prenatal factors
- Birth – perinatal factors
- Postnatal factors
- Environmental influences on child health
- Inequalities in health care

There are many factors which can affect children's health before birth (pre-conceptual and prenatal), during birth (perinatal) and after birth (postnatal). They are a combination of inherited conditions and environmental influences on health. Children are the product of their parents and may be affected by any pre-existing conditions or by an unhealthy lifestyle. All children deserve to be healthy and well and most children are, despite the enormous, sometimes negative, influences on their health.

Knowing how these environmental factors may affect children should help childcare workers to understand the need for providing settings which promote and support children's health and development. It will also increase awareness about strategies for modifying the environment to promote good health for children.

Pre-conceptual factors

Because the embryo develops rapidly in the first twelve weeks after conception, it is vital that parents give serious consideration to their health before pregnancy begins. The influence of many factors which could potentially affect the health of the child are operating before a pregnancy begins and in its very early stages. Doctors, midwives and health visitors provide pre-conceptual advice and may offer clinics for offering specific health care advice before pregnancy.

The main areas to be considered before pregnancy are the following.

Contraception

The contraceptive pill should be stopped at least three months before pregnancy is attempted to allow the menstrual cycle to re-establish itself. Knowing the exact dates of the last menstrual period (LMP) helps to ensure that the length of the pregnancy is measured accurately and appropriate care is offered at the right time.

Diet

A well-balanced diet before pregnancy begins should ensure that the developing embryo (and later fetus) receives the necessary nutrients for good health. Daily intake from the four food groups should ensure a balanced diet.

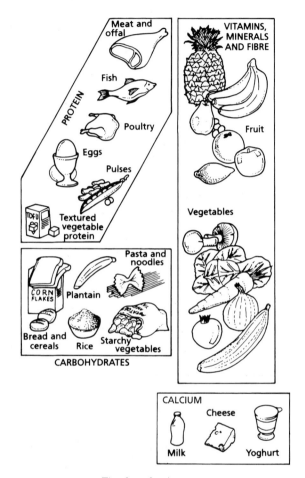

The four food groups

Folic acid

Women are advised to take folic acid tablets (the recommended dose is 0.4mgs daily) for three months before pregnancy begins and for three months into the pregnancy. This vitamin is important in the formation of the brain and spinal cord and it is believed to prevent spina bifida and neural tube defects which occur in the early weeks of pregnancy. Dietary advice before pregnancy should also include warnings about pâté and soft cheeses which may carry listeria. This bacteria can cross the placenta and damage the baby in its early development. Toxoplasmosis is caused by a protozoa found in undercooked meat and cat faeces. It may be prevented by cooking foods thoroughly and wearing gloves for gardening and dealing with cat litter trays.

Drugs

Any substance which is used for its effects on the way the body works is a drug e.g. insulin for diabetes. The term 'drugs' includes nicotine in tobacco, prescription medicines, over-the-counter medicine, glue and solvents, and illegal drugs e.g heroin, cocaine, ecstasy etc. Drugs cross the placental barrier and affect the baby – it is preferable to discontinue their use before pregnancy begins unless the well-being of the mother and fetus is dependent on them. Staff in a pre-conceptual clinic can advise future parents about services which are available to treat addictions and offer support and guidance.

Immunity

Checking immunity for rubella (german measles) before pregnancy begins enables women to have the necessary immunisation if they do not have antibodies to the virus. Pregnancy should be avoided for at least one month after immunisation.

Health

Blood tests can be offered to assess haemoglobin levels which will check for low amounts of iron in the blood. This is a cause of anaemia which can be treated with iron tablets and an iron rich diet. Immunity to rubella can be checked with a blood test and if there are no antibodies, rubella immunisation will be offered. Sexually transmitted diseases such as syphilis and gonorrhoea can be treated before pregnancy to prevent the infant being affected. A blood test for AIDS (Acquired Immune Deficiency Syndrome) may be performed with the mother's consent if she thinks that she or her partner may have been in contact with the Human Immunopathic Virus (HIV) or have been at risk. A medical check up will provide a base-line before pregnancy begins and also highlight any area(s) which need treatment or attention e.g. if a woman is overweight before pregancy begins, the pregnancy will be a potential risk to her health. Strategies for reducing weight need to be discussed with the doctor or practice nurse. General health care includes attention to overall well-being e.g. exercise, sleep and rest routines.

> **Remember**
> The embryo develops rapidly before pregnancy is confirmed. Attention to health before pregnancy is therefore of vital importance to try to ensure the healthy growth and development of the embryo and fetus.

Genetic counselling

Couples with a family history of any inherited condition can be referred to a genetic counselling unit, where they are informed of the potential risks to their future pregnancy and the services provided for prenatal testing.

Radiation

Work-based risks should be discussed with the GP who may refer a couple to environmental health or their workplace health and safety officer.

Progress check

1 Why is pre-conceptual attention to health important?
2 Which aspects of the diet should be given special consideration before pregnancy and why?
3 Which blood tests may be offered to check for the immunity status and the health of a woman before pregnancy?

Case study

Susan is 17 years old and lives with her foster parents. She smokes 20 cigarettes a day and enjoys socialising with her friends. Susan became accidentally pregnant but had a miscarriage after 10 weeks. She had confirmed the pregnancy with a test from Boots, and had not been to see her doctor at all. Although the pregnancy was not planned, she was beginning to get used to the idea – and now thinks that it would be nice to have a baby. She thinks that she would be able to offer the baby the love and stability that she was deprived of during her early years.

1 What reasons would you give to Susan to encourage her to attend for pre-conceptual care before getting pregnant again?
2 What aspects of her health would be considered at a pre-conceptual care clinic?
3 What are the most important lifestyle changes for Susan to improve her health?
4 How do you think she could be helped to achieve these?

Pregnancy – prenatal factors

The health of the fetus during pregnancy has long-term effects on its future health and development.

About one third of all disabilities present at birth are thought to be caused in the first three months of pregnancy and about one third of these causes are negative environmental influences. The increasing emphasis of health promotion on pre-conceptual and prenatal health is attempting to reduce these numbers. Improving the outcome of pregnancy is a priority area and health professionals offer preparation for parenthood, access to genetic counselling, family spacing advice, advice on alcohol, smoking, diet and safe-eating programmes in an attempt to improve the health of the child.

Congenital disorders

These are conditions that have developed during pregnancy and can sometimes be prevented.

A tendency to a particular disorder may also be inherited and this may be triggered by adverse conditions in the environment e.g. spina bifida may be caused by a genetic predisposition which can be triggered by low levels of folic acid in the maternal diet.

Genetics

Inherited (genetic) conditions

These are passed from parent(s) to child and are present from the time of conception. As the product of our parents, we bear physical resemblances to them. Some diseases and disabilities may be inherited and carried via the chromosomes and genes.

Dominant inheritance

One parent carries a dominant gene for a particular disorder. There is a 1 in 2 chance of this being passed on with each pregnancy.

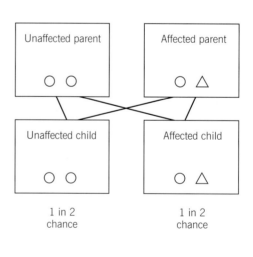

Examples:
Tuberous sclerosis
Achondroplasia
Huntington's chorea
Neurofibromatosis
Marfan's syndrome

Dominant gene defects

Recessive inheritance

Both parents carry a defective gene for a particular disorder e.g. cystic fibrosis, sickle cell disease and thalassaemia. There is a 1 in 4 chance of the disorder being passed on with each pregnancy.

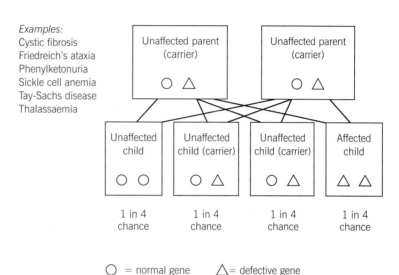

Examples:
Cystic fibrosis
Friedreich's ataxia
Phenylketonuria
Sickle cell anemia
Tay-Sachs disease
Thalassaemia

Recessive gene defects

Sex-linked inheritance

Sex-linked or X-linked disorders are passed from mothers to their sons, e.g. haemophilia, duchenne muscular dystrophy and colour blindness. With each pregnancy, mothers who carry an affected gene on their X chromosome have a 1 in 2 chance of each boy being affected and a 1 in 2 chance of each girl being a carrier.

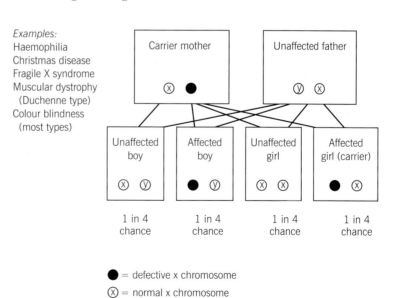

Examples:
Haemophilia
Christmas disease
Fragile X syndrome
Muscular dystrophy
 (Duchenne type)
Colour blindness
 (most types)

X-linked gene defects

Chromosomal abnormalities

Conditions which result from defects in the chromosomes result in a general pattern of characteristic abnormality. Down's syndrome is a well known chromosomal abnormality.

The chromosome pattern of a male infant with Down's syndrome. Note the presence of the extra number 21 chromosome, Trisomy 21.

Chromosomal pattern of Down's Syndrome

Maternal health

Diabetes, heart disease and other chronic conditions which affect the health of the mother can also affect the health and development of the fetus and baby e.g. there is a higher incidence of congenital abnormalities in babies born to mothers with diabetes.

Pre-eclampsia and eclampsia

This condition only occurs during pregnancy and pre-eclampsia is characterised by high blood pressure, swelling of the tissues (oedema), protein in the urine and excessive weight gain. Eclampsia is the onset of convulsions and is fortunately rare, but it can occur if treatment for pre-eclampsia is not given, or if it is ineffective and the condition is especially severe.

Pre-eclampsia usually occurs after the 28th week of pregnancy and is most common in first pregnancies, in teenage mothers and those over 35 years of age. It can result in poor fetal growth and low birth weight. The condition is only relieved with the birth of the baby. Severe cases will result in a premature birth to prevent the condition worsening and risking the life of the mother and baby. The health of the baby will be affected if it is delivered in poor condition after a period of delayed growth caused by placental insufficiency (the placenta is damaged as a result of high blood pressure and as a result it cannot nourish the fetus adequately).

Infection

Infections in pregnancy can pass through the placental barrier to affect the embryo/fetus. Rubella, toxoplasmosis and listeriosis are examples of pathogenic organisms that can have a catastrophic effect on the future health of the child.

Rubella

Rubella infection during the first twelve weeks of pregnancy can cause blindness, deafness, heart disease and possibly cerebral palsy.

Toxoplasmosis

Toxoplasmosis in early pregnancy can result in blindness and damage to the developing brain. It may cause epilepsy and delayed intellectual development. Many European countries routinely screen for this condition in pregnancy.

Listeria

Listeria is a bacteria found in pâté and soft cheeses and can be transferred to the fetus causing damage.

Cytomegalovirus

Cytomegalovirus may cause flu-like symptoms and cross the placenta to infect the fetus. The baby may develop hepatitis, inflammation of the brain and blindness. The developing child will usually have delayed motor skills and severe learning difficulties. Infected babies will excrete the virus in the urine for months and years and may infect pregnant women.

HIV

HIV can be passed from mother to child. The incidence of infected mothers having HIV infected babies is about 14 per cent. There is no evidence to suggest that the virus affects the embryo/fetus in the developmental stages. There is high risk associated with breast feeding and mothers who are known to be HIV positive or have AIDS are advised to bottle feed their infants.

Sexually transmitted diseases

Sexually transmitted diseases such as gonorrhoea, herpes and syphilis may affect the fetus during pregnancy or infect the baby during the birth process.

> ## Good Practice
>
> All women should check their immunity to rubella before becoming pregnant. Childcare workers are more vulnerable to infections than most other adults, because of their prolonged contact with children. Establishment managers should encourage staff to have their rubella antibody status checked and if necessary have the rubella immunisation.

Smoking

Smoking is associated with a large number of problems for children both before and after birth. Tobacco releases nicotine into the body which affects the growth and development of the baby. During pregnancy it can affect the developing embryo and foetus, causing the baby to weigh less at birth than it would have done if the mother had not smoked. There is also evidence to suggest that babies of smokers have reduced intellectual ability and are at a higher risk of sudden infant death syndrome (SIDS) or cot death, ear disease and admissions to hospital for respiratory illness. Smoking may also cause fires in the home and be related to increased risk of adult diseases like cancer and heart disease.

It is difficult to determine whether exposure to smoking before or after birth is most significant and also whether the negative outcomes are the result of associated social factors. There is a higher incidence of smoking in the lower social classes for whom this habit may be a response to severe life stresses.

Children of smokers are more likely to smoke as adults. This reduces their chance of good health.

Alcohol

Alcohol in pregnancy is best avoided. Moderate drinking in pregnancy can result in an increased risk of miscarriage, minor malformations and slower development in childhood. Heavy, 'binge' drinking episodes can result in 'fetal alcohol syndrome' – this condition affects fetal growth and causes delayed development, learning difficulties and congenital abnormalities.

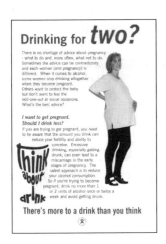

Alcohol in pregnancy is best avoided

Drugs

Drugs in any form should be stopped during pregnancy because of their potential effect on the fetus. Prescribed medicines should be taken only if the doctor and pharmacist have ensured their safety in pregnancy. Some drugs, which can normally be taken safely can, if taken during pregnancy, cause deafness, cleft lip and palate or masculine features in female babies.

Non-prescibed or illegal drugs such as heroin, cocaine or barbiturates cause addiction in the baby, and require careful 'weaning off'. They may result in all-round (global) developmental delay and epilepsy in the child.

Diet

Healthy eating should be continued as detailed under pre-conceptual factors (see pages 38–9).

Deficiencies in the diet may cause certain congenital malformations e.g. lack of sufficient folic acid in the first 12 weeks may result in a neural tube defect such as spina bifida.

Liver is best avoided in pregnancy because too much Vitamin A can cause fetal abnormalities.

Irradiation

Exposure in early pregnancy may have a harmful effect on the developing fetus and result in a higher risk of cancer in childhood. Abnormalities may occur in the next generation if the reproductive cells in the embryo/fetus are affected.

✅ *Progress check*

1 What is the difference between an inherited condition and a congenital disorder?
2 Explain recessive and dominant inheritance.
3 Which infections can cross the placental barrier and what are the possible results?
4 Why is smoking discouraged in pregnancy?
5 How can babies and children be affected by their parent(s) smoking after birth?
6 What can result from heavy alcohol consumption in pregnancy?
7 What are 'drugs' and why should they be stopped during pregnancy?
8 Why is it best to avoid foods which are rich in vitamin A in pregnancy?

Activity

Research into the provision of antenatal care in your area. You could arrange to talk to a midwife or health visitor to find out about the different services available such as:

■ who provides care and where
■ the types and methods of offering health advice
■ what sort of examinations and tests are performed
■ how often women are examined
■ the choices available for delivery.

Birth – perinatal factors

Birth is much safer today than it was 50 years ago, but there are inevitable risks associated with the process. Adverse events at delivery can be:

■ fetal distress usually caused by lack of oxygen – anoxia – which can cause damage to the brain. To relieve the condition, the baby should be delivered quickly with an assisted delivery
■ effects of analgesia (pain killers) and anaesthetics which, if used too close to the birth, can result in a floppy baby who is slow to breath and requires resuscitation
■ abnormal presentations resulting in a longer labour which tires the baby and may result in anoxia.

Postnatal factors

Postnatal factors are those which affect a child from birth onwards. Everything that happens to a child throughout childhood can affect the progress they make. This section describes some factors which are necessary for a child to maintain healthy growth and development and to be able to fight infection. It should be read in conjunction with 'Meeting needs' in Chapter 1 (see page 23) which describes the health needs of children.

Hormones

A hormone is a chemical substance which is made in one part of the body and carried in the bloodstream to act on tissues or organs in another part. It is a chemical messenger. Hormones are usually produced in *endocrine* (ductless) glands; these glands pass their secretions directly into the bloodstream, for distribution around the body, to their 'target' organ.

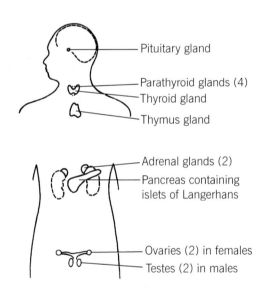

Endocrine glands

Infection

Several childhood illnesses can affect growth and development. Some of them are controlled by the childhood immunisation programme i.e. diphtheria, tetanus, whooping cough (pertussis), meningitis, polio, measles and mumps (see page 77).

Before birth, a baby is protected by the mother's immunity: her antibodies to infections pass through the placenta into the baby's bloodstream. After birth, babies need to develop their own immunity which depends upon their own immune system.

Infectious illnesses can affect health, not only for the duration of the illness but sometimes for the rest of a child's life (see 'Chapter 3, Preventing infection' and 'Chapter 8, Infectious diseases'.)

Endocrine glands			
GLAND	**HORMONE**	**FUNCTION**	**EFFECTS OF TOO MUCH OR TOO LITTLE**
Pituitary – the master of the orchestra of endocrine glands. It secretes hormones which control the activity of the other endocrine glands	Growth hormone Gonadotrophic hormone ACTH Lactogenic hormone (prolactin)	Controls: ■ the rate of growth ■ the development of the reproductive organs and secondary sexual characteristics ■ blood pressure ■ urine production	Giantism or dwarfism if too much or too little growth hormone is produced
Thyroid	Thyroxine	Stimulates: ■ general growth rate ■ bone development ■ the nervous system ■ muscle development ■ circulation ■ the function of the reproductive organs	■ Congenital hypothyroidism is the result of too little thyroxine before birth ■ poor growth ■ slow movements and clumsiness ■ intellectual delay ■ large and protruding tongue
Parathyroid	Parathyroid hormone	To control the use of calcium and phosphorous. These are vital for: ■ healthy bones and teeth ■ for efficient muscle action ■ blood clotting	Too much parathyroid hormone causes softening of the bones and weak muscles Too little parathyroid hormone causes painful muscle cramps
Pancreas	Insulin	To control the amount of sugar in the bloodstream	Insufficient insulin causes diabetes mellitus
Adrenal	Adrenalin – the 'fight or flight' hormone Cortisone	Provides: ■ the strength to fight or the energy to run away ■ control of certain body minerals affecting growth ■ assistance to sexual maturation	Too much cortisone leads to *Cushing's syndrome* which can lead to death. Too little cortisone leads to *Addison's disease* which results in male characteristics in females and female characteristics in males.
Ovaries	Oestrogen Progesterone	To control the development and functioning of the reproductive organs in females	Failure to develop the secondary sexual characteristics
Testes	Testosterone	To control the development and functioning of the reproductive organs in males	Failure to develop the secondary sexual characteristics

<table>
<tr><td>

Remember

Parents' decisions about infant feeding should always be treated with respect.

</td></tr>
</table>

Breast feeding

Although mothers should choose their preferred method of infant feeding, breast feeding has undoubted benefits to the health of the baby and child, such as:

■ reduced risk of infection due to the presence of antibodies in the breast milk

- reduced risk of juvenile diabetes
- protection against allergic diseases such as asthma and eczema
- reduced risk of SIDS (sudden infant death syndrome).

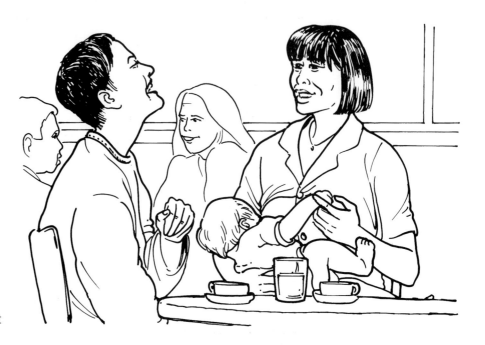

Breast feeding is convenient

Diet

Well-balanced diets contain protein, carbohydrates, fat, minerals, vitamins and water. Children should be offered a wide variety of foods from the different food groups to ensure that all the necessary nutrients are given in acceptable quantities.

Children from poor families tend to have diets which are high in saturated fats and sugars, combined with inadequate amounts of minerals, vitamins and iron. This is because parents receiving state benefits may find it increasingly difficult to supply a healthy, nutritious diet on their low income. They may offer cheap, filling foods such as chips and bread. This will affect their children's general health and their growth and development – inadequate amounts of protein in early life may result in delayed learning. The results of a diet that does not contain all the essential nutrients may be:

- poor growth including growth of the brain
- recurrent infections such as colds and respiratory tract infections
- health problems such as anaemia
- impaired intellectual development
- delayed physical development
- emotional difficulties.

> ## Good Practice
>
> Meals provided in childcare establishments should always be of high nutritional value. They should offer choices for children who are on particular diets due to their culture, religion or medical condition.

Current dietary concerns

Some diet-related conditions which may originate and become apparent in childhood are as follows.

Dental disease

Fifty per cent of children have dental disease before their second teeth appear.

Nutritional anaemia

This is due to insufficient intake of iron, folic acid and vitamin B12.

Obesity

This may lead to high blood pressure and raised blood cholesterol which are risk factors for coronary heart disease. Being overweight in late childhood is likely to lead to obesity in adult life.

Inadequate bone mass

Weakened bones will result from poor intake of calcium and lack of physical exercise. This may lead to osteoporosis (softening of the bones) in later life.

Cancer

Thiry-five per cent of all cancers may be diet related. Low intake of fruit and vegetables, especially in childhood, increases the risks of cancer of the colon and breast in adulthood.

Intellectual performance

There is some evidence to suggest that poorly nourished children perform less well at school.

Dental care

Dental caries (tooth decay)

This is the main dental disease affecting children and the one which will probably continue into adult life. Although there have been improvements to dental health over the last few decades, there is still the potential for further reduction in the incidence of dental caries.

- Forty per cent of 5-year-old children have active dental decay.
- Five-year-olds have, on average, two teeth affected by tooth decay.

- Children who attend the dentist only as emergencies have a higher rate of diseased teeth than those who attend regularly for check-ups.
- There is a higher rate of dental disease in children from the lower social classes.

Ways of reducing the incidence of tooth decay
- Sugar is the most likely cause of tooth decay, so reduce the number of times it is eaten or drunk during the day and avoid sweet snacks and drinks between meals.
- Fluoride in the water supply and in toothpaste reduces the incidence of dental decay.
- Regular dental checks are advised from babyhood – twice a year is the recommended frequency.
- Brush the teeth thoroughly in the morning, before bed and after meals if possible.

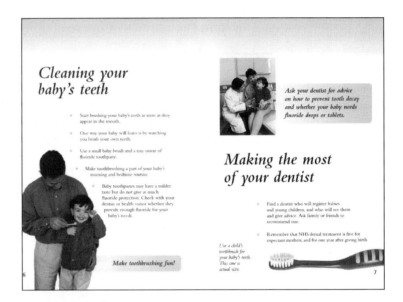

A Health Education Authority leaflet gives advice about dental care

---

Good Practice

Children should be offered the opportunity to clean their teeth after meals in childcare establishments. By using their own tooth brushes with adult supervision the children are encouraged to develop a habit for life.

 Progress check

1 What may affect the health of the baby at the time of birth?
2 What is a hormone?
3 Which hormones affect growth and development?
4 What may be the result of a deficiency of any of these hormones?

5 How can infection affect the health of a child?
6 What are the benefits of breast feeding for the health of the infant?
7 Why is a nutritionally balanced diet important for children?
8 What are the possible results of a diet which does not contain all the essential nutrients?
9 Why are some children likely to have tooth decay?
10 What can be done by childcare workers to prevent tooth decay in young children?

Case study

Hamish was born after a long and difficult labour at 34 weeks of pregnancy. His mother, Alison, tried to breast feed him but stopped after 48 hours because Hamish would not fix onto the nipple properly. When he was given a bottle instead, he gained weight steadily and was thriving. At 4 months Alison tried to wean him but he refused the spoon and cried for his bottle. When he was 9 months old the health visitor conducted a routine screening check after his hearing test – his weight had increased by only 300 grams in 8 weeks and his mother explained the difficulties she was having in feeding him.

The health visitor advised and supported Alison with Hamish's feeding and he began to take food from a spoon, but only if it was very sweet. Alison went back to work, leaving Hamish in a local private day nursery, where he started to drink cows' milk at 12 months, refused savoury dinners, enjoyed his puddings and took the occasional piece of toast and sucked it. He continued to enjoy honey on his dummy, learning to dip it into the pot himself. Hamish was constantly suffering from coughs and colds in his second year and he had several ear infections. Alison was shocked when his front two teeth (upper incisors) rapidly decayed.

1 What factors influenced Hamish's health?
2 How could Hamish have been encouraged to eat a nutritious diet?
3 What caused his tooth decay?
4 How could his dental health be improved?
5 Which professionals may be able to help this family to improve their health?

Environmental influences on child health

This section highlights important external influences which can affect child health.

There are many factors in the physical and social environment which have the potential to affect children's health and welfare. A person's environment includes their total surroundings: the family and the community including their culture, religion and education. The environment however, is more than the immediate surroundings and extends to include the town or city, county, country, continent and even the world in which we live. Children should always be seen in the context of their family and total environment (see Chapter 1). Laws and policies passed by various governments will ultimately have an effect on the health of the population in that country and may spread further afield, e.g. the aims of the The World Health Organisation (WHO).

Nature and nurture

The amount of potential given to a child is decided by heredity (nature) and the environment determines the extent to which that potential develops (nurture). If a child has the genetic information to grow to 150cm, the outcome will not be affected by however much food, care and stimulation is provided; but these contributory factors will determine whether or not a child achieves their maximum i.e. the best they can. By offering children the opportunity to fulfil their potential, in all areas of growth and development, they are given a good basis for life.

Mortality rates

Statistics are gathered yearly to assess the death rates for a range of conditions i.e. the numbers of people dying from various causes. These figures are collated by the Office of Population, Censuses and Surveys (OPCS) and provide important information about the health of the nation. The rates which apply to children are defined below.

Stillbirth rate

The stillbirth rate is the number of babies born after 24 completed weeks of pregnancy with no signs of life. The number is calculated per 1,000 total births.

Perinatal mortality rate

The perinatal mortality rate is the number of babies dying in the first week of life. The number is calculated per 1,000 total births (this figure includes the number of stillborn babies).

Neonatal mortality rate

The neotal mortality rate is the number of babies dying in the first 28 days of life. The number is calculated per 1,000 live births.

Post-neonatal mortality rate

The post-neonatal mortality rate is the number of babies dying after the first 28 days and before the first birthday. The number is calculated per 1,000 live births.

Infant mortality rate

The infant mortality rate is the number of babies dying in the first year of life. The number is calculated per 1,000 total births. The infant mortality rate is an indicator of the health of the population. There are many countries which have lower mortality rates than the UK, so it seems that there are many improvements which could be made.

A hundred years ago only 6 babies out of 10 survived to adulthood. Today the death of a child is usually unexpected and constitutes a great tragedy.

Activity

Find out what the different mortality rates are nationally and in your health region. This information is published annually by OPCS and should be available in your local library or in the college learning centre.

Poverty

The main causes of poverty are low wages or living on state benefits. People are most likely to be poor if they are unemployed, disabled, living in single-parent families, members of minority cultural groups or elderly. The disadvantages associated with poverty, such as poor housing and overcrowding, have not been eradicated and social conditions continue to have negative effects on health today.

Since the beginning of this century links have been made between poverty and its negative influences on child health. Damp, inadequate and dangerous housing leads to poor health, illness, accidents and encourages the spread of infection because adequate hygiene is difficult.

Although overall death rates have fallen this century, there continues to be a higher mortality rate among babies and children born to parents in social class 5. Social class is based on the Registrar-General's classification of occupations ranging from social class 1 (professional) to social class 5 (unskilled).

A baby born into social class 5 is twice as likely to die between the end of the first month and the first birthday than a child born to parents in social class 1.

A male child with unskilled parents compared with the son of a professional person is:

- 4 times more likely to die before his first birthday
- 7 times more likely to be killed in a road accident
- 10 times more likely to die before 14 from an accident concerning fire, falling or drowning.

Pollution

Environmental pollution can seriously affect children's health. The most serious pollution occurs where there are large cities and many factories. Children who live in inner-city areas are more at risk from the pollution from car exhausts, industrial processes and dangerous discarded items. Children's bodies are quicker than adults' to absorb toxic substances, and slower to get rid of them. This, combined with the fact that children breath in twice as much air per pound of body weight than adults, makes them very vulnerable to pollution.

- Chemical pollution has been linked to cancers in children – it can be caused by the fertilisers and insecticides, used by farmers, polluting the air and water supply.
- Air pollution from factory chimneys and fumes from car exhausts can damage health and affect intellectual achievement in children. Road traffic is the fastest growing cause of air pollution and since 1993 all cars have been built with catalytic converters to reduce the levels of nitrogen oxide, carbon monoxide and hydrocarbons which they excrete.
- Radioactivity, mainly associated with nuclear energy, creates many risks to health, in particular the disposal of radioactive wastes and the effects of catastrophic accidents such as Chernobyl in 1986.

Pollution can act as a trigger for asthma and can worsen an existing condition. The rate of admissions to hospital is affected by pollution levels.

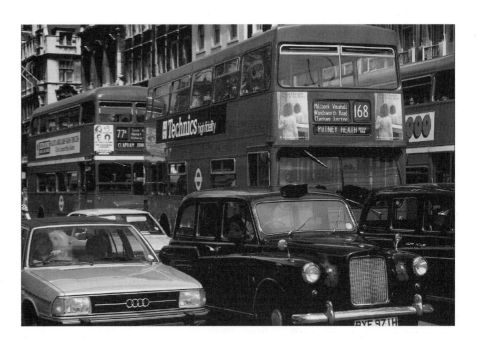

Inner-city pollution can affect child health

Unintentional (accidental) injury

Unintentional injuries are the commonest cause of death and injury to children. Calling them accidents implies that they are acts of God and that we cannot do anything to prevent them. This is not the case – with more care many 'accidents' would not happen.

More children aged 1 to 4 years are killed or injured in road accidents – either as passengers in motor vehicles or as pedestrians – than in any other type of accident. This is closely followed by fire and flame accidents, drowning, inhalation and ingestion accidents, falls, suffocation and poisoning. The causes of unintentional injuries are directly related to:

■ the developmental age/stage of the child
■ the child's changing perception of danger
■ the degree of exposure to different hazards at various ages.

Social class can affect the chances of an accident occurring, some injuries are up to six times more common in the poorest areas compared to the most affluent.

Attitudes to child care can affect, for example:

1 how much independence children are allowed
2 supervision travelling to and from school
3 opportunities to play safely outdoors – children may be allowed to play on the street and to cross the road before they are old enough to judge traffic safely.

The table below highlights the most common accidents with general ideas for prevention.

TYPE OF INJURY	PREVENTION
Road accidents – passenger	Children should travel in seats or restraints which comply with BSI safety standards
Road accidents – pedestrian	Children should be supervised on the roads at all times. Safe play areas, traffic-free areas, safe journeys to school
Tricycle/bicycle accidents	Safety helmets for all children, no access to roads until a cycling proficiency test has been passed
Fire and flame and scalds	Smoke alarms fitted in all homes. Coiled flex on kettles. Reducing thermostat on hot water tanks
Drowning	Parent education about bath dangers. Covered and fenced ponds and pools. Swimming lessons for 4–7 year olds
Suffocation and strangulation	Nuts, small sweets, plastic bags etc. should be kept away from small children. Safe disposal of old fridges and other appliances which children can 'hide' in
Poisoning	Continuing improvement in child-proof packaging for medicines and domestic chemicals. Locked cupboards out of reach to children
Falls	Window catches and bars, safe balconies. No furniture near windows to climb on. Safe surfaces in playgrounds
Glass injuries	Safety glass and safety membranes covering glass doors and windows
Dog attacks	Education for parents and children about the dangers of dogs. Dogs should be trained and cared for
Sunburn and heatstroke	'Slip, slap, slop': Tee-shirt, hat and high factor sun cream

Good Practice

Childcare workers have a continuing responsibiltiy to keep the children in their care safe. This means:

■ thorough inspection of the environment for safety hazards
■ constant vigilance by a watchful adult
■ awareness of the particular dangers at various stages of development.
■ ability to predict and avoid dangerous situations.

Non-accidental injury

Research shows that child abuse does not occur entirely at random, but is more likely to happen in some situations rather than others. There is a wide variety of predisposing factors to abuse, these may include an adult's personality and background, some kind of difficulty and stress in the adult's life or environment and factors relating to the child. Abuse is usually the result of a series of these factors occurring together but in each case there will be a different combination of factors, and their relative importance will also vary.

Children who are abused will probably experience long-lasting effects on their health and development e.g. failure to thrive, inability to make relationships and to play, leading to withdrawal and depression, behaviour difficulties, low self-esteem, learning difficulties and symptoms of stress.

Sudden infant death syndrome (SIDS)

The number of babies dying as a result of SIDS or cot death (see page 190) has been falling over recent years, especially due to the research conducted by the Foundation for the Study of Infant Deaths (FSID), which resulted in the publication of information about the following avoidable hazards:

- **Smoking** – no smoking in the same room as the baby. Parents should not smoke at all, but if this is impossible they should smoke outside.
- **Overheating** – cot quilts should not be used – a sheet and blankets is preferable so that layers can be removed or added.
- **Sleeping position** – babies should sleep on their back, or supported on their side. Their feet should be at the bottom of the cot to prevent slipping down under the covers.
- **Breast feeding** – may be a protective factor. It may be the feeding intention which is more important because it indicates an awareness of the baby's needs.

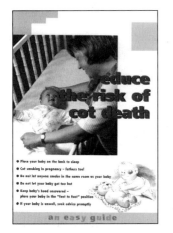

Recent research has increased knowledge about how to reduce the risks of SIDS

Case study

Jamie lives near the centre of a large industrial city, with commuter and commercial traffic filling the air with smoke and fumes. He is an asthmatic child who was diagnosed when he was 2 years old after a year of repeated chest infections. At times his mother says she can smell and taste the pollution. This area has one of the highest rates of asthma in the region and 17 children per 1,000 are admitted to hospital each year with severe respirarory problems associated with asthma. Only 10 children per 1,000 from a nearby leafy suburb are similarly affected. In the heat of the summer the air is heavy, the heat of the sunshine acts on polluting gases to form a summertime smog.

1 Why do you think this area has such a high rate of childhood asthma?
2 How do you think the air quality in inner-city areas could be improved?

> ✓ **Progress check**
>
> 1 What does the child's environment include?
> 2 Explain the difference between nature and nurture.
> 3 What are mortality rates and why are they collected?
> 4 How can poverty have a negative influence on children's health?
> 5 Why do you think that there is a higher mortality rate in children from social class 5?
> 6 Why are children in inner city areas more vulnerable to the effects of pollution?
> 7 Give an example of each of the main types of pollution.
> 8 What are the causes of accidental injuries related to?
> 9 Why do you think that social class can affect the risk of a child being involved in an accident?
> 10 Which factors may predispose to child abuse?
> 11 What are the avoidable hazards which have been associated with SIDS?

Activity

Using the table of types of the most common accidents on page 57, and your own research, complete an 'Accident Prevention' report which includes the following information about each type of injury.

1 What may cause this type of accident?
2 Which age group is the most vulnerable?
3 Why do you think this is?
4 Prepare a 24-hour safety routine to prevent children from being at risk of any of these injuries:

- at home
- in their childcare establishment.

Inequalities in health care

Although the health service is available to the whole population, regardless of social class and status, it is not used to the same extent by everyone. It is generally the educated middle-classes who are aware of their entitlement to health care and who access the services offered most regularly. It is this group who are more likely to respond to advice offered during health education campaigns and as a result of personal contact with health professionals. In areas with the most sickness and death, GPs have larger caseloads and less hospital support. Hospital doctors have heavier workloads with less staff and equipment than in the healthiest areas.

Remember

The inverse care law: the availability of good health care tends to vary inversely with the need of the population served.

The groups most in need of support are the ones who are usually the least likely to take advantage of the available services and resources. This is known as the 'inverse care law' – the amount of health care and advice available and accepted is inversely proportional to the level of need. This combines with other social factors to produce inequalities in health and health care.

Poor take-up of health services may be due to the following.

- Social isolation – could be due to personality problems or language or cultural barriers.
- Language difficulties – in spoken or written language. This will make the service appear frightening and inaccessible.
- Cultural background – health services that do not respect and value differences between cultural groups are not 'user friendly'.
- Low self-esteem – people who do not value themselves will not value good health either.
- Lack of awareness of the importance of health care – parents who have not experienced positive health care themselves may be unaware of its importance for their families.
- Previous negative experience.
- Mistrust of professionals who are seen as 'interfering' and authoritarian – poor educational experiences and clashes with 'authority' in the early years may continue throughout life unless an effort is made by health care workers to build positive relationships.

Race issues in health

Many black people in Britain tend to live in deprived inner city areas. The factors affecting the health of black people in Britain are related largely to their socio-economic circumstances i.e. family income due to low pay and unemployment, housing conditions, lack of safe play areas in a deprived physical environment, social tensions and racial abuse and attack. The health of black and ethnic minority children will also be affected if health service providers fail to ensure that the child health service is appropriate for them.

Most of the health services offered to families are based on white, middle class needs such as screening for 'white' conditions such as phenylketonuria (PKU) which affects 1 in 14,000 white people. Sickle cell anaemia which affects 1 in 400 African-Caribbean people and thalassaemia are not always routinely screened for despite their higher incidence within certain racial groups.

Development checks are based on the average progress of white middle-class children and do not reflect the differences between the races. Reaction to toys and the ability to build with bricks are often central to development tests. Children from ethnic minorities may have limited experience of these toys and will perform accordingly. Assessment of hearing for speech and verbal reasoning are usually carried out in English, often by English health workers. Children for whom English is not the first language will be disadvantaged. These tests could be described as culturally racist.

Health care and childcare workers should be trained to recognise and appreciate the differences between cultural groups, and accept alternative child-rearing practices with sensitivity and understanding.

Social disadvantage

People are described as disadvantaged if they do not have the equal opportunity to achieve what other people in society regard as normal. About two and a half million children live in poverty in Britain today. There is a well-established link between ill health and social deprivation which can lead to low achievement at nursery and mainstream school. Children born into families in the lower social classes are less likely to attend for screening services and their mothers are less likely to have received adequate antenatal care during pregnancy. Because children cannot learn the necessary skills to generate good health from their parents, they copy the poor example of the previous generation. Disadvantage is influenced by:

- low income
- poor housing
- large family **or**
- single-parent family

but, of course, not all families with some of these social conditions are disadvantaged.

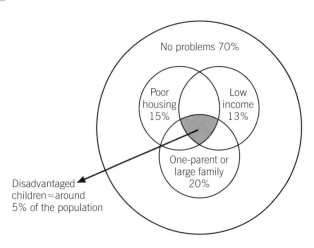

Circles of social conditions

Remember

Poverty is not only about having no money – poor people experience deprivation and disadvantage in most areas of their lives. Poverty is more common in inner-city areas and children may be affected by 'multiple deprivation'.

The members of a family who are disadvantaged are more likely to become ill because they have fewer personal and physical resources to cope with illness and are less likely to receive medical care. National studies of child development have found that the children of disadvantaged families are on average 4cm shorter than other children of the same age.

- **Education** – children may lack a home environment which stimulates development.
- **Health** – inner-city areas are usually poorly serviced with doctors. People may not be aware of their rights from the Welfare State. Poor diets lead to ill health.

- **Housing** – accommodation may be damp, unheated or modern high-rise accommodation. There may be bleak areas with few play areas, dangerous roads, high crime rates and social problems.
- **Shopping** – having no car makes large supermarket shopping difficult. The small local shop is expensive. Poor people can buy only small quantities which are expensive. They may need credit and pay high interest charges.
- **Family life** – poverty increases family problems such as depression, despair and hopelessness, which may lead to arguments and violence.

Case study

George and Rachel Miller and their three children had been rehoused in a high rise block of flats after their house had been repossessed. George was a coal miner but had been unemployed for six years since the pit was closed. His local council could not provide the necessary accommodation so the family had moved to a large town several miles away from their extended family. The children were aged 10, 6 and 2 years. The youngest was born while the family lived in the flats and she had never been well, suffering from recurrent ear and chest infections. Money was tight and there never seemed to be enough for everything, food was expensive from the local shops and the supermarket was two miles away. George and Rachel sometimes went without meals so that the children could eat. Rachel was depressed about having no money and George seemed to have given up looking for work. The family did not go out together any more and the stress of their situation lead to friction and arguments. Lack of space to play meant that when the two eldest children went out, Rachel was glad to have some peace and quiet.

1 What problems associated with deprivation are this family experiencing?
2 Why are the two eldest children at risk when they go out?
3 What factors are affecting the health of this family?

The role of the childcare worker

These families need extra care and support from helpful and empathetic people. The role of the childcare worker is to liaise with other professionals in the health care team and social services and to offer the highest standards of care in a non-judgmental way, whilst maintaining confidentiality. This involves recognising the value and dignity of every human being, irrespective of their socio-economic group, ethnic origin, gender, marital status, religion or disability. The childcare worker may be able to refer the family to other agencies which can offer specific help in times of need or crisis and can provide a focus for other parents/carers to support each other.

The relationship with the parents should be on equal terms with the aim of creating an environment where the parent and child can develop as individuals with increased confidence. The parents' wishes should be respected, not least because they know their children best. The parents will then be able to make appropriate decisions about their children's health and care.

 Progress check

1 Explain what the *inverse care law* means.
2 Which factors may influence the rate of use of health services?
3 How can race affect the health care available to families?
4 What can be done to increase equality of health care for black people?
5 What is social disadvantage?
6 What effects can poverty and disadvantage have on child health?
7 Which factors may predispose towards social disadvantage?
8 What is *multiple deprivation* and what areas of life may be affected?
9 How can childcare workers support families who are disadvantaged?

Key terms

You need to know what these words and phrases mean. Go back through the chapter and find out.

chromosome	mortality rates
congenital	nature and nurture
contraception	neonatal mortality
dental caries	non-accidental injury
dominant inheritance	perinatal
drug	pollution
eclampsia	postnatal
endocrine	pre-conceptual
folic acid	pre-eclampsia
genetic counselling	prenatal
genetics	recessive inheritance
hormone	sex-linked inheritance
immunity	social disadvantage
inequalities in health	sudden infant death syndrome
inverse care law	

Chapter 3 Preventing infection

This chapter includes:

- Disease-causing organisms
- How infection is spread
- Natural defences against infection
- Terms used in relation to infection
- Immunity
- Immunisation in childhood
- The role of the childcare worker in immunisation
- Providing a hygienic environment

All childcare workers have an important role in preventing the spread of infection and trying to reduce the incidence of disease in children. To understand how this can be achieved effectively they need an insight into the types of micro-organisms which cause disease, and knowledge about how they are transmitted from person to person. A child's natural defences to infection must be enhanced by both scrupulous attention to personal hygiene and high standards of care in the workplace. Other methods of prevention, such as immunisation and health education, are important tools in preventing infection and the consequences of illness. Because children are vulnerable to infections they need the protective care of responsible adults to enable them to grow and develop in a healthy environment.

Disease-causing organisms

Microscopic organisms (micro-organisms) which enter the body and cause illness or discomfort are called pathogens – this word is derived from the Greek *patho* meaning suffering and disease. Pathogenic micro-organisms are commonly known as germs and generally divided into three groups: bacteria, viruses and fungi.

However, not all micro-organisms are harmful – we use fungi in the form of yeasts and moulds to make bread, wine and cheese. Bacteria and fungi are used to make antibiotics.

Bacteria

These cells vary in size and have a tough outer wall. In favourable conditions bacteria divide into two to reproduce and quickly form large colonies. They need:

- warmth
- moisture

- food
- time

for successful reproduction. The human body supplies all these requirements. When conditions are less hospitable, bacteria form thick-walled spores which can survive for years as dust, only beginning to reproduce when the conditions become favourable.

Examples of diseases caused by bacteria are whooping cough, food poisoning and ear infections.

Bacteria can be successfully treated with antibiotics.

Viruses

Viruses are much smaller than bacteria and are true parasites – they need to invade a living cell (host) and then make hundreds of copies of themselves. When the affected host cell dies the new viruses are released and the process continues.

Diseases caused by viruses include chicken-pox, measles, the common cold, influenza and AIDS (acquired immunodeficiency syndrome) caused by the human immunodeficiency virus (HIV).

There is currently no effective drug treatment to combat viruses, but there are methods of dealing with the symptoms of the diseases they cause.

Fungi

There are only a few fungi which are harmful to humans. Fungal diseases are spread by:
- airborne spores
- contact with infected people
- walking bare-foot on infected floors and mats.

A common fungal disease is ringworm which causes a circular swelling on the skin and also can attack the scalp and the groin. Athlete's foot and thrush are also caused by fungal infection.

Human parasites

There are other organisms that cause disease which are large enough to be visible to the human eye, for example roundworms such as threadworms, flatworms such as tapeworms, fleas, scabies and head lice. See Chapter 11 for more detailed examinations of these.

Roundworms are round when cut in cross-section and are pointed at both ends. Roundworms live in soil, in fresh and salt water and are parasites of most vegetable and animal life. About 40 different species are parasites of human beings, the commonest in the Western world being the threadworm.

Threadworm

The threadworm looks like a small, white thread and may be seen in freshly passed stools. It lives in the bowel and lays its eggs around the

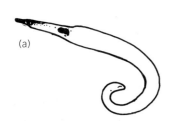

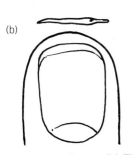

(a) The threadworm (b) The threadworm is not much bigger than the width of the little fingernail

anus, usually at night, causing severe itching around the bottom and when the child scratches her/his bottom the eggs are caught under the finger nails. It is transmitted via unwashed vegetables, soil, towels, bedding and less than scrupulous hygiene.

Drug treatment is available which, together with thorough hand washing, nail scrubbing and attention to laundry hygiene, is generally effective.

Tapeworms

These worms have flattened bodies and belong to a group of animals known as flatworms. They are, fortunately, rare in Britain, and are prevented by efficient sewage disposal. Imported meat should be carefully inspected for worms which can be seen with the naked eye.

Scabies

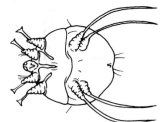

These external animal parasites are also known as itch mites because of the intense itching they cause. They prefer areas where the skin is thin and the female burrows under the skin where she lays her eggs. These hatch and more mites crawl out of the burrow to mate with the males on the skin surface.

Scabies are transmitted by skin-to-skin contact and via clothing, bedding and towels.

Scabies

Fleas

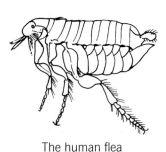

Fleas are small insects which are able to bite through skin and suck blood. Some fleas may carry other germs which they pass from person to person during feeding. Fleas cannot fly but they can jump from person to person and, although very small, can be clearly seen with the human eye.

Children may be bitten by fleas which usually infest cats and/or dogs.

Fleas can transmit typhus, bubonic plaque and anthrax.

The human flea

Head lice

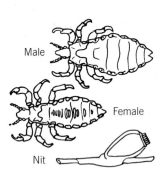

Unlike fleas, lice complete their life cycle on the host. They lay eggs – called nits – cemented onto the hair shaft, near to the scalp. Nits look like dandruff, but are impossible to brush off as they remain firmly attached to the hair. The eggs hatch leaving an empty shell, still cemented to the hair. Children who have been infested for some time will have a series of nits in varying stages of development down the hair shaft towards the root.

Male

Female

Nit

The male and female head louse and nit

Because head lice bite the skin to suck blood they can cause itching. Any child scratching their head repeatedly should be checked. Long-term infestations can cause lack of sleep, reduction in energy and vitality – the phrase 'feeling lousy' resulted from the effects of the louse.

The best prevention is regular combing or brushing of the hair, preferably straight after school or nursery as well as morning and evening. This breaks the legs of the louse and makes it incapable of laying eggs. Regular inspections of the head by parents and carers will spot infestations early – the hair behind the ears and at the back of the head /neck are the most likely areas.

✓ Progress check

1 What is the name given to microscopic organisms which cause disease?
2 What conditions do bacteria need to reproduce?
4 Give three examples of diseases caused by bacteria.
5 How do viruses multiply?
6 Give three examples of diseases caused by viruses.
7 How are fungal diseases spread?
8 What is the most common roundworm in the Western world?
9 What do scabies, fleas and head lice have in common?

How infection is spread

Pathogenic micro-organisms can enter the body in several ways. They can be:

■ inhaled – breathed in through the nose or mouth
■ ingested – eaten via the mouth
■ inoculated – entering through a break in the skin.

The ways that diseases are transmitted are almost endless; every time an epidemic occurs scientists try and find the source of the infection and how it is spread. Recent outbreaks of meningitis have resulted in microbiologists, pathologists and other health staff trying to detect the cause.

Direct and indirect contact

Diseases can be spread by direct or indirect contact.

■ **Direct contact** – physical touch such as kissing, contact with infected skin or sexual contact, is required for the disease to be transmitted.
■ **Indirect contact** – some pathogens can live for a while outside the body, and infected people may leave germs behind on objects which they have handled. These objects then become potential sources of infection by indirect contact.

The following are the most usual means of transmission with examples of diseases spread in that way.

Droplet infection

The actions of talking, singing, coughing and sneezing release tiny droplets of moisture from the nose and mouth. When we sneeze, about 20,000 droplets of moisture are released into the atmosphere and can

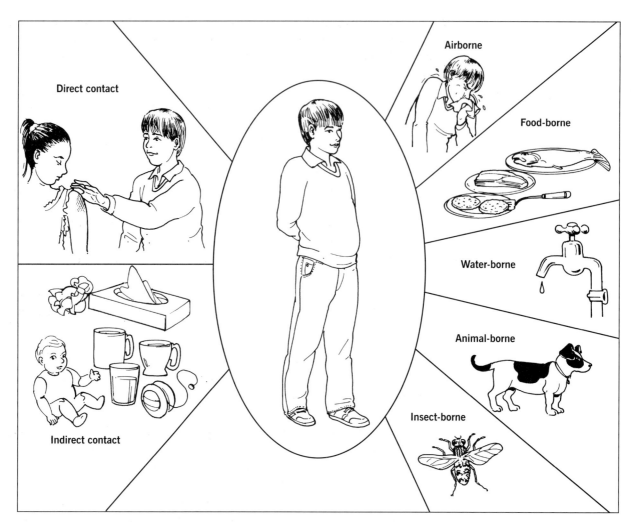

Direct contact

Airborne

Food-borne

Water-borne

Animal-borne

Indirect contact

Insect-borne

Sources of infection

eventually fall up to 4 metres away, usually floating in the air for some time. If these droplets are infected with bacteria or viruses, anyone who inhales the air may become infected. This method of transmission is responsible for spreading the common cold, flu, diphtheria, pneumonia, whooping cough, measles and many other infectious diseases.

Good Practice

Encourage children to wash their hands regularly and to cover their nose and mouth when they cough and sneeze. These simple precautions provide the most effective methods of preventing the spread of infection in childcare establishments.

Food and water

There are many ways by which food and drink can become contaminated and potentially very dangerous. There are two main categories of diseases spread by food.

- Food poisoning is the result of eating food which has been infected with bacteria which are normally found in the bowel of humans and animals. Large colonies of these bacteria in food will present serious symptoms in children.
- Food-borne infection refers to specific diseases caused by infected food such as typhoid, cholera, enteric fever and amoebic dysentery. BSE (referred to as 'mad cow disease' in the media) is thought to be responsible for the increase in Kreutsfeldt Jacob disease in humans.

Preventing contamination from food and water
The following simple precautions will prevent the majority of cases of food poisoning and food borne infections.

1 Hands can become contaminated after visiting the toilet, assisting children with toileting or attending to other bodily functions. If they are not washed thoroughly before handling food they may infect the food with bacteria.
2 Cuts, grazes and infected skin conditions should be covered before preparing food. It is preferable for people with skin infections to avoid contact with children's meals and snacks.
3 Avoid touching the nose or mouth and coughing and sneezing when preparing food.
4 Uncovered food may be contaminated by flies who have visited decomposing waste and faeces. They carry germs (and sometimes tapeworm eggs) on their legs.
5 Food storage is important e.g. covering food which is standing, checking the temperature of the fridge and freezer, storing cooked meat above raw meat in the fridge, chilling and refrigerating cooked food.
6 Cooking food thoroughly prevents most types of food poisoning. Food should be thoroughly defrosted prior to cooking, and cooked thoroughly to the centre. Special care should be taken with chicken and meat.
7 Primitive or inefficient sewage arrangements can result in diseases being spread via drinking water.

Animals and insects

Houseflies carry germs on their feet (see above), bodies and in their digestive systems. They spread typhoid, dysentery, cholera and tapeworm eggs.

Insects which suck blood can carry disease from one person to another e.g. malaria from the mosquito, and from animals to humans e.g. the bubonic plague can be spread from rat to flea and flea to human.

Terrapins spread salmonella food poisoning. Rabies is spread by dogs, foxes and wolves.

Healthy carriers of disease

All humans carry some bacteria in and on their bodies. Some people 'carry' pathogenic bacteria in the nose, throat and hands without showing any symptoms of disease. They are not aware that they are in this

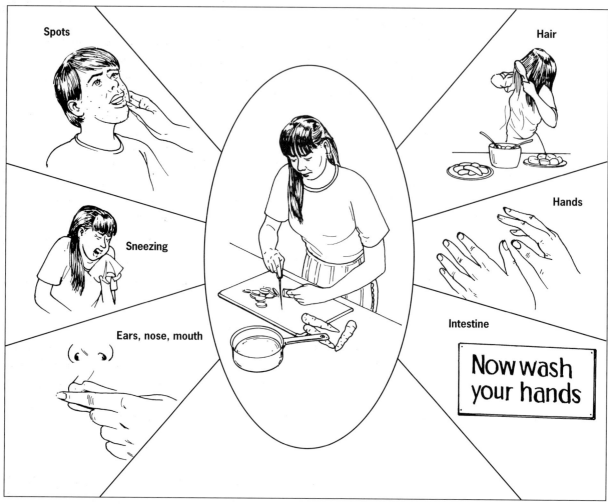

Spots

Sneezing

Ears, nose, mouth

Hair

Hands

Intestine

Now wash your hands

People often pass bacteria onto food

Remember

Some organisms can remain on objects which have been touched, sucked or contaminated by droplets from infected children or adults.

condition and can spread these germs to others causing mysterious outbreaks of disease. Strict hygiene precautions for all people, especially those working with, or in contact with, young children should prevent infection spreading.

✔ **Progress check**

1 How can pathogenic micro-organisms enter the body?
2 What is the difference between direct and indirect contact in the spread of infection?
3 Explain how droplets can spread infection.
4 What are the two main categories of disease spread by food?
5 Give five methods of preventing contamination from food and water.
6 Which animals and insects spread disease, and how?
7 How can humans be healthy carriers of disease?

Case study

Seagrave House Family Centre provided lunch-time meals for several children and their parents. Daphne the kitchen supervisor was not feeling very well, she was coughing and sneezing and constantly blowing her nose. Another member of staff was off with a sickness bug and so Daphne felt that she must go in to work or she would be letting the children down. When she got to work she found that the chicken had been left out all night; someone had forgotten to put it back into the cold store the previous day after taking out some pork. It had been a cool night, so Daphne decided to use the chicken anyway. She prepared chicken curry and rice with freshly cooked blackberries and apples for dessert. Several of the children complained of tummyache that afternoon and evening and many had bouts of diarrhoea and vomiting.

1 What are the possible causes of the outbreak of diarrhoea and vomiting?
2 What should Daphne have done to prevent this outbreak?

Natural defences against infection

Children are vulnerable to infections and need the protection of caring and responsive adults who encourage their healthy growth and development, recognise the early signs of illness and seek professional medical help when necessary.

A healthy body has many defences against infection.

The skin

The skin, when unbroken, acts as a barrier to the entry of germs. It secretes oily **sebum** which is a bactericidal substance (prevents the growth of bacteria) and prevents the drying of the skin to maintain its suppleness and resistance to water.

Mucous membrane

All the external entrances to the body (the mouth, nose, vagina, urethra etc.) are lined with mucous membrane which secretes mucous to trap germs and other particles carried in the air. Some mucous membrane, such as that in the respiratory passages, contains **cilia** – fine hair-like projections – which waft mucous, germs and dirt outside the body. The back-and-forth movements of the cilia in the respiratory passages carry the mucous, trapped dirt and germs to the back of the throat where they are swallowed and rendered harmless by the digestive juices.

The stomach

The stomach contains powerful hydrochloric acid and digestive enzymes which are usually successful in killing any germs that enter the digestive system.

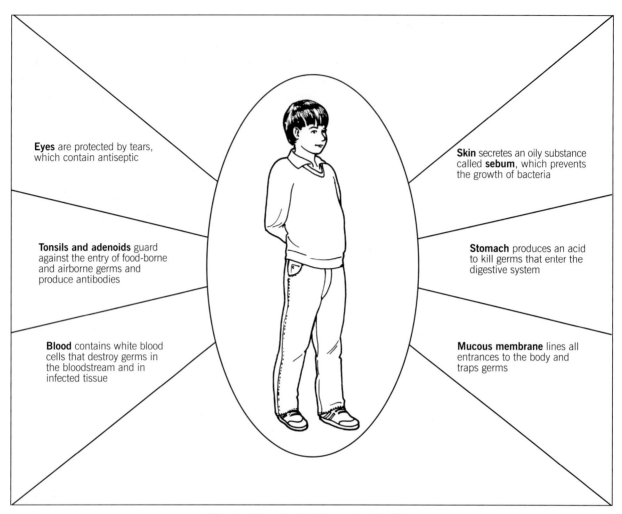

Eyes are protected by tears, which contain antiseptic

Tonsils and adenoids guard against the entry of food-borne and airborne germs and produce antibodies

Blood contains white blood cells that destroy germs in the bloodstream and in infected tissue

Skin secretes an oily substance called **sebum**, which prevents the growth of bacteria

Stomach produces an acid to kill germs that enter the digestive system

Mucous membrane lines all entrances to the body and traps germs

The body's natural defences to infection

Tears

The eyes are protected by antiseptic **tears** which contain lysozymes, an anti-bacterial enzyme, to help to prevent infection. The continual production of tears in the tear glands, combined with blinking, ensures that the eyes are bathed constantly to wash away germs and dust.

Tonsils and adenoids

Tonsils and adenoids form a protective ring of lymphoid tissue which guards against the entry of germs in food and in the air. They are large in early childhood when the risk of infection is greatest and shrink in late childhood and teens. Doctors' reluctance to remove tonsils and adenoids is mainly to do with their protective role in preventing and fighting infection.

White blood cells

White blood cells (leucocytes) circulate in the blood stream and act as defenders of the body. They try to destroy invading bacteria and viruses by leaving the blood vessels, surrounding the invading germs and ingesting them. When an infection is present, the body manufactures more white blood cells to fight it.

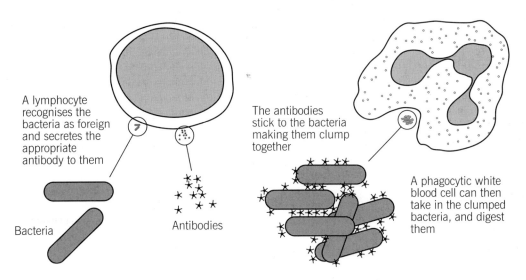

A lymphocyte recognises the bacteria as foreign and secretes the appropriate antibody to them

Bacteria

Antibodies

The antibodies stick to the bacteria making them clump together

A phagocytic white blood cell can then take in the clumped bacteria, and digest them

Phagocytosis: how white blood cells destroy bacteria

There are two particularly important types of white blood cells which fight infection:

■ phagocytes – surround, engulf and destroy bacteria. They are not effective against viruses.

■ lymphocytes – produce antibodies in response to foreign proteins (antigens) in the blood. They have a 'memory' and can recognise antigens they have been in contact with before; they produce the antibodies which are effective against a particular antigen. This is called immune response (see 'Immunity', pages 74–5)

The lymphatic system

The lymphatic system is involved largely with immunity and protecting the body when it is invaded by pathogenic organisms. The lymph glands are spread all over the body to cope with the various entry points of germs. They help to prevent infection from entering the bloodstream by filtering and destroying the germs. Lymphocytes produce antibodies to specific infections.

The lymph glands may swell when there is an infection present (see pages 148–9).

Terms used in relation to infection

It is important to read, understand and try to remember the following definitions of words and phrases commonly used in relation to infection.

- **Communicable disease**. A disease which is passed from one person to another by direct or indirect contact.
- **Infectious disease**. A disease which is caused by a specific organism and results in the same signs and symptoms. It can be transmitted by direct or indirect contact.
- **Incubation period**. The time between the organism entering the body until the appearance of the first signs and symptoms.
- **Quarantine**. Isolating an infected person until it is clear that they have or have not contracted a disease. Animals entering this country are placed in quarantine for the incubation period for rabies, to prevent rabies affecting our animal population.
- **Epidemic**. Outbreak of a disease in an area where many people are affected at the same time.
- **Endemic**. A disease which keeps recurring in a particular area or locality.

✓ *Progress check*

1 What are the natural defences to infection?
2 How are all the external entrances to the body equipped to fight infection?
3 Why are doctors reluctant to remove tonsils and adenoids from young children?
4 What is the role of white blood cells in protecting the body from infection?
5 What is the role of the lymphatic system in preventing infection?
6 What is the incubation period?
7 Explain what quarantine means.
8 What is an epidemic?

Immunity

There are many different types of immunity, the table below describes some of the ways that children can develop and acquire immunity to some diseases.

Immunity may not be effective for a whole lifetime, especially in the cases of passive immunity and active acquired immunity. Lymphocytes may lose the 'memory' of how to make a particular antibody. The most effective immunity results from having the disease itself, but many diseases have side-effects which it is preferable to avoid if possible.

ACTIVE IMMUNITY

The body is ACTIVE and works to produce antibodies – this is the **immune response**, the way the body deals with the invasion of pathogenic organisms. There are two main types of active immunity.

TYPE OF IMMUNITY	DESCRIPTION	EXAMPLE
Active natural immunity	This is the immune response to a naturally occurring infection – when a child has had a particular disease	If a child has had chickenpox, the body will have formed specific antibodies Each subsequent time the child is in contact with the disease the body will make the right antibodies to prevent the illness occurring again
Active acquired immunity	This is the immune response to an artificially introduced antigen as part of an immunisation programme	The polio vaccine which is given to children as part of the childhood immunisation schedule. This is much 'weaker' than the actual pathogen

PASSIVE IMMUNITY

The body is PASSIVE and relies on the antibodies which have been created in another organism and introduced into them. The body does not have to do any work. This type of immunity lasts only for a fairly short time

TYPE OF IMMUNITY	DESCRIPTION	EXAMPLE
Passive natural immunity	This naturally occurring immunity is the result of antibodies being passed from mother to child: ■ across the placenta in pregnancy ■ in breast milk during breast feeding – especially in the first milk, colostrum	Babies are born with a degree of immunity naturally acquired from their mother during pregnancy. e.g. measles and polio
Passive acquired immunity	Antibodies are transferred from one organism to another via injection	Many of the childhood immunisations contain 'ready-made' antibodies and provide this type of immunity e.g. diphtheria, tetanus

Herd immunity

It is not always necessary to immunise the whole population to protect all children. Some diseases such as diphtheria, where the disease is passed directly from one person to another and the immunisation is effective, can be almost eradicated with immunisation of 80 per cent of the total population. Immunising one group can therefore protect another.

Herd immunity is the phrase used to describe the status of the whole population where enough people are immunised to prevent the spread of the disease.

High rates of immunisation are required to ensure that the population is protected from certain diseases and their side-effects.

> **Remember**
>
> The immunisation of all children who can safely be immunised may result in herd immunity. This will offer some protection to other children who have not been immunised because of their medical condition.

Progress check

1 What is active immunity?
2 Give an example of active natural and active acquired immunity?
3 Describe passive natural immunity.
4 What is passive acquired immunity?
5 What are the benefits of herd immunity?

Completed primary vaccinations (all antigens) by 12 months and 24 months in the UK, January–March 1996

	% coverage at 12 month	% coverage at 24 month	% Health Authorities reaching at least 90% coverage by 24 months	% Health Authorities reaching at least 95% coverage by 24 months
Diphtheria	93	96	98	75
Tetanus	93	96	98	75
Pertussis	92	94	91	43
Polio	93	96	98	73
Hib	93	95	95	70
MMR	n/a	91	73	9

Herd immunity should be achieved when over 90 per cent of children receive their primary immunisations

Source: PHLS, CDSC

Pertussis notifications to ONS and vaccine coverage figures for children by their second birthday
England and Wales (1940-95)

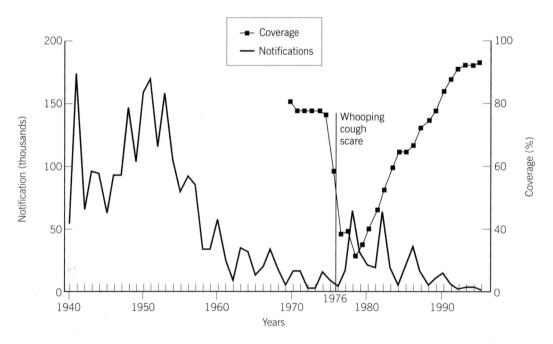

Immunisation in childhood

Immunisation is the use of vaccines to protect people from disease. The vaccines contain either:

■ minute weakened parts of the virus or bacteria which cause the disease (active acquired immunity) OR

■ small parts of the toxins that they produce (passive acquired immunity).

They have been treated to prevent the actual disease occurring, but stimulate the body to make the relevant antibodies.

Because babies and children are very vulnerable to infection the following schedule of childhood immunisations is given to children with their parents' written consent. Immunisation protects children from serious diseases and protects other children by preventing diseases from being passed on. Children who have not been immunised are at more risk.

AGE	IMMUNISATION	METHOD
2 months	HIB (meningitis) diphtheria, whooping cough, tetanus polio	1 injection 1 injection by mouth
3 months	HIB (meningitis) diphtheria, whooping cough, tetanus polio	1 injection 1 injection by mouth
4 months	HIB (meningitis) diphtheria, whooping cough, tetanus polio	1 injection 1 injection by mouth
12–15 months	measles, mumps, rubella (MMR)	1 injection
3–5 years pre-school booster MMR booster	diphtheria, tetanus polio measles, mumps and rubella	1 injection by mouth 1 injection
11–14 years	BCG (Bacillus Calmette-Guerin) vaccine to protect against TB (tuberculosis). All children are HEAF tested first to check their immunity.	1 injection
15–18 years leaving school booster	diphtheria, tetanus polio	1 injection by mouth

Care after immunisation

Some children may have a mild reaction to their immunisations.
- They may be irritable, unwell or have a fever for a while. If this occurs they should be given plenty of fluids to drink and kept cool, some paracetamol elixir may be suggested by the practice nurse, health visitor or doctor. This must be given in the correct dose for the age of the child. Some professionals advise that paracetamol is given to all infants after an immunisation.
- The site of the injection may become red or swollen. This should gradually disappear.
- Any serious symptoms, such as convulsions or a high temperature that does not come down after treatment with fluids and paracetamol, should be reported to the doctor immediately.

> ### *Good Practice*
>
> Babies and children who have been immunised should be observed carefully for 24 hours. If the temperature rises, extra fluids should be given and paracetamol elixir can be offered if the doctor and parents consent. If the temperature does not fall as a result, the doctor should be called.

Possible reasons for reduced uptake of immunisations

Although there are very few reasons why immunisation should not be given to particular children, there is still a reluctance amongst some parents to have their children immunised. There are a number of reasons.

- Parents may give immunisations low priority because many of the diseases immunised against are rarely seen in this country. However, measles and whooping cough (pertussis) are very distressing and still kill children every year. Mumps is the commonest cause of aseptic meningitis and also can cause hearing loss in children.
- Low advertising and resource budget. Other aspects of childcare are constantly in the media e.g. child abuse and acute illnesses, and to allay public concerns these take resources at the expense of the immunisation programmes.
- Negative publicity – media reports of side-effects from immunisations cause immediate reductions in the numbers of children having immunisation. A lot of children have not been immunised against pertussis because of media scares about children suffering from brain damage as a direct result of the immunisation. Research data suggests that children who have not been immunised against pertussis are more likely to be intellectually disadvantaged by the age of 5.
- Incorrect information about contra-indications – parents and some professionals may believe that certain conditions, such as eczema and asthma, mean that children should not be immunised. Access to reliable advice should provide the correct information to everyone.

Benefits of immunisation

The main advantages of childhood immunisation are listed below. Immunisation:

- prevents a child from suffering from a particular disease
- reduces the risks of side-effects
- protects children who are unable to receive immunisation (herd immunity)
- is cost effective. In financial terms it is cheaper to immunise the community than to care for those who have the disease and suffer from its complications (side-effects).

Contra-indications

Occasionally children are not immunised because there are contra-indications (reasons why something should not be done). Usually these contra-indications mean that the immunisation should be postponed and not necessarily that it should never be done.

Sometimes the immune system may not work because it has been attacked and is prevented from producing antibodies. This happens when AIDS (acquired immune deficiency syndrome) has occurred. AIDS is the disease which results from infection with the human immune deficiency virus (HIV).

Good Practice

Childcare workers should always show respect for the wishes of parents not to have their child immunised, whatever the reason for their decision.

Homeopathic alternatives to immunisation

Occasionally parents prefer not to have their children immunised with traditional vaccines. Homeopathic alternatives are available, but statistics suggest that children who are given these are more likely to contract the actual disease. However they are less likely

- to be severely ill as a result AND
- to have the disease at all

than if they had not been immunised.

Some GPs offer a homeopathic immunisation programme, usually for children who are unable to have the usual regime. Qualified homeopaths may also provide this service.

 Progress check

1. What types of immunity do immunisations provide?
2. Why is it important that babies and young children are immunised against diseases?
3. What is the immunisation schedule from birth to 5 years?
4. What care should be offered to children after immunisation?
5. What reasons may parents/carers give for not allowing their children to be immunised?
6. How could these arguments be resolved?
7. What are the benefits of immunisation?
8. What are homeopathic alternatives to immunisation?

The role of the childcare worker in immunisation

Professional childcare workers have a responsibilty to the children in their care to keep them well by preventing accidents and minimising the risks of infection and illness by communicable diseases.

Understanding how diseases are spread and how to reduce the risks of cross-infection are essential if children are to be cared for safely and healthily. Knowledge of the childhood immunisation schedule is also important so that appropriate advice can be offered to parents.

Childcare workers could implement the following good practice points to increase awareness of immunisation issues:

- invite a health visitor to speak to groups of parents about preventive health and the importance of immunisations
- prepare displays to inform parents about the values of immunisations
- know where to seek advice locally and advise parents to seek professional medical advice
- be well informed about the immunisation schedule – keep up to date about any changes which occur
- be enthusiastic and emphasise the benefits of immunisation
- keep a record of individual children's immunisation status.

Childcare workers must also be aware of their own immunisation status. It is important to check that all immunisations are up to date especially polio and hepatitis.

Remember

Childcare workers are often consulted by parents about a range of subjects related to child care. It is important to be up to date with the information provided and/or to know where to refer parents to gain professional help.

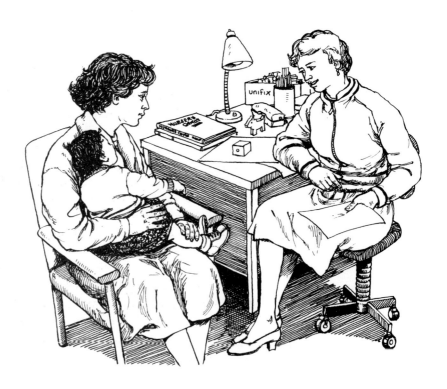

Childcare workers should be able to inform parents about where to obtain advice

> ✅ ***Progress check***
>
> 1 Why is it important for childcare workers to be informed about immunisations?
> 2 How can childcare workers promote immunisations positively to parents?

Activity

1 In a small group plan a display to promote the benefits of childhood immunisations. Include information about:
   - the effects of the relevant illnesses on children who have not been immunised.
   - where immunisations are carried out in your area.
2 Participate in a role-play activity with one person taking the part of a childcare worker discussing immunisations with parents/carers. The following examples provide some fairly common attitudes:
   - anxious parent who is concerned about any harmful effects on their child
   - parent who cannot see the value of having their child immunised because 'these diseases are not around any more'
   - parent who was not immunised herself because of asthma and believes that her child should not be immunised for the same reason
   - parent who 'is much too busy to go to the clinic – it's a waste of time anyway'.

Providing a hygienic environment

Hygiene means the study of health and involves all aspects of keeping children well and healthy including promoting cleanliness and safety and preventing the spread of infection.

Children are extremely vulnerable to infection, and diseases can spread very quickly in a childcare establishment. Infection can be transmitted via child to adult contacts (such as parents and childcare workers) as well as between the children themselves. Children are more likely to develop infections for the following reasons.

- Their immune systems are not fully developed and they cannot fight infection as effectively as a healthy adult.
- Childcare settings mean that many children are close together in enclosed environments for fairly long periods of time – increasing the risks of infection spreading from child to child.
- Children's behaviour is not naturally hygienic – they need to be taught and reminded often about ways to prevent the spread of infection e.g. hand washing.

> ### Remember
>
> Children are more vulnerable to infection because of their immature immune systems, their developmental stage and behaviour. Close contact with many other children in childcare establishments increases the risks of infection.

- Normal developmental progress makes children vulnerable e.g. putting objects and hands in the mouth can introduce infection; grazed hands and knees after falls create breaks in the skin through which infection can enter.

Establishing routines is the most effective way of ensuring that hygiene requirements are provided for. Basic workplace routines can prevent diseases being spread if they are carried out efficiently, thoroughly and regularly.

Three important areas of routine hygiene in the childcare establishment are:

- personal hygiene
- environmental hygiene
- disposing of waste materials.

Personal hygiene

Good personal hygiene routines involve regular and thorough cleaning of the skin, hair, teeth and clothes.

Keeping a high standard of personal hygiene is important for these reasons:

- it directly prevents the spread of infection
- it provides a positive role model for children to follow
- being clean and fresh helps people feel good about themselves and may result in a more positive manner and attitude.

Hands

Hand washing is especially important because it is the single most effective means of preventing the spread of infection.

- Childcare workers should ensure that they wash their hands often throughout the day especially after going to the toilet, cleaning up after children's accidents, before handling food, making feeds for babies etc.
- It is more difficult to keep long nails clean, so nails should be kept short to prevent infection and to avoid injuring children. Nail varnish should not be worn – bacteria grows where the varnish is chipped.
- Disinfect nailbrushes and other equipment used for washing the hands.
- Use disposable paper towels or hand dryers to dry the hands. If this is not possible make sure that hand towels are washed daily in a hot wash to destroy any pathogenic organisms.
- Cover any cuts and abrasions on the hands with a waterproof plaster.
- Wear gloves when changing nappies or dealing with any situation involving blood or any other body fluid.

Hair

- Hair should be kept clean, brushed often and tied back.
- Check regularly for head lice and treat if found.

Environmental hygiene

A clean childcare setting is not only more welcoming but it is also less likely to contain harmful pathogenic organisms. Although children should not be expected to be paragons of cleanliness there are basic routines which, if followed, will help to reduce the spread of infection.

There is a wide range of methods of reducing the number of pathogens which may come into contact with young children.

Disinfectants

Disinfectants kill all micro-organisms. They can be used to clean floors, walls, toilets and drains. Avoid contact with the skin, as they can burn.

Antiseptics

Antiseptics prevent the growth of germs without necessarily killing them all. Savlon and Dettol are antiseptics which may be used to clean toys. Do not use antiseptics to clean skin, as children may have a severe reaction to the chemical.

The use of the above chemicals combined with the following routine care of the childcare establishment can prevent the spread of infection by diminishing the amount of pathogenic micro-organisms in the environment.

- Sunlight kills pathogenic organisms, so doors and windows should be opened if possible. Children should be encouraged to play outside.
- Ventilation – keeping a window open can reduce the number of pathogens in the air, ensuring adequate oxygen levels
- Regular supervised toileting of children where they are shown and encouraged to use the correct handwashing techniques is important.
- Avoid overcrowding – strict guidelines in the Children Act 1989 stipulate how much floor space is required by children within each age group.
- Separate rooms for babies and toddlers and separate areas for different age-groups minimises the risk of cross-infection.
- Consistency of staffing the different areas will enable childcare workers to build positive relationships and identify illness in a child sooner.
- Laundering facilities should be kept away from the kitchen area to prevent contamination of food preparation areas.
- Disinfect toys and play equipment regularly. Toys should be washed and disinfected daily if the children are under 12 months and still at the oral stage of development.
- Provide damp dusting daily.
- Use cloths and mops only in their designated areas e.g. floor mops for the toilet area only or playroom only.
- Clean up spills and accidents immediately.
- Use paper towels and tissues and provide covered bins for their disposal.
- Regularly check and clean the toilet/bathroom areas.
- Liquid soap is less likely to harbour pathogens than bars of soap.

- Wash and sieve sand.
- Discourage parents from bringing children who are unwell into the establishment. Children with a raised temperature and specific signs and symptoms should be excluded, whatever their age. Written advice to parents when the child starts at the establishment may prevent misunderstandings and resentment.
- Ensure that the class pet is clean and well cared for – regular feeding, cleaning of the cage/tank, changing of bedding etc is important.

Good Practice

Attention to environmental hygiene includes giving children plenty of opportunity to benefit from fresh air. Open windows and access to outdoor play areas in all seasons will improve health and help to reduce the spread of infection.

Hygiene in food preparation

- Use a separate area for preparing food with disinfected work surfaces.
- Wear an apron or kitchen overall, tie the hair back and wash hands before beginning to prepare food.
- Avoid touching nose or mouth, or coughing and sneezing in the food preparation area.
- Kitchen cloths should be disinfected and changed regularly.
- Tea towels should be replaced daily, and dried between use.
- Sterilising bottles, teats and feeding equipment is essential for babies under one year of age.
- All food in the kitchen area should be covered.
- Food can be stored safely in a refrigerator at 0°C–5°C and in the freezer at −18°C to −25°C.
- Food should be cooled quickly before placed in the fridge or freezer.
- Defrost food thoroughly before cooking unless the manufacturer recommends cooking from frozen.
- Ensure that all food is thoroughly cooked, especially meat dishes e.g. chicken, sausages and joints of meat.
- Cook eggs thoroughly so that the yolk and white are firm.

Outdoor hygiene

- Check the outdoor play area for animal excrement and hazards such as broken glass and other refuse.
- Ensure that the play area is secure with fencing and a childproof gate.
- Ensure that all equipment used is safe and does not present a hazard.
- Provide the opportunity for outdoor play.

> ## *Case study*
>
> Adelphi Playgroup runs for four sessions a week. It is held in the hall at the community centre which is also used by several other local groups at other times in the week – morning, afternoon and evening. The playgroup staff have recently been having several problems since the community association was re-elected. Some days the kitchen is in a deplorable condition with a dirty sink, unwashed cups and saucers, stale milk and cutlery lying on the floor.
>
> The toilets are often unflushed and the soiled sinks are overflowing with no soap or paper towels for hand washing. The children usually play in the outside yard area with a small grassy area, but this has been difficult lately because the gate is sometimes left unlocked and the area is fouled with dog excrement, empty beer cans and used contraceptives. The playgroup leader has decided to attend the next meeting of the community association.
>
> 1 How are the children potentially at risk from this environment?
> 2 What policies and procedures could the playgroup workers suggest to the community association to improve health and hygiene standards for all the community centre users? Relate your answer to these areas:
>   ■ kitchen hygiene
>   ■ toilet facilities
>   ■ outdoor area.

Disposing of waste material

All waste materials should be disposed of carefully with consideration of their:
■ re-cycling value **and**
■ potential to spread infection.
All childcare establishments should have a health and safety policy with regard to the disposal of body fluids. Hepatitis B virus and human immunodeficiency virus (HIV) are present in the bloodstream of infected people, and hepatitis A virus is present in the faeces of infected people. Care must be taken with all bodily waste to prevent the transmission of these diseases. Because these infections can be present without showing signs and/or symptoms, the hygiene policy must be strictly maintained.

The following guidelines should be implemented.
■ Skin injuries should be covered with a waterproof dressing.
■ Staff should wear disposable latex gloves when in contact with bodily waste i.e. blood, faeces, urine.
■ Blood should be covered with a 1% hypochlorite solution to destroy the virus – it can then be wiped up with a disposable cloth.
■ Hands should be washed with an antiseptic soap.
■ Nappies, dressings, disposable cloths and used latex gloves should be placed in a sealed bag before placing in the appropriate bags for incineration in a covered bin.

> ### Remember
>
> To create a suitable childcare environment consideration must be given to the following:
> - noise
> - light
> - cleanliness
> - equipment
> - space
> - ventilation
> - temperature.

- There should be designated areas with covered bins for different types of waste.
- If body fluid should contact damaged skin encourage the wound to bleed and wash the area immediately with an antiseptic solution. Urgent medical aid will be required.

✓ Progress check

1 Why are children more likely to develop infections?
2 What is the most effective way of ensuring that hygiene requirements are provided for?
3 Why is it important to maintain high standards of personal hygiene?
4 Explain how the care of the hands can help to prevent the spread of infection.
5 What is the difference between an antiseptic and a disinfectant?
6 Describe how routine care of the childcare establishment can prevent the spread of infection.
7 What particular care should be given to food preparation areas?
8 At what age is it safe to discontinue sterilising feeding equipment?
9 What are the optimum temperatures for safely storing food in a fridge and freezer?
10 What precautions should be taken in the outdoor play area?
11 Which diseases can be transmitted in body fluids?
12 Describe the precautions that should be taken to prevent the spread of infection by contact with body fluids.

Activity

Using the information contained in this chapter and Chapter 6, prepare an information sheet for parents explaining why the nursery prefers children who are unwell to stay at home. Include:
- details of signs and symptoms which may indicate illness in their child
- why children are vulnerable to infection
- descriptions of nursery routines to prevent the spread of infection.

Key terms

You need to know what these words and phrases mean. Go back through the chapter and find out.

active immunity	**fleas**
antibodies	**fungi**
antiseptic	**head lice**
bacteria	**herd immunity**
cilia	**homeopathy**
disinfectant	**hygiene**

immunisation

immunity

leucocytes

lymphoid tissue

micro-organisms

mucous membrane

passive immunity

pathogen

roundworm

scabies

sebum

tapeworm

threadworm

virus

Chapter 4 Screening

This chapter includes:

- Screening
- Hearing
- Vision
- Hip tests
- Child Health Records
- The role of the childcare worker in screening and child health surveillance

Child health surveillance and screening is a system of reviewing children's progress. It involves observing babies and children and conducting developmental assessments in order to detect early signs of ill-health and/or developmental difficulties. This is carried out by health care professionals, usually health visitors, midwives, community paediatricians, school health nurses and general practitioners. Surveillance comes within the area of health promotion (see Chapter 1) and includes formal screening tests and regular reviews which are performed on all children at critical periods of childhood. Childcare workers have a role in surveillance and screening. Their skills in observing children as individuals and in groups highlights areas of progress and also areas of concern, enabling referral to other agencies if individual children are not achieving their potential.

For children to grow and develop healthily, needs must be met.

Screening

Screening in childhood is the checking of the **whole population** of children at **specific ages** and looking for abnormalities. These checks identify apparently well and healthy children who may have a disease, and those who probably do not. Screening tests do not necessarily diagnose diseases but they do pick out those children who need further investigation, for example routine hearing tests detect children who need more sophisticated tests, they do not provide a definite diagnosis.

Screening is performed by trained professionals because even the most astute parents may be unaware of a problem e.g. hip tests on babies to detect congenital dislocation. Routine reviews of children give parents the opportunity to discuss their worries – they may be unsure of what to do to follow up concerns they may have about their child.

Although the potential for screening tests is great, childhood screening concentrates on:

- development
- hearing
- vision
- specific medical conditions.

Why is screening important ?

- Parents value knowing about the health of their child and feel that they have a 'right to know' if there is anything of concern related to their child.
- If screening does detect an abnormality, early intervention and treatment can improve the outcome for the child and family by dealing with the condition.
- It provides the opportunity for genetic counselling, if this is appropriate, before another child is born.
- Quality of life can be improved by enabling the family and their child to cope with the disability with the support of the available services such as health, education and social services.
- Access to education and social services in the pre-school period can be arranged to help individual children to achieve their potential.

Recommended child health screening programme

The table on pages 90–91 shows the screening time-table used by some health authorities. This programme is the result of national recommendations and although there may be local variations amongst health authorities, the differences will be minor.

The screening procedures are best performed at the recommended ages, but if this is not feasible they should be done as soon as possible afterwards.

This programme is performed by members of the primary health care team – the health visitor and general practitioner usually in the child health clinic and occasionally at home. In some areas community paediatricians are available in clinics. The school health service (school nurses and doctors) take over the responsibility for child health when a child reaches statutory school age i.e. the beginning of the first term after the fifth birthday.

Screening tests

Screening tests are ideally performed on **all** children throughout their childhood with their parents' consent. For screening tests to be useful and effective they should be simple to perform but provide an accurate result.

> **Remember**
> Screening tests do not diagnose conditions. They detect children who need further investigations.

AGE	SCREENING PROCEDURE	HEALTH PROMOTION
	These procedures are performed by midwives, doctors and health visitors throughout childhood	Health visitors discuss the following issues with parents and carers to heighten their awareness of important issues affecting their child at critical ages. Health education is offered appropriately and tactfully
Birth	FULL PHYSICAL EXAMINATION: **usually performed by a hospital paediatrician before the mother and baby are discharged home. If the baby is born at home the general practitioner will conduct the examination:** ■ weight ■ heart and pulses ■ hips ■ testes ■ head circumference ■ eyes ■ Guthrie test (after 6 days of milk feeding) to test for phenylketonuria (PKU), hypothyroidism and cystic fibrosis ■ sickle cell and thalassaemia test if suspected	Cot death (SIDS) prevention Feeding techniques Nutrition Baby care Crying Sleep Car safety Family planning Passive smoking Dangers of shaking baby Sibling management
10–14 days	**Health visitors perform these checks, usually at the birth visit in the home.** Review of birth check Assess levels of parental support	Nutrition Breast feeding Cot death (SIDS) prevention. Passive smoking Accident prevention: bathing, scalding and fires Explanation of tests and results
6–8 weeks	**All babies receive this check performed by the GP and health visitor.** REVIEW: Parental concerns, e.g. vision, hearing, activity Risk factors including family history of abnormalities FULL EXAMINATION INCLUDING: ■ weight ■ head circumference ■ length ■ hip check ■ testes ■ eyes: squint, movement, ■ tone and general development ■ heart and pulses ■ Guthrie test result given to parents	Immunisation Nutrition and dangers of early weaning Accidents: falls, fires, over-heating, scalds Hearing Recognition of illness in babies and what action to take e.g. fever management Crying Sleeping position Cot death (SIDS) prevention Passive smoking Review of car safety
2–4 months	**Health visitor check.** Parental concerns Hip check	Weighing as appropriate Maintain previous health promotion Promotion of language and social development Hearing Discourage future use of baby walkers

AGE	SCREENING PROCEDURE	HEALTH PROMOTION
6–9 months	**Health visitor check.** Hip check Distraction hearing test Discussion of developmental progress – asking about vision, hearing and language development Check weight and head circumference Observe behaviour and look for squints	Parental concerns Nutrition Hearing Accident prevention: fires, choking, scalding, burns, stair and door gates, fire guards etc Review of car transport Dental care Play and development needs
18–24 months	**Health visitor check.** Parental concerns – behaviour, vision and hearing. Observation of gait (walking posture) Emphasis on value of comprehension and understanding of spoken and non-verbal communication in relation to speech development Height measured and plotted	SAFETY: Accident prevention, falls from heights, drowning, poisoning, road safety DEVELOPMENT: ■ language and play ■ management and behavioural issues ■ promotion of positive parenting ■ toilet training ■ diet, nutrition and prevention of iron deficiency
3 years 3 months to 3 years 6 months	**Health visitor check.** Enquiry and discussion of vision, squint, hearing, behaviour, language development and referral to other professionals as necessary Discussion of education needs and choices Notification of any special educational needs Height measured Testes checked if necessary Hearing test if hearing impairment suspected	SAFETY: ■ Accident prevention, burns, falls from heights, drowning, poisoning, road safety DEVELOPMENT: ■ language and play, socialisation ■ management of behaviour ■ issues ■ school readiness ■ toilet training ■ dental care ■ diet, nutrition and prevention of iron deficiency
5 years school entrant	**School nurse check. School health doctor if necessary.** SCHOOL ENTRANT REVIEW: Review of pre-school record Discuss parents and teachers concerns Height – compared with previous measurements Weight Hearing sweep audiometry test Snellen vision test Observation of gross and fine motor skills	Consent for planned programme of health checks Access to school health service surveillance programme Sleep Friendships/settling in at school Accident prevention, road safety, stranger danger Dentist Dietician Management of medicines at school Care in the sun
Year 3: 7–8 years	**School nurse check.** Teacher concerns Review of records Height, weight, vision General health check Issues raised by the child	Accident prevention, road safety, safety at play, stranger danger Friendships Exercise, nutrition and dental care Care in the sun

Criteria for screening tests

Screening tests must comply with the following characteristics.

Important condition

The condition being sought (tested for) must be an important one. Serious disorders can affect development and life chances e.g. detecting congenital dislocation of the hip (CDH) results in treatment which will enable a child to walk and develop gross motor skills unimpaired. Screening for hearing loss will detect deaf babies who can be offered treatment to improve their hearing capacity or enable them to use other forms of communication.

Screening for verrucae or colour blindness or nappy rash will not have such dramatic results.

Tried and tested treatment

There should be a tried and tested treatment which is successful in either:
■ curing the condition
■ relieving the symptoms.
Not all conditions which are found as a result of screening are curable e.g. cerebral palsy (CP).

However, knowing that a child has a particular condition will enable the relevant services to offer appropriate help and to support the family, for example in providing equipment, preventing secondary conditions and helping the child to achieve their full potential.

An early stage of detection

There should be an early stage of the disease when it can be detected and symptoms are absent or slight. Congenital dislocation of the hip (CDH) was a fairly common cause of walking difficulties and limping before rigorous screening of all babies was applied. If correct early treatment is offered the hip develops normally.

An acceptable test

An acceptable test should be available. The test should be suitable for the condition which it is trying to detect. Any discomfort should be outweighed by the importance of finding and treating the disease e.g. the heel prick used for the Guthrie test for phenylketonuria (PKU) is uncomfortable but parents accept that it is important. By contrast, testing all 2-year-olds for anaemia by taking blood would not be viewed as important enough to outweigh the pain of the test. It may well be unacceptable to parents.

Well understood process of the disease

The process of the disease should be well understood. It must be clear that treatment makes a difference to the long-term effects of the condition, so that screening is effective. There is little point in implementing a full screening programme for conditions for which there is no effective treatment. This is very clear in the treatment of congenital dislocation of the hip and phenylketonuria – early detection and treatment means that an affected child can continue to grow and develop normally.

General agreement about who to treat

There should be general agreement about who to treat. Although there may be minor differences in treatment schedules in different areas of the country, most children are offered treatment as soon as an abnormality is detected.

Cost effective

The test should be cost effective. This means that the cost of the test and early treatment should be less than late detection and treatment. Balancing the financial cost against the personal cost of disease or abnormality is very difficult. However, cost **is** a factor in screening, and in all health promotion programmes, the benefits are measured in financial terms as well as in improvements to health.

Developmental screening

Screening for development does not always meet all the above theoretical criteria for a screening programme. This is developmental surveillance – based on observing children, asking relevant questions about their development and having some background knowledge or information about environmental, social and health factors influencing their development (see Chapter 2 for factors affecting health).

Health visitors usually know their families very well and have the advantage of insight into their personal circumstances. Their professional opinion about the development of a particular child is usually made with the benefit of a lot more information than a doctor would have –who may only see the child on one occasion.

Good Practice

Childcare workers have an important role to play in developmental surveillance. They see the same children regularly and can observe their development and note any areas of less than average progress. Childcare workers should:

- keep records of children's development and achievements
- work in partnership with parents to promote development and share information
- be aware of the recommended child health screening programme
- know the local methods of referral to health professionals for children who are causing concern.

✔ Progress check

1 Explain what childhood screening is.
2 Which important areas does screening in childhood concentrate on?
3 Which health care professionals conduct screening procedures?

4 Why is screening in childhood important?
5 Which aspects of health education are discussed during the first year?
6 What are the criteria for screening tests?
7 What is developmental screening and surveillance and why is it important?

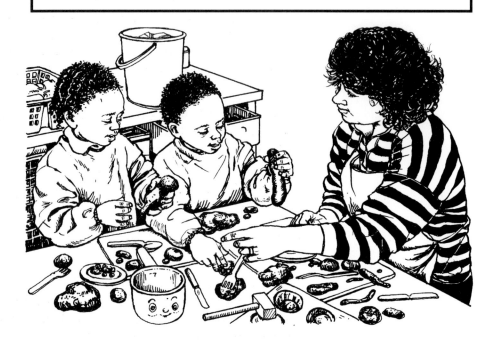

Childcare workers see children often and can assess their progress

Screening in pregnancy

Screening takes place in the antenatal period as well as after birth. Most of the antenatal tests and investigations are performed with the aim of checking the health of the baby. They also detect any abnormalities in the embryo/fetus. Parents will be offered the option of terminating the pregnancy if a potentially serious abnormality is detected.

Common screening tests during pregnancy

Common pregnancy screening tests are as follows.

Serology
Serology will detect syphilis (a venereal disease), which can be treated to prevent damage to the baby.

Haemoglobin
Haemoglobin, the iron content of the blood, is recorded at monthly intervals. All mothers of African, Asian or Mediterranean descent have their blood tested for sickle cell disease and thalassaemia.

Rubella
Blood is tested for rubella antibodies.

Serum alpha-fetoprotein (SAFP)

This test is taken at 16 weeks of pregnancy when a raised level of SAFP indicates that the baby may have spina bifida. After a detailed ultrasound scan, an amniocentesis is offered to mothers with a raised SAFP.

Triple test

This blood test may be offered to women over 35 years of age, or it may be requested. The blood test calculates the risk of the baby having Down's syndrome. By measuring the levels of human chorionic gonadotrophin (HCG), SAFP and oestriols (placental hormones) in conjunction with the mother's age, the test can indicate whether further tests are necessary.

Ultrasound scan

The ultrasound machine is an echo-sounding device which uses high-frequency sound waves. It can be used to:

- check the position of the fetus in the uterus
- measure the size of the fetus
- find the position of the placenta
- detect and confirm multiple pregnancies
- diagnose some fetal abnormalities.

At 18 weeks of pregnancy women are offered a detailed scan for doctors to look at the structure of fetal organs in detail.

Placental function tests

A healthy placenta is essential for a fetus to grow and develop normally. It is possible to test the health and strength of the placenta by checking the amount of pregnancy hormones it produces.

Hormones are carried in the blood and then excreted in the urine. Blood or urine tests, to test the presence and amount of hormone, will indicate how well the placenta is working.

Amniocentesis

Amniocentesis involves the removal of a small sample of amniotic fluid from the uterus, via the abdominal wall. It may be performed after the 16th week of pregnancy, when it is possible to check that the chromosomes, including the sex chromosomes, are normal.

Amniocentesis may be offered to women who have:

- a history of chromosomal abnormalities, such as Down's syndrome
- raised SAFP
- a history of sex-linked disorders, such as Duchenne muscular dystrophy
- passed the age of 35 years (the risk of chromosomal abnormalities, especially Down's syndrome, increases with age).

Chorionic villus sampling (CVS)

CVS is carried out between 8 and 11 weeks of pregnancy. With the help of an ultrasound scan to find the position of the placenta and the fetus, a small sample of placental tissue is removed via the cervix. CVS is used to detect inherited disorders such as:

- Down's syndrome
- haemophilia

- thalassaemia
- sickle cell disease
- cystic fibrosis.

It can also be used to detect the sex of the fetus if there is a family history of sex-linked conditions.

If a disorder is recognised that will have an effect on the health and development of the baby, the parents may be offered a termination of pregnancy. Whatever their decision, they will need a great deal of support and empathy from all the professionals involved in their care.

Does early detection of abnormality matter?

Some screening tests are potentially harmful because of the unnecessary worry they produce. False positives can lead to referrals to other professionals and unnecessary medical procedures.

Thinking about the test results and waiting for them to arrive creates anxiety and worry. Parents continue their high anxiety levels for a long time after a test shows the baby to be normal.

Doctors should be able to offer treatments, change or improvement as the result of detecting a condition after a screening test. In pregnancy this usually means termination. Parents may feel obliged to participate in screening programmes because it is expected of them, even when they have no intention to terminate under any circumstances; so having some antenatal investigations such as chorionic villus sampling and amniocentesis is of limited value for them. If parents do not accept the value of certain tests, they must be given the opportunity to opt out of them. However, testing can reassure parents if nothing abnormal is found. If a particular condition is detected in pregnancy, time is allowed for physical and emotional preparation for the arrival of a child with special needs into the family.

The quest for the 'perfect' baby

For thousands of years, human beings have rejected defective babies. The Spartans used to leave their disabled babies outside to die. Some parents still reject babies with severe defects – but wilful killing of infants is against the law. Abortion is within the law and it is common practice for abnormal fetuses to be aborted; even those people who are generally against abortion may agree that in these cases the procedure is justified.

All parents want a 'normal' baby. But what is 'normal'? Every baby is unique and very different from other babies whether or not they have what society considers to be a disabling condition. Generally, these conditions are what able-bodied people consider to be a disability e.g. Down's syndrome, cerebral palsy etc. People who have managed to lead worthwhile lives with the particular disability would often disagree that it is a valid reason to terminate a pregnancy. Antenatal testing can put pressure on parents to conform and do the expected thing, there may be subtle pressures to abort when the test results are known. As society strives for perfection, disabled groups feel that this society marginalises them, making them feel like

> **Remember**
>
> Screening in pregnancy is performed to check the health of the mother and fetus. Parents should be given careful explanation of the reasons for particular tests, and also detailed information about what the results mean for their baby.

second-class citizens, by aborting fetuses with conditions which are considered (by able-bodied people) to affect the quality of life.

However, the parents have to make a choice in the light of their knowledge and experience. No pressure should be put on them to make one choice instead of another. A decision to abort is not easy, whatever the circumstances, and neither is the decision to continue with a pregnancy knowing that caring for a disabled child and adult places a huge burden on the family and ultimately a financial burden on society.

Good Practice

All professional carers should show that they value all people regardless of their level of ability or social status. They should show respect for individuals and enable them to achieve their potential by offering support, compassion and practical assistance.

Progress check

1 Which blood tests are used during pregnancy?
2 What is chorionic villus sampling?
3 When is an ultrasound scan offered to all pregnant women and what can it detect?
4 Do you think that early detection of abnormalities is important and if so, why?
5 Why do you think that disabled people sometimes feel marginalised in view of the emphasis on antenatal testing?

Case study

Geraldine is a 35-year-old teacher of the deaf who is expecting her first baby. She agreed to have the triple blood test to find out whether she is a high risk for having a baby with Down's syndrome. The results have shown that the risk is above average for her age group and she has been advised to have an amniocentesis to check the baby's chromosomes. Geraldine has worked with several children with Down's (hearing loss is common in this condition), and has found them to be generally responsive and loving children who enjoy life and develop some independence skills. She and her partner realise that caring for such a child would be hard work but very rewarding. Geraldine feels that if the baby has Down's and she terminates the pregnancy, it would be difficult to face the parents and the children she works with. She believes that termination would be like saying that children with Down's are of less value than children who do not have the condition, which is not her attitude at all. They are not sure that they would terminate the pregnancy if the condition was confirmed but would find it difficult to refuse the test.

1 Why do you think that Geraldine and her partner feel under pressure to have the amniocentesis?
2 If they decide to have the test, how could the knowledge of the child's condition – affected or not – help them?
3 Why do you think that Geraldine feels that having a termination would be reducing the value of the children she works with?

Hearing

All babies are born with the parental expectation that they have the capacity to grow and develop within 'normal' parameters. However, areas of development are dependent upon the ability of the body to receive sensory stimulation especially hearing and vision.

Can your baby hear you?

Tick if response present

Shortly after birth
Your baby should be startled by a sudden loud noise such as a hand clap or a door slamming and should blink or open his eyes widely to such sounds.

☐

By 1 month
Your baby should be beginning to notice sudden prolonged sounds like the noise of a vacuum cleaner and she should pause and listen to them when they begin.

☐

By 4 months
He should quieten or smile to the sound of your voice even when he cannot see you. He may also turn his head or eyes toward you if you come up from behind and speak to him from the side.

☐

By 7 months
She should turn immediately to your voice across the room or to very quiet noises made on each side if she is not too occupied with other things.

☐

By 9 months
He should listen attentively to familiar everyday sounds and search for very quiet sounds made out of sight. He should also show pleasure in babbling loudly and tunefully.

☐

By 12 months
She should show some response to her own name and to other familiar words. She may also respond when you say 'no' and 'bye bye' even when she cannot see any accompanying gesture.

☐

> Your health visitor will perform a routine hearing screening test on your baby between seven and nine months of age. She will be able to help and advise you at any time before or after this test if you are concerned about your baby and his development. If you suspect that your baby is not hearing normally, either because you cannot answer yes to the items above or for some other reason, then seek advice from your health visitor.

Hearing – a checklist of some of the general signs to look out for in a baby's first year

Hearing loss is a hidden disability, there is no outward sign that a new baby may be deaf or have a mild to profound hearing loss.

A useful checklist for parents has been devised to inform them of the signs to look for to confirm that their baby is hearing during the first year of life (see page 98).

Deaf babies are often very skilled at picking up non-verbal clues to understand situations and often appear to be behaving normally.

Children may develop hearing problems in childhood – possibly as the result of ear infections, general illness or injury.

Detection of hearing loss

Neonatal screening

Parents are usually aware of their baby's ability to hear sounds. Babies respond to sudden loud noises by stiffening, blinking, opening the eyes widely, crying and/or the Moro reflex (the baby's arms stretch out with fingers curved and are then brought back across the chest as if in an embrace). They may also quieten to listen to the sound of the mother's voice, and respond to prolonged low tones by becoming still and quiet.

Babies at risk of hearing loss will be offered sophisticated and complex hearing tests such as auditory response cradle or the brainstem evoked response audiometry, which are conducted by highly skilled personnel. Babies who are at risk of hearing loss are as follows:

■ suspected or confirmed rubella during pregnancy
■ born at less than 33 weeks gestation or weighing less than 1500grams at birth
■ intensive care after birth for more than 48 hours
■ family history of genetically transmitted hearing loss
■ chromosome defects e.g. Downs syndrome.

Distraction hearing test

All babies between 6 and 9 months of age are assessed with a distraction hearing test.

This test relies on the ability of the baby to turn its head to locate sounds. The baby must be able to sit with support and to have achieved head control, 6 to 9 months is the optimum age to test because most babies have achieved this level of development. By 8 months 95 per cent of babies can locate a sound accurately and will participate when sounds are repeated, responding as if to a new sound each time. By 10 to12 months most babies have developed the concepts of object and person permanence and will turn to look for the tester when no new sounds are made – this makes testing very difficult. Deaf babies have learnt to make 'checking' turns which sometimes results in their apparent satisfactory performance in the test.

Performance of the distraction test
A quiet room, preferably sound-proofed to prevent sounds from outside distracting the baby and making the test difficult.

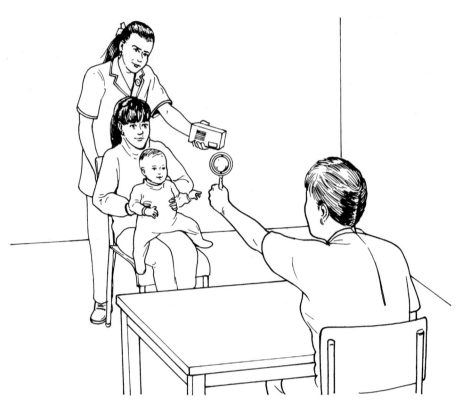

The distraction hearing test

The room is set out with a chair for the carer in front of a small table. The light source should be behind the table to avoid shadows.

Two people are required, both of whom have been trained in the delivery of the hearing test. The **tester** makes the sounds. The **distractor** keeps the babies attention to the front.

The baby sits on the front of the carer's knee facing the distractor who sits or kneels at a small table, talking quietly to the baby and playing with a colourful small spinning top or similar moving toy, to attract the baby's attention. When the baby's attention is riveted on the toy, the distractor slowly covers it and avoids eye contact with the baby. At this moment the tester (who is standing behind the carer and baby) introduces a sound at one metre from the baby's ear on the right or left side, but not within the baby's range of vision. Ideally, the baby should turn to investigate the sound (this is **localising** the sound). The distractor pulls their attention back to the front and the test continues.

Each ear should be tested for the range of sounds, which are required for normal speech development, at 35 decibels which is very quiet. A satisfactory test is one in which the baby responds clearly to two high and two low sounds on each side.

Sounds used include the Manchester rattle, 'ssss ssss', 'ooo ooo' and warble tones produced by an electronic device.

Common difficulties with the distraction test
When completing the test it is difficult to:
■ keep the baby's attention for long enough to complete the test

- decide between random movements and genuine responses to the sounds
- keep the test sounds quiet enough – there can be a temptation to 'increase the volume' to get a response.
- work in a noisy room – health centres are often situated on bus routes, and are busy places in their own right!

Failed tests

Many babies fail to perform adequately for their first test. It could be because they are in an unsuitable behavioural state because they are:

- tired
- generally unwell
- developmentally immature.

However, if there is any concern at all about the baby's ability to hear, s/he should be referred for expert assessment. All babies who fail two hearing test should be referred for further investigation.

Speech discrimination test

Language development may be delayed or behaviour difficulties may indicate the possibility of hearing loss. If there are suspicions that there is a hearing problem between 2 and 5 years children can be tested using the speech discrimination test.

Remember

Hearing loss is a hidden disability. There is no outward sign that a baby has a hearing loss, so parents and childcare workers should be vigilant to detect the first signs of hearing difficulties.

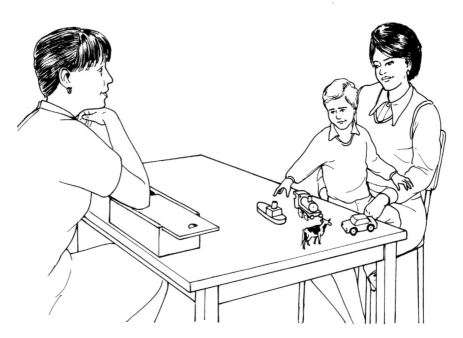

The speech discrimination test

This test involves using a set of small toys, all with a single syllable name e.g. plane, plate, shoe, spoon, tree, key, house, horse, duck, cup etc., which will test the child's ability to hear different consonants like p, g, d, m, s, f and b. The child must be gently encouraged to co-operate with the tester and together they name the toys with a normal voice. The child is then asked to find the toys with decreasing voice intensity. For example 'show me the duck', 'put the plane in the box', 'give the cup to mummy'. Each ear is tested through the range of sounds.

Sweep audiometry test

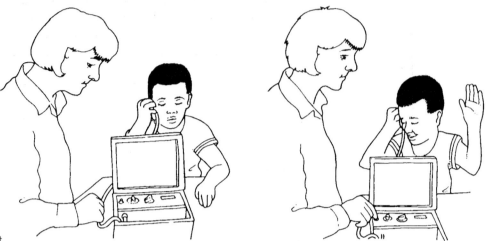

The sweep test

All school entrants have the sweep test which is a simplified version of pure tone audiometry. It involves the child in wearing a pair of earphones and listening for tones produced by an audiometer. The tones cover the range required for speech and each ear is tested separately.

Special cases for access to hearing tests

- If a parent is concerned at any time. There should be access to expert hearing testing because parents are usually right about their children and when they suspect a hearing loss there is a high chance that they are correct.
- Children under 5 years who have had meningitis.
- Children who have had measles or mumps infections.
- Children at high risk of 'glue ear' e.g. those with Down's syndrome, cleft palate or with recurrent ear infections.

✔ *Progress check*

1 Which babies are at risk of hearing loss?
2 Which tests may be offered in the neonatal period?
3 Describe the performance of the distraction hearing test.
4 Why do some babies fail the distraction test and what should be done about their performance?
5 What may indicate that a child has hearing difficulties between 2 and 5 years of age?

> ## *Good Practice*
>
> **Any childcare worker who has a concern about a child's hearing should discuss their observations with the senior worker or teacher in the establishment. Speaking to the parents may reveal that they have similar worries. The health visitor, if the child is pre-school age, or the school nurse if the child is at school, will be able to arrange a hearing test.**

Activity

Prepare a display for use in a day nursery which will inform parents, and other childcare workers, about:

- the signs of normal hearing in the first year of life
- the development of speech
- signs of hearing loss.

Vision

The following checklist, offered to parents, highlights some of the signs of normal visual development to be noted during the first year.

Can your baby see?

Tick if response present

At birth
Your baby will briefly look at your face. ☐

Age 1 month
Your baby will watch your face intently when being fed and will follow your face as it moves from side to side. ☐

Age 3 months
Your baby will follow dangling toys held in front of his face. He will follow your movements around the room and start looking at his own fingers. ☐

By 6 months
Your baby can recognise you across the room. He can see small objects (like a Smartie) and try to pick these up from the floor or table. If you notice a squint (or turn) of the eye, please tell your health visitor. ☐

By 9 months
Your baby can now recognise his toys across the room. He can see tiny crumbs on the floor and try to pick them up. He can find objects that are hidden while he is watching. ☐

> Your Health Visitor and Clinic Doctor examine your child's eyes at regular intervals. If, however, you are worried about your child's vision at any age, or if you think there is a squint (the eyes not looking straight at you) please tell your Health Visitor and she will arrange for you to see the doctor or orthoptist.

Sight – a checklist of some of the general signs to look for in a baby's first year

Parents are usually the first ones to detect a visual abnormality and any concerns voiced should be taken seriously and investigated. Minor visual problems are common – between 5 to 10 per cent of children have a squint and/or a refractive error. Early diagnosis is important because:

- some conditions need early treatment e.g. cataract and glaucoma
- eye defects can be associated with other abnormalities which may need treatment
- genetic causes must be found to avoid the birth of another affected child
- visual defects affect all areas of development and may result in emotional and behavioural problems.

Squint

This means that the eyes do not work together properly, one eye seems to be looking in another direction. There are different types of squint.

Latent squint

Latent squint is only present when the child is under stress i.e. tired or ill. Children with this type of squint usually do not need treatment.

Manifest squint

Manifest squint is present all the time. This is never regarded as normal and needs treatment.

Alternating squint

Alternating squint means that the child fixates with each eye alternately.

Pseudosquint

Pseudosquint is the appearance of a squint caused by broad epicanthic folds – a wide bridge to the nose.

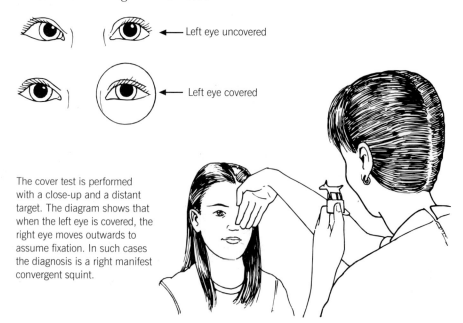

Left eye uncovered

Left eye covered

The cover test is performed with a close-up and a distant target. The diagram shows that when the left eye is covered, the right eye moves outwards to assume fixation. In such cases the diagnosis is a right manifest convergent squint.

The cover test

Refractive errors

This phrase means that the eye is not functioning as a perfect visual system. There may be a degree of short-sightedness (myopia) or long-sightedness (hypermetropia) or a structural defect in the eye resulting in a distorted image (astigmatism).

Testing vision

For accurate testing a degree of co-operation is required from the child, and an ability to report what they see – this is obviously difficult in babies and very young children. By the age of 2 to 5 years some co-operation can be achieved. The following gives guidance on the range of vision testing in childhood.

Birth–6 weeks

The midwife checks the eyes and the doctor uses an opthalmoscope to check for cataracts – a condition where the lens of the eye is cloudy and not transparent as it should be.

6 weeks–6 months

The health visitor and doctor observe any signs of a squint. This can be tested using a cover test and the corneal reflection test.

2–5 years

Because children are now more able to co-operate, distance vision can be assessed using single letters with a letter matching chart, so that the child does not have to name the letters. Each eye is tested separately using a patch to cover one eye. The tester uses a mirror placed three metres away or stands at that distance and holds up a letter, then the child points to the letter on their chart.

A child with normal vision is said to have 6/6 vision.

> ### Remember
> Parents are the experts about their child. Any concerns they have should be taken seriously and investigated.

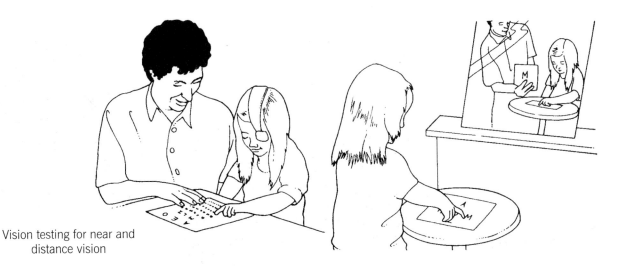

Vision testing for near and distance vision

School entry

Vision is tested by the school nurse at the school entrant review. Colour vision may be tested at secondary school age.

 Progress check

1 What are the signs of normal visual development in the first year of life?
2 What are the different types of squint?
3 How is vision tested during childhood?

Hip tests

The hips are checked regularly throughout infancy to exclude congenital dislocation and instability of the hip joint. In an unstable hip the head of the femur slips in and out of the pelvic socket – the acetabulum.

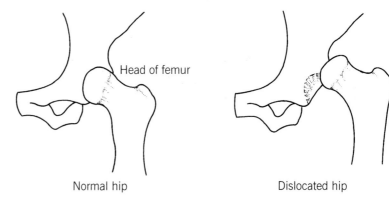

Congenital dislocation of the hip

Normal hip   Dislocated hip

Head of femur

It can be difficult to identify this condition at times, so carers and health professionals must observe the child until they are walking normally.

Risk factors

- breech presentation at delivery (bottom and/or legs first)
- family history in a close relative
- abnormalities of the foot
- babies born by caesarian section.

Testing the hips

- *From birth–8 weeks* the test used is the modified Ortolani/Barlow manoeuvre, the baby's legs are abducted (turned outwards) by the examiner and the click/clunk can be heard as the head of the femur slips back into the acetabulum.

- The child is examined visually to see if the groin and thigh creases are in the same position in both legs. If a hip is dislocated one leg will be shorter than the other and the skin creases will not be symmetrical. When the legs are straightened by the examiner the knees will not be level if there is a dislocation. These signs are easier to see after 8 weeks of age.
- The gait must be observed when the child is walking. A limp or awkward walking posture should be referred for medical opinion. Children with bilateral dislocation (both hips dislocated) may walk at the usual time but will have a waddling gait.

Good Practice

Parents and childcare workers should observe babies for signs of congenital dislocation of the hip. Although not conclusive signs of CDH, the following signs should be investigated:
- refusal to weight bear
- delayed walking
- waddling gait.

Treatment

This depends upon the severity of the condition. The baby will be referred for ultrasound scanning of the affected hip to confirm the diagnosis. Doctors will then decide which type of splinting to use.

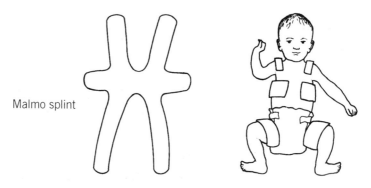

Malmo splint

Splints for congenital dislocation of the hip

 Progress check

1 What are the risk factors for CDH or instability of the hip?
2 What methods are used to test the hips?
3 How is CDH treated?

Case study

Jade was born at 39 weeks gestation by caesarian section for a breech presentation. She weighed 3.46 kgs and was discharged home after a 24 hour stay in hospital. Her mother was delighted that the birth check performed by the hospital paediatrician was completely normal, as she was concerned that the baby's hips may be a problem because her sisters children had both had treatment for congenital dislocation of the hip. Jade was breast fed and seemed to be thriving. She attended clinic for the 6 week check and all her immunisations. Each time her hips were checked they seemed to be stable.

The family moved to another area when Jade was 6 months old, but pressure of time prevented the family from registering with a new GP until Jade was 14 months old. By this time she was walking and her mother thought her wide-legged waddle was due to wearing terry nappies.

The health visitor called at the home to welcome the family to the practice and noticed that Jade had an abnormal gait. She was referred to the GP and then to the hospital where it was discovered that she had bilateral dislocation of the hips. It will take several operations to correct this problem.

1 When could this CDH have been detected earlier?
2 What other screening tests and checks did Jade miss?
3 What else could have been detected had she attended for all of these?
4 How could this late diagnosis have been avoided?

Child Health Records

In most parts of Great Britain each child's main surveillance record – the Personal Child Health Record (PCHR) – is held by the parents. Parents welcome this system and although concern was originally expressed about the safety of the record, parents are in fact no more likely to lose it than the professionals! It is probably safer.

The records are usually distributed by midwives in late pregnancy or soon after the birth of the baby. S/he explains the use and contents of the booklet. Since its introduction in 1990 the many anticipated benefits of using the PHCR have been recognised.

- It is a very positive way of involving parents with their child's surveillance programme and encourages openness between parents and professionals.
- It will go with the child when they have a hospital appointment, start school, change general practitioner or move to another area of the country. Children who are adopted, fostered or taken into care will take their record with them.

■ Information is easily accessible to parents and communication between health professionals involved with the child is simplified. Before this record was developed, hospital and community staff exchanged information only by letter or telephone conversations making it difficult to keep up to date with a child's progress and /or treatment.

■ It reduces the duplication of records held by different health departments e.g. GP, health visitor, hospital services, speech therapist, dietician, physiotherapist etc.

Child Health Checks

Your doctor or health visitor will do some simple routine checks on your baby. These include blood tests and various other checks and reviews, for example checks of your child's hips, hearing, eyesight and development.

– Checks or reviews done in this way are called screening tests.
– Screening tests have to be safe and acceptable to your baby/child.
– Screening tests can never by **absolutely 100%** accurate.
– Sometimes a screening test may cause a 'false alarm'.
– Sometimes a screening test may miss a problem.
– Occasionally a new problem may occur after your child has had a 'screening test'.

All these mean that it is very important that *whenever* you think your baby has a problem – you should seek further advice.

Contents

Contents page of a Personal Child Health Record

Contents of the Personal Child Health Record

■ Records of every contact/consultation with health service professionals is recorded.

■ The books are regularly updated to ensure that all information in the PCHR is in line with current recommendations.

■ Parents have a copy of every screening test and every surveillance check and are reminded that screening is not 100 per cent perfect.

- Health advice includes hints for parents in detecting hearing and visual defects, stages of language development, accident prevention, reducing the risk of cot death (sudden infant death syndrome – SIDS) and general advice about managing a crying baby and childhood ailments.
- Health promotion information is offered throughout the book in the developmentally appropriate section e.g. 6 to 9 months review section reminds parents about the need for fire-guards and to start brushing teeth as soon as they appear.

Growth charts

Information about the child, taken from the PCHR is stored on computer systems. This is to ensure that each child receives their development/ health checks and immunisations at the appropriate age and so that information may be used for service and research purposes. All information stored in this way is completely confidential and only released to parents, health care professionals working with the child, the local health authority and the Family Health Services Authority (FHSA).

Translation pages are available for families whose first language is not English.

 Progress check

1 What are the benefits of the PCHR?
2 What information is contained in the PCHR?
3 Why is information from the PCHR stored on computer data bases?

Case study

Tristan's father Jack travels all over the country working for a national supermarket chain as a relief manager. Each job lasts 3 to 6 months and although they keep the family home, Tristan and his mother prefer to travel with Jack. The firm pays for family accommodation with each job so Tristan can benefit from being with both parents during his early years. In each new area Tristan's mother makes contact with a GP and health visitor and shows them the PCHR.

1 How does the PCHR benefit this family?
2 Which screening and surveillance checks might Tristan have missed in the first year without the PCHR?

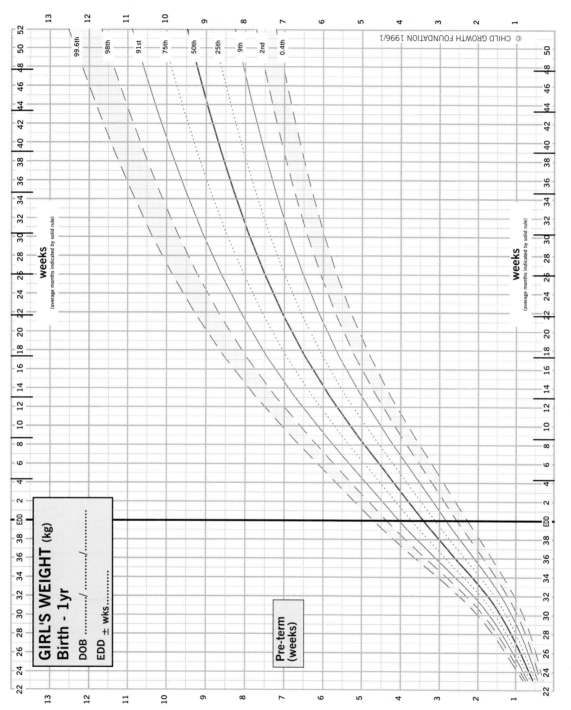

Percentile chart for a girl's weight

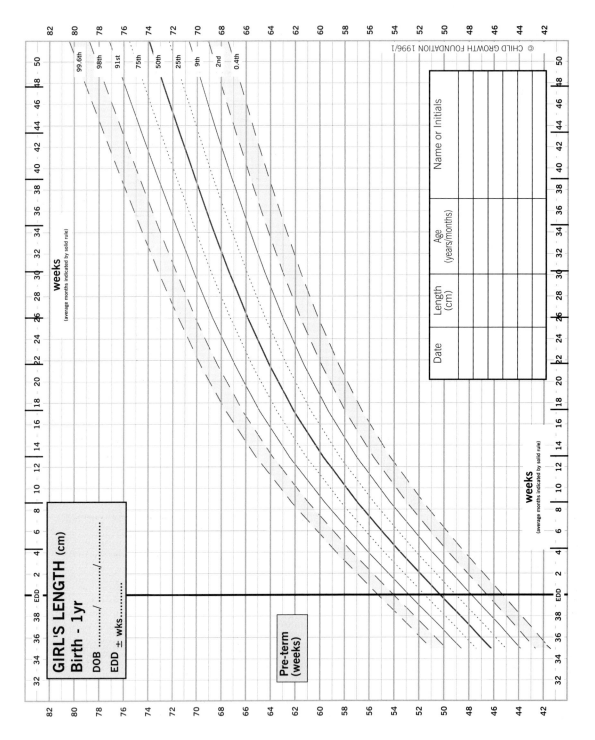

Percentile chart for a girl's length

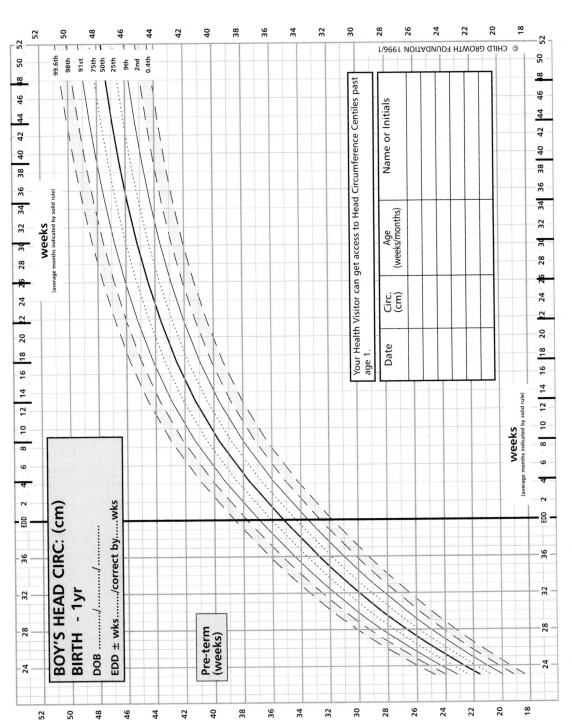

Percentile chart for a boy's head circumference

Activity

1 Investigate the use of the Personal Child Health Record (PCHR) in your area. Interview:

■ two parents and

■ a health visitor

about the values of the PCHR to them.

2 Request permission from a health centre practice manager to visit a child health clinic. Talk to the parents and staff about the screening and surveillance programme. Find out:

■ which screening checks are performed in your area

■ at which ages they are performed

■ who routinely carries out the screening checks

■ how parents are notified that a screening check is due

■ what happens if the child does not attend the clinic for a check.

The role of the childcare worker in screening and child health surveillance

Childcare workers have a role to play in the detection of any deviations from the norm in child development. They are often in daily contact with the same children and are ideally placed to perform opportunistic screening and surveillance of children who may not have regular health checks. People trained to Level 3 in childcare and education are prepared for monitoring progress in the babies and children in their care because they are:

■ aware of the holistic (whole child) approach to assessing child development

■ aware of referral procedures if there are concerns about a child

■ able to stimulate development with accessible and appropriate activities

■ willing to offer reassurance and practical help to parents, for example where to access help, the importance of screening

■ educators of parents and children about relevant health education issues such as travel safety, value of immunisations, safe sun etc.

■ an effective role model of positive health.

> **Remember**
>
> Professional childcarers are trained to detect developmental abnormalities in their very early stages.

The professional child watcher

Trained childcarers are excellent observers of children who have insight and knowledge about child development. They are aware of 'normal' and 'abnormal' patterns of development and have skills in listening, observing and asking relevant questions. Knowledge of a particular child and the factors that may affect their health and development are valuable tools in surveillance. All of this forms the basis for interpreting children's behaviour in order to make professional judgements.

The 'skill-mix'

More and more health authorities and health visitors are recognising the particular skills of nursery nurses/childcare workers and their value in child health programmes. Several areas employ nursery nurses to assist health visitors in clinics and to perform home visits. They have become a vital part of many primary health care teams. Skill-mix involves looking at the needs of the community and trying to meet them by employing people with appropriate skills and a positive attitude.

With some extra training childcare workers are able to:

- do child development checks
- take weight and height measurements and record them
- do distraction hearing tests
- give childcare advice to parents/carers e.g. about toilet training, weaning management, sleeping difficulties etc.
- visit family homes and support parents and children
- support families of children with special needs and provide some respite care when parents need to go out
- set up and manage toy libraries
- run crèches and playgroups in the child health clinic.

 Progress check

- Which skills do professionally qualified childcare workers use to monitor developmental progress in babies and children?
- Why are professionally qualified childcare workers ideally placed to monitor development?
- What is the 'skill-mix'?
- Given some extra training, what tasks may childcare workers be able to perform in the field of child health?

Key terms

You need to know what these words and phrases mean. Go back through the chapter and find out.

amniocentesis	**Personal Child Health Record**
child health surveillance	refractive errors
chorionic villus sampling	screening
congenital dislocation of the hip	speech discrimination test
distraction hearing test	squint
Guthrie test	sweep test
hip tests	ultrasound scan

This chapter includes:

- The primary health care team
- Roles in the primary health care team
- The role of the health visitor in child health
- Child health clinics
- The school health service
- Education services providing support for children and their families
- Hospital-based services

This chapter should be read in conjunction with 'Chapter 4, Screening'.

The National Health Service (NHS) provides health care for the whole population on the basis of need. This chapter identifies the range of professionals and services in the NHS who are involved in the care of children at home, at school and in hospital. The roles of teams and individual workers is identified and explained, so that childcare workers can develop an understanding of the services available. They will then be well informed and able to advise parents, if necessary, in the process of accessing health care for their children.

The primary health care team

The people involved with primary health care are those who are based in the community and are the first point of contact for the parents/carers. The primary health care team (PHCT) is made up of a range of professionals, each with specific training and skills which complement each other, enabling the health needs of children and families to be provided for. Every member of the team recognises and understands the roles of the other members.

A single general practitioner (GP) or GP practice (group of GPs) forms the basis for the PHCT. All the patients registered with a particular doctor have access to a health visitor, practice nurse, district nurse and community midwife. Sometimes a social worker is attached to a GP practice. This team meets regularly with the aim of co-ordinating the care they offer in order to give the patients the best possible service. They are often based in the same health centre, which improves access for their patients and makes it possible for them to see each other on a regular basis.

The role of the team is to care for people who are unwell and also to prevent ill health by offering health promotion services such as health education, surveillance and screening. The services offered by the PHCT may include some or all of the following:

- child health clinics (see page 122)
- antenatal clinics
- family planning services
- immunisation clinics
- specialist clinics e.g. for diabetes, asthma etc.

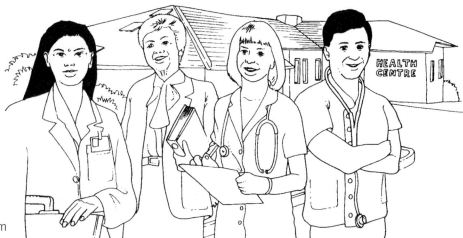

A primary health care team

The health centre

As well as a base for the PHCT a local health centre may also contain the following.

Community dental service

Community dentists usually carry out school dental examinations and a comprehensive screening examination. They offer selective treatment to school children at least three times during their school years – the target ages are 4 years +, 8 years +, 11 years + and 14 years +. They also provide dental care to children with special needs on an annual basis.

Chiropody service

Chiropodists treat problems with the feet such as corns, calluses and ingrown toenails. Chiropody under the NHS is available to the elderly, pregnant women, disabled people and children. GPs refer patients for this service as necessary.

Speech therapy

Speech therapists identify, assess and treat communication disorders in adults and children; they may work with children who have language problems on a one-to-one basis or in group work. Their work is aimed at building up language ability on a systematic basis, so they need to involve parents and carers in daily programmes which can be conducted at home or in nursery/school.

Community dietician

Qualified dieticians may become involved with children who have feeding difficulties, food refusal or a medical condition requiring a special diet. They also have an important role in health education with people on low incomes and those who need help in ensuring a balanced diet for themselves and their children. They may be consulted in a health centre and sometimes do home visits.

Community physiotherapists

Some areas provide a community physiotherapy service, although physiotherapists are usually hospital-based. They are able to provide exercises and physical activity programmes to encourage gross motor skills and co-ordination and to prevent the disabling effects of illness or accidents.

Community occupational therapists

Occupational therapists are usually based in the local authority social services department. They visit homes to assess disability and advise about coping with daily living. They may recommend aids and equipment for families with a disabled child.

Community psychiatric nursing service

This service provides support and counselling to people with mental health problems, so that they can continue to live in the community. Community psychiatric nurses usually become involved as the result of GP referral, but some areas accept direct referral from people in need or their families.

> **Remember**
> Health centres usually offer a full range of health services, with the aim of providing a network of support to everyone who is registered with the GP's practice.

 Progress check

1 Which health care professionals are members of the PHCT?
2 Which services may be offered by the PHCT?
3 What other support services may be situated in the health centre?
4 What is the difference between a physiotherapist and an occupational therapist?

Roles in the primary health care team

General practitioner

The GP is a doctor who has completed extra training in caring for people in the community. Since 1983 doctors have had to complete two years of hospital practice and undergo a year of training in general practice, before they can become a GP. They are independent practitioners who have a contract to provide services within the NHS. They have a key role

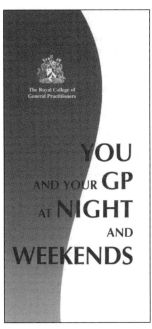

An information leaflet explaining the role of the GP

in health care, as the family doctor is usually the first person to be consulted when there is a health concern, and they are responsible for:

- diagnosing and treating conditions
- referring patients for specialist treatment
- organising other members of the PHCT to become involved as appropriate
- consulting other agencies e.g. social services if necessary
- implementing health promotion.

Health visitor

The health visitor (HV) is a qualified nurse who has completed midwifery or obstetric training, as well as extra training in preventive health care. Health visitors are primarily involved with the promotion of health and the prevention of ill health in the community, and with families of children under 5 years. They may be GP attached or cover a geographical patch, visiting people in their own homes and conducting a variety of clinics and group sessions in health centres and elsewhere, such as church halls, doctors' surgeries etc. They also organise and participate in health education sessions in schools, shopping centres, factories, offices – in fact anywhere where people may be receptive to a health education message such as safe sex, coping with stress, the benefits of immunisation, parentcraft, weight control etc.

Health visitors are not always exclusively involved with care of the under-fives, some specialist HVs concentrate on care of the elderly or people with special needs.

For the role of the health visitor in child health see page 121.

Practice nurse

Employed by GPs, a practice nurse is a trained nurse who is responsible for performing practical treatments in the surgery or health centre. The role of the practice nurse is constantly changing and expanding and some are employed as nurse practitioners, who may be able to prescribe treatments and medicine for minor ailments.

With the necessary training they may:

- see and examine patients and decide whether or not they need to see the GP
- carry out practical treatments such as changing dressings and doing cervical smears
- provide immunisations
- offer family planning advice and counselling
- run well-person clinics.

District nurse

These trained nurses are involved with the care of patients in their own homes, usually after they have been discharged from hospital or because they are too elderly or infirm to cope at home.

They carry out a wide range of practical care such as:

- changing dressings
- administering drugs and injections
- helping patients to bath or providing bed baths
- enabling patients who are terminally ill to be cared for at home by relatives and friends.

Community paediatric nurse

Some areas may provide a community paediatric nurse who specialises in the care of sick children at home. Children are often discharged early from hospital because they recover more quickly at home in a familiar environment. A trained children's nurse can support parents to provide specialised individual care.

The best place for sick children is at home, if specialist care can be provided. The aims of the community paediatric nursing service are to shorten hospital stays and avoid hospital admissions if possible.

Four main categories of patient are supported by community paediatric nurses.

- Terminally ill children whose parents wish to care for them at home. Nurses can offer physical care, assess the need for pain relief and support the whole family.
- Chronically sick and disabled children whose parents need support and/or advice.
- Children having long-term treatments e.g. for leukaemia or other malignancies, or cystic fibrosis.
- Children with acute (short-term) conditions.
  The role of the community paediatric nurse also includes:
- support for parents to encourage them to be as independent as possible
- teaching parents and students
- liaison with other staff in the community e.g. health visitors, district nurses, GPs, social workers, and teachers.

Community midwife

Community midwives are trained to provide care throughout pregnancy, childbirth and during the postnatal period – for a minimum of 10 days and up to a month after the birth. All midwives are practitioners in their own right which means that they do not have to refer to a doctor if a pregnancy is progressing normally. They can prescribe and administer some drugs during the birth or if an emergency arises.

Community midwives are usually attached to a health centre or a group of GPs. They see expectant mothers regularly during the pregnancy, offering support to families and practical help and advice. They may be involved with the birth if the baby is born in a GP unit, at home or as part of the 'domino' (domiciliary-in-out) scheme where the midwife accompanies the mother in labour to hospital, delivers the baby and accompanies them home after about 6 hours. In most areas they are responsible for introducing the parents to the parent-held Child Health Record, and explaining its use and value.

Case study

Jane and David Ricks have three children – Joshua is 3 years old, Jack is 2 and Sophie is 13 months. Jane and David are both carriers of the gene for cystic fibrosis and Jack was diagnosed with this condition when he was 6 months old. Joshua has recently been admitted to hospital with diabetes and will be discharged shortly. Jane has discovered that she is pregnant again.

Using the information contained in this chapter answer the following questions.

1 How do you think the members of the PHCT can help this family?
2 What other services may they require?
3 How can the skills of the health visitor be used to support the parents and children?

 ### Progress check

1 What is the role of the GP in the PHCT?
2 Explain the difference between the roles of the practice nurse and the district nurse.
3 Describe the role of the health visitor in health promotion.
4 What is the role of the community midwife?

The role of the health visitor in child health

Most health visitors involved with child health are based in the community, but some hospital trusts employ paediatric liaison health visitors to support families with children in hospital and to communicate with the PHCT, especially the family health visitor.

Health visitors have a very important job to do to promote health with families and children in a non-threatening and non-judgmental manner.

Their role is mainly educational and advisory, providing a resource for all families to promote good health and prevent ill health. Because they have contact with families over quite a long period of time, they can build up a relationship of trust and mutual respect, resulting in parents/carers valuing their involvement and contacting them with a variety of concerns. They participate in every health promotion activity, screening, surveillance and health education (see Chapters 1 and 4). They:

■ have a statutory (legal) obligation to visit all new babies, usually taking over from the midwife 10 to 12 days after the birth. They do not have the right of entry into a home, but are obliged to try

- concentrate on children under 5 years and continue to visit and monitor the child until they go to school
- offer advice on child care, child development and children's needs
- conduct child health clinics, weighing and measuring babies and offering appropriate advice, such as safety, immunisations, feeding practices, behaviour, toilet training and all aspects of childcare and development
- perform developmental assessments in clinic and at home
- conduct hearing tests
- support families through times of crisis
- refer children and/or families for specialist help e.g. speech therapy, social services etc
- are independent professionals who decide whom to visit and how often – they accept referrals from outside the NHS
- may closely monitor cases of suspected child abuse.

> **Remember**
>
> The health visitor is the only member of the PHCT who visits and has contact with every family with children under 5 years of age, regardless of their health status.

Good Practice

Parents and childcare workers can consult the health visitor about any issues related to young babies and children. Health visitors are an invaluable resource for health promotion and advice. They will visit childcare establishments to talk to groups of staff, children and parents about any health issue. Their primary role is to try to prevent illness and promote good health through health education.

 Progress check

1 How does the health visitor promote child health?
2 What legal obligation does the health visitor have?
3 What is unique about the role of the health visitor in the PHCT?
4 Explain the values of health visiting in your own words.

Child health clinics

Child health clinics are usually conducted by health visitors and health care assistants. A doctor is often present – this may be the GP if they have an interest in child health, or a community paediatrician. The clinics may be weekly, fortnightly or monthly depending upon where they are held – the premises and geographical area. They may be held in health centres, GP surgeries or another convenient location – in a rural area it could be the village hall, a church hall, etc.

Wherever it is held, the clinic should be clean, warm and welcoming and contain the following provisions:

- changing area with changing mats, bin for used nappies, etc.
- weighing area with scales
- safe floor play area with toys for babies
- seats for parents/carers in a waiting area
- toys – some areas employ a play leader who provides activities for the older children
- a toy library may be available where toys can be borrowed and exchanged regularly
- a room for parents to talk to the health visitor about any health, development or caring concerns
- consultation room for the doctor to examine babies and children and discuss any issues with parents in confidence
- health promotion leaflets
- noticeboard / display area about child health issues
- provision for breast feeding.

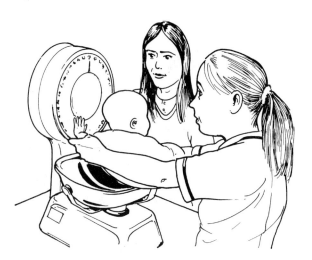

The baby clinic

Clinic routine

A member of the team welcomes parents and children to the clinic.

The health care assistant or nursery nurse usually weighs the babies, enters the recording in the Personal Child Health Record and asks the parent/carer if they want to see the doctor and/or the health visitor. They should be informed of an approximate waiting time – some clinics provide timed appointments and encourage parents to book beforehand.

Adults are encouraged to sit and chat together while they wait for their appointment. Babies and children should be able to play – a play leader or nursery nurse may encourage older children to investigate some of the activities offered. This makes a visit to clinic more fun and can be informative for parents about how to provide appropriate play materials for their child/ren.

A visit to clinic can be a social event as well as an important opportunity for health assessment and advice.

Clinic services

Services provided by child health clinics are:
- routine developmental surveillance
- screening
- medical examinations
- immunisations
- health promotion advice.

Activity

Prepare an A4 sized leaflet for parents about child health clinics. Explain the procedure at the clinic, what sort of provision is available and how often parents can attend with their child(ren).

Incorporate the benefits of screening and surveillance contained in previous chapters. See 'Chapter 4, Screening'.

Progress check

1 which health care staff are present at child health clinics and what are their responsibilities?
2 How can parents and children benefit socially from CHCs?
3 What services are available at child health clinics?

Case study

Sandra, Dale and their 8-month-old son Warren have been placed in bed and breakfast accommodation in an inner city area of the Midlands after their house was repossessed by the building society. They experienced severe financial difficulties after the factory where the couple worked was closed, the company went into liquidation and Sandra found out that she was pregnant. They have been regular attenders at the CHC since Warren was born – sometimes they go together, but often take it in turns to take him.

1 Why do you think this family enjoy their visits to the CHC?
2 What benefits will Warren experience as a result of regular attendance at the CHC?

The school health service

The first school doctor and nurse were appointed more than 100 years ago, but there were no standardised routines or procedures then for monitoring and promoting children's health.

The Education Act in 1944 stipulated that each local education authority (LEA) must provide a school health service. In 1974, when the NHS was reorganised, the responsibility for school health was taken over by each district health authority. The Court Report published in 1976 stressed the need to provide a service that is both preventative and curative, staffed by specially trained school nurses. In 1980 the school nurse training was formalised.

The 1981 Education Act widened the school nurse's role further with the integration of children with special needs into mainstream schools.

The school health team liaise closely with the PHCT to ensure that information received is accurate.

Aims of the school health service

- To ensure that children are physically and emotionally fit so that they can benefit fully from their education and achieve their potential.
- To prepare them for adult life and to help them achieve the best possible health during the school years and beyond.

Responsibilities of the school health service

Health staff working in schools have a responsibility to children and their families to:

- enthusiastically participate in health promotion programmes
- conduct regular surveillance of school-age children
- arrange or refer for investigation and/or treatment where necessary
- inform school and the local education authority about the effects of a particular condition on a child's education
- accept referrals from parents and other agencies
- liaise with PHCT and school staff
- work closely with medical, teaching and social work colleagues in the management of children with social, emotional, learning and medical problems.

Members of the school health team

The school health service is staffed by nurses, doctors, dentists and technicians.

School nurse

School nurses for the primary sector are usually responsible for several schools, and they may be assisted by health care assistants (who usually have a childcare qualification). They are aware of all children in their allocated schools, because health records are transferred from the health visitor to the school health service when a child reaches school age. Each school nurse is informed about every child beginning school or transferring in from another school.

They usually visit each school weekly, or as often as possible, to conduct the routine health appraisals. Because they have contact with children throughout their primary years they are able to get to know the children well and build up trusting relationships with them and their families.

They regularly meet the headteacher and other staff to discuss any children who are causing concern; medical examinations with the school doctor can then be arranged if necessary. They encourage parents to consult them about any concerns they have.

School nurses regularly provide the following (see 'Chapter 4, Screening'):

- growth measurements – height and weight
- vision testing
- audiometry – hearing tests
- immunisation
- management of health conditions, for example children with special needs or long-term health problems may require support; and teachers often need guidance about the management of particular conditions in the classroom
- referral to other professionals/agencies as appropriate – some children may need speech therapy, specialised hearing assessment, etc
- health care advice and information – this may include health education sessions with groups of children and parents on topics such as dental health, use of cycle helmets to promote safety, sun safety, etc
- enuresis (bed-wetting) advice. This is a relatively common problem in school-age children (1 in 10 children wet the bed at the age of 6 years). The school nurse can offer practical advice and support for children and families, including an enuresis alarm if the condition persists.

School doctor – community paediatrician

School doctors are responsible for the routine health care and screening of the children in their allocated group of schools. They see children for a medical consultation when a problem has been highlighted by parents, teachers or the school nurse. Routine health appraisals are performed by school nurses who inform the doctor if they are concerned.

Role of parents

Parents/carers should be able to discuss any concerns about their child with the school nurse and doctor. The comprehensive screening and surveillance routines (see Chapter 4) should reassure them that their children's health needs are being provided for. To ensure an efficient and accurate service, the parents should:

- complete health details about their child on the appropriate forms sent to them and return them to the school

> **Remember**
> School nurses have an important role in the screening process. They see all the children who attend their allocated schools regularly and are responsible for health surveillance programmes. Any health concerns about a child at school should be discussed with the school nurse and the parents.

- contact the school nurse or their child's teacher if they are worried about any aspect of their child's health
- try to attend medical check-ups with the school nurse or doctor
- check hair for head lice once a week.

✔ **Progress check**

- What are the aims of the school health service?
- How is the school nurse informed about the children attending the school(s) s/he is responsible for?
- Which screening and surveillance checks does the school nurse conduct?
- What are parent's responsibilities in relation to the health care of their children at school?

Case study

Rose is a school nurse. She used to work in the paediatric wards of the local hospital and then worked as a district nurse until she started a family. When her children started school she decided that school health was where she could use her special skills for the benefit of children. Life was certainly busy in her new job. She had seven primary schools in her case-load and three of them had nurseries attached. This week she was going to perform 18 health appraisals on new school entrants, conduct audiometry sessions at two of her schools and talk about the role of the school nurse at an information giving evening for new parents at one of her schools. She was also due to attend school medicals with a community paediatrician. Rose needed to discuss the identified health problems of three children with the headteachers at three of her schools and liaise with the education social worker. One headteacher had asked her to talk to a group of parents about head lice this week, and she was programmed to participate in her regular health education lessons for years 5 and 6 pupils.

1 How does Rose participate in health promotion?
2 Why do you think it is important to provide a regular school nurse for each school?

Education services providing support for children and their families

Children may experience difficulties which could affect their health and well-being, which require the specialist involvement of services provided by local education authorities. These services are available to all local authority nurseries and schools and accept referrals from teachers, social services, GPs and the school health service.

School psychological child guidance service

This service is a specialised agency administered by the local education authority. The team is concerned with children's problems as they appear within school, often as challenging or unusual behaviour. The team is composed of social workers, educational psychologists, psychotherapists and specialist tutors who are qualified teachers. Child psychiatrists may be available for consultation and become involved with individual cases. Because they provide such intensive involvement with children and their families they have a relatively small number of cases at one time. Parental involvement in therapy is encouraged.

Child guidance clinic

Children and their families may be given an appointment in a child guidance clinic based in a child development centre, hospital or education offices. They may be seen by the range of professionals involved in the child guidance service with an emphasis on family therapy.

Educational psychologist

The educational psychologist (EP) is primarily concerned with the assessment of children's learning difficulties. The EP is allocated a number of secondary schools and the feeder primary schools, and may provide some therapy for referred children.

Educational psychologists are also involved with the assessment of a child's special needs. They can scientifically test educational ability and consider the most appropriate type of school to meet the child's individual needs.

Parents must give their consent for the intervention of an EP.

The education welfare service

The education welfare service is a specialised agency usually administered by the local education authority. Parents have a legal obligation to educate their children – usually at full-time school. When this does not happen the education welfare service will be informed by the school, after they have tried to encourage parental co-operation. An education social worker will become involved with the case (see below). The education welfare service also provides financial help in the form of grants for essential school clothing, travel allowances and free school meals for children from low income families.

Education social worker (formerly educational welfare officer, EWO)

The education social worker (ESW) is primarily concerned with school attendance. It is the ESW's job to find out why children are constantly absent from school, or attending irregularly, and to offer appropriate help. The ESW may also become involved if there is a suspicion that a child is working illegally.

The ESW may also talk to teachers about particular children who are presenting problems; and may be able to inform school staff about the difficulties experienced by some families at home.

✓ *Progress check*

1 Which professionals are involved in the school psychological child guidance service?
2 What is the role of an educational psychologist?
3 When may the education welfare service become involved in the life of a child?
4 What is the role of the education social worker?

Hospital-based services

Admission to hospital is a fairly common experience for children – 1 in 4 children under 5 years will be admitted to hospital, and about two and a half million will be examined in the accident and emergency department each year.

Hospital staff share the responsibility for child health promotion as there are many opportunities for promoting health in hospital practice. These range from giving immunisations to children who are hospital in-patients to following up cases from the casualty department after children's accidents.

Accident and emergency department

Some hospitals have a separate accident and emergency (A & E) department for children. This is preferable because the environment can be geared to provide for the needs of children. Play leaders can provide play opportunities more effectively. A & E departments should have:

■ separate waiting areas and treatment rooms for children
■ paediatric nurses on duty at all times
■ doctors who are trained in the care of children
■ play leaders to support sick children.

In-patient care

Details of care in hospital are given in Chapter 15.

Outpatients department

Many children are seen in outpatient departments for a variety of reasons every year. Some hospitals have a paediatric clinic solely for babies and children. Play leaders should be available to give children the opportunity to play and cope with their anxieties.

Child development centre

Each regional health authority should provide a child development centre (CDC) or child development unit (CDU) to provide specialised assessment, support and treatment for chronically ill or disabled children. These centres are staffed by a highly trained multi-disciplinary team composed of paediatricians, nurses, nursery nurses and play therapists, physiotherapists, occupational therapists, speech therapists, psychologists, dieticians and many others who are skilled in assessing development and providing the required stimulation and practical help to enable progression. Together with the parents they will plan the most suitable treatment and therapy to enable individual children to fulfil their potential. The aims of the team are to:

- diagnose the child's condition and its most likely outcome (prognosis)
- consider the genetic factors – whether there is a chance that this condition may occur in future children
- decide which adaptations may be required in the home to make life easier, such as ramps, rails, etc. or consider other accommodation
- provide access to mobility aids such as wheelchairs and other special equipment such as computers
- consider the most suitable form of education for each individual child
- plan the treatment and therapy the child will need
- consider other associated difficulties e.g. hearing or vision
- ensure the family applies for and receives all the social security benefits they are entitled to
- provide or arrange respite care as necessary.

The benefits of a child development centre

Families caring for a very ill child will experience the many advantages of care and assessment from a highly skilled team of therapists. Each child and family is allocated a link worker who is available to translate if the first language is not English and to advise the team about important cultural factors. Other benefits include:

- a friendly and caring multi-disciplinary staff team who relate to each child and family as individuals
- an opportunity to meet other families and share experiences. Parents sometimes join voluntary support groups and even begin new ones as a result of contact with others at the CDC
- playgroups, parent and toddler groups and day care is sometimes available which encourages interaction between adults and children. It may be possible to leave the child for a short time in the capable hands of a professional, giving parents some time for themselves
- CDCs should be accessible for families. This is not always the case, but transport can be arranged when necessary, for example for families without a car or if children have particular mobility problems.

Paediatric intensive care

There are less than 500 paediatric intensive care cots and beds in the UK. 12,000 children each year need intensive care, half of them are aged under 2 years. Several beds are situated in an adult intensive care unit and the staff are not necessarily trained in caring for children's individual needs. The Department of Health recommends that all areas train staff and that there should be specialised paediatric intensive care available in all district general hospitals.

 Progress check

- How can accident and emergency departments in hospitals meet the specific needs of children?
- What are the aims of a child development centre?
- What are the benefits of a child development centre?
- How can play leaders in hospital help children to cope with their experience?

Useful terminology

cardiology	The study of the heart and how it works.
endocrinology	The study of the endocrine organs.
gynaecology	The treating of diseases which occur only in women i.e. of the female reproductive system.
haematology	The study of the nature, functions and diseases of the blood.
neonatology	The study and treatment of the baby within the first month of life.
neurology	The study of the nervous system i.e. the brain, spinal cord and nerves.
obstetrics	The branch of medicine dealing with pregnancy and labour.
occupational therapy	Treatment with interesting activities to re-educate and co-ordinate muscles in physical defects.
oncology	The branch of medicine dealing with cancer.
ophthalmology	The study of the eye and its diseases.
orthopaedics	The correction of deformities of the bones and skeleton.
paediatrics	The branch of medicine dealing with diseases of children.
physiotherapy	Treatment of muscular and skeletal conditions by natural forces e.g. massage, exercise, heat, light etc.
psychiatry	The branch of medicine which deals with disorders of the mind and thinking processes.
radiography	Examination by X-rays.
radiotherapy	Treatment of diseases by radium, X-rays etc.
renal	Relating to the kidney.
speech therapy	Treatment of speech disorders.
urology	The study of the diseases of the urinary tract.
X-ray	Electro-magnetic waves which can be used to make images of the body to aid diagnosis. They are also used to treat disease.

Key terms

You need to know what these words and phrases mean. Go back through the chapter and find out.

child development centre
child guidance
child health clinic
chiropodist
education social worker
educational psychologist
health visitor

occupational therapist
paediatric nurse
physiotherapist
practice nurse
primary health care team
school health service

Part 2: The Sick Child

Childcare workers usually care for children who are fit and well. However, children can become ill very quickly, so it is vitally important that the earliest signs of illness are recognised. Chapter 6 explains the range of signs and symptoms which children may display, and the action that should be taken by carers. Symptom charts provide a guide to action to be taken in certain circumstances. The following chapters describe conditions which affect particular systems and/or parts of the body.

The format of Chapters 7 to 14 follows a common theme using the following headings to explain each condition: 'What is . . .?', 'What causes . . . ?', 'How to recognise . . .', 'Immediate action', 'Ongoing care', 'Possible complications', and 'Further information'. This structure enables the chapters to be used as easy reference tools, as well as for more in-depth study. Brief details of the specific caring role of parents and carers are given with each condition. Detailed care of ill children is given in Part Three.

Chapter 6 Recognising illness in a child

This chapter includes:

- Signs and symptoms: definitions
- Pyrexia (high temperature)
- General malaise (feeling unwell)
- Swollen glands
- Coughing
- Pain
- Behaviour changes
- Vomiting
- Changes in bowel habits
- Diarrhoea
- Appetite loss
- When to call the doctor

People who work with children must be familiar with the signs and symptoms of a range of illnesses and should also be aware of their significance. This means being able to distinguish between minor problems and those which require immediate attention. Children are not always able to tell their adult carers that they feel unwell, so carers must be able to recognise signs of illness at an early stage and take the appropriate action.

They are also responsible for accurately reporting their concerns about changes in the child's physical condition and/or behaviour promptly and sensitively to the child's parent or main carer. To do this reliably and effectively childcare workers know individual children well and are skilled observers, realising when a mild change in the child's health may develop into something more severe and consequently paying scrupulous attention to their well-being. Accurate recording of a child's condition is important – for instance when they last ate or drank, when they urinated or had their bowels open, if they have slept etc.

Calling the doctor may be necessary – parents should be contacted prior to this if possible, but there are occasions when this is difficult. Emergencies require childcare workers to seek medical assistance first and to contact parents when the initial danger has resolved.

Day care circumstances are different – a nanny in sole charge in the parents' absence may be expected to seek medical aid as part of her/his duties. Staff caring for a child in a mainstream nursery or infant setting may only call the doctor in an emergency.

This chapter aims to highlight the main signs and symptoms of illness, with suggestions for the cause and when parents and/or the doctor should be contacted.

Signs and symptoms: definitions

Sign

A sign of illness is one that can be seen by an observer such as a rash, change in skin colour etc. It is therefore objective and can be measured. It is not based upon personal involvement.

Symptom

A symptom of illness is something experienced by the individual concerned e.g. pain or discomfort or general feelings of illness. These are subjective and rely upon description by the person who is complaining of illness.

Generalised signs and symptoms

Systemic (affecting the whole body system and not confined to a particular part) signs and symptoms are usually associated with increased body temperature and feeling generally unwell.

Pyrexia (high temperature)

A body temperature of 38°C or above is a sign of infection by a virus or bacteria and is usually accompanied by other signs and symptoms of illness. See the chart on pages 138–139. A pyrexia in a child may be recognised by:
- a flushed appearance
- feeling hot to the touch
- complaints of thirst
- irritable or unusually subdued behaviour.

Children can develop high temperatures very quickly and it is important to control the temperature to avoid any complications e.g. febrile convulsions.

Activity

Prepare a display for your placement to draw the attention of staff and parents about treatment for children who develop a high temperature.
- Include the signs and symptoms of pyrexia and the treatment which can be offered to reduce the temperature. Remind parents that they will be contacted to take their child home if they develop a temperature whilst in the childcare establishment.
- Include information about when a doctor should be called to a sick child.

How to take a temperature

The normal body temperature range is between 36–37°C. A temperature of more than 37.5°C is abnormal and means that the child has a fever – a pyrexia.

A temperature of 35°C or below means that the child is too cold and is suffering from hypothermia (see pages 191–3).

There are several different types of thermometer.

- Mercury thermometer: this is the classic type used in most establishments and homes. It is made of glass and contains mercury, which is a poison. Great care must be taken to ensure that the thermometer does not break. It should **never** be placed in a child's mouth. Taking the temperature with a mercury thermometer takes about 5 minutes. Before it is used it must be shaken down, so that the mercury is below 35°C. It takes some practice to be able to read a mercury thermometer reliably.

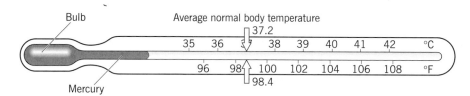

A mercury thermometer

- Digital thermometer: this thermometer gives a very quick readout of the temperature and is much safer than a mercury thermometer.
- Temperature strip: this heat-sensitive strip takes the skin temperature. Although it is easy to use, it lacks sensitivity

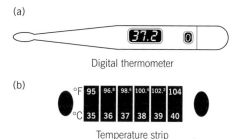

(a) A digital thermometer and (b) a temperature strip

The axillary temperature

The temperature of a child should be taken in the axilla (armpit). Qualified doctors and nurses may take a young child's temperature in the rectum.

Taking a child's temperature

FEVER IN CHILDREN

Fever – a temperature above 38°C (100° F) – is usually an indication of viral or bacterial infection; however, fever can also be caused by overheating. If your child seems unwell, take his or her temperature and note any other symptoms that might help the doctor to make a diagnosis.

START HERE

Go to chart
RASH WITH FEVER
(pp. 146-7)

Does your child have a rash?

- RASH
- NO RASH

Does your child have any of the following symptoms?

- SORE THROAT OR REFUSING SOLID FOOD
- COUGH
- RUNNY NOSE
- NONE OF THE ABOVE

How would you describe your child's breathing?

- UNUSUALLY NOISY
- UNUSUALLY RAPID
- NORMAL

Does your child seem very unwell and does he or she also have any of the following symptoms?

- STIFF NECK
- HEADACHE
- ABNORMAL DROWSINESS
- UNUSUAL IRRITABILITY
- NONE OF THE ABOVE

POSSIBLE CAUSES

TONSILLITIS (see p. 293)

ACTION NEEDED

MEDICAL HELP
If your child is no better after 24 hours, consult your doctor.

SELF-HELP
See *Good Practice: Reducing a raised temperature* (pp. 140-1); *Comforting a sore throat* (pp. 294-5).

POSSIBLE CAUSES

CROUP (see p. 184) or ASTHMA (see p. 300)

ACTION NEEDED

MEDICAL HELP
⊕ URGENT! Phone your doctor immediately!

SELF-HELP
See *Good Practice: Management of an asthma attack* (p. 302).

POSSIBLE CAUSES

A COMMON COLD (p. 289) or INFLUENZA (p. 290). MEASLES (p. 205) is also a possibility.

ACTION NEEDED

MEDICAL HELP
If there is no improvement within 48 hours, if symptoms worsen, or if other symptoms develop, phone your doctor immediately.

SELF-HELP
See *Good Practice: Reducing a raised temperature* (pp. 140-1); *Soothing a cough* (p. 151); *Easing a cough in a baby* (p.187).

POSSIBLE CAUSES

PNEUMONIA (p. 299)

ACTION NEEDED

MEDICAL HELP
⊕ URGENT! Phone your doctor immediately!

SELF-HELP
See *Good Practice: Reducing a raised temperature* (pp. 140-1); *Soothing a cough* (p. 151); *Easing a cough in a baby* (p.187).

POSSIBLE CAUSES

MENINGITIS (see p. 208)

ACTION NEEDED

MEDICAL HELP
✚ **EMERGENCY!** Call an ambulance.

Does your child have a swelling between the ear and the angle of the jaw on one or boths sides?

- **SWELLING**
- **NO SWELLING**

POSSIBLE CAUSES

GASTRO-ENTERITIS (see p. 175 [babies]; p. 252 [older children])

ACTION NEEDED

MEDICAL HELP
Get medical advice within 24 hours.

SELF-HELP
See Good Practice: Preventing dehydration in children (p. 163).

Does your child have any of the following problems?

- **EARACHE**
- **TUGS AT EITHER EAR**
- **WAKES UP SCREAMING DURING THE NIGHT**
- **NONE OF THE ABOVE**

POSSIBLE CAUSES

MUMPS (see p. 200)

ACTION NEEDED

MEDICAL HELP
Make an appointment to see your doctor.

SELF-HELP
See Good Practice: Reducing a raised temperature (pp. 140-1).

Does your child have any of the following symptoms?

- **PASSES URINE MORE FREQUENTLY THAN USUAL**
- **PAIN OR BURNING SENSATION WHEN PASSING URINE**
- **VOMITING WITH OR WITHOUT DIARRHOEA**
- **NONE OF THE ABOVE**

POSSIBLE CAUSES

OTITIS MEDIA (see p. 282)

ACTION NEEDED

MEDICAL HELP
Get medical advice within 24 hours.

SELF-HELP
See Good Practice: Reducing a raised temperature (pp. 140-1); Relieving earache (p. 283).

POSSIBLE CAUSES

URINARY TRACT INFECTION (p. 156)

ACTION NEEDED

MEDICAL HELP
Get medical advice within 24 hours.

SELF-HELP
See Good Practice: Reducing a raised temperature (pp. 140-1).

POSSIBLE CAUSES

Your child may have become overheated.

ACTION NEEDED

MEDICAL HELP
If the self-help measures do not succeed in lowering your child's temperature within 1 hour, phone your doctor immediately.

SELF-HELP
See Good Practice: Reducing a raised temperature (pp. 140-1).

Has your child been outside in the sun or in a hot room for several hours?

- **OUT IN THE SUN**
- **IN A HOT ROOM**
- **NEITHER**

If you cannot identify your child's problem from this chart, phone your doctor at once.

Source: Valman, Bernard, *The British Medical Association Children's Symptoms*, Dorling Kindersley, 1997

Remember

Always seek medical help within 24 hours for a child with a temperature which does not respond to treatment.

Follow this procedure when taking a child's axillary temperature.

1   Explain to the child what is going to happen.
2   Find a book together or some small toys that the child can play with while sitting on the carer's knee.
3   Collect the thermometer.
4   Take the child's top layer(s) of clothing off (to their vest) and sit them on your knee.
5   Place the thermometer under the armpit and hold the arm in position gently to prevent dislodging the thermometer (see figure).
6   A digital thermometer will stop rising fairly quickly and provide an accurate temperature recording. A mercury thermometer will take up to 5 minutes to 'cook' so the child will need to be distracted to prevent boredom.
7   Write the temperature in the child's records with the date and time.
8   Decide if the parents should be contacted if the temperature is raised.

Good Practice

Reducing a raised temperature

The following action points should be put into practice promptly if a child has a raised temperature.

1   Offer cool drinks.
2   Remove excessive clothing. Reduce bedding to a cotton sheet if the child is in bed.
3   Give paracetamol elixir, e.g. Calpol, if parents have provided the medicine and given their consent that it should be used in case of such an emergency. If not, contact the parents and get their verbal consent – arrange for them to collect the child as soon as possible and suggest that a doctor's advice is sought. Always follow the instructions on the container and give the correct dose.

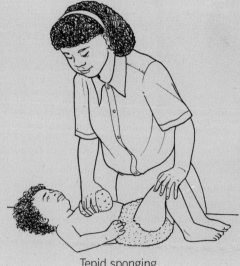

Tepid sponging

4 Lower the room temperature, if possible, to about 15°C (60°F).
5 Fan the child if possible.
6 Provide tepid sponging.

Removing the child's clothes and sponging them with tepid (lukewarm) water will reduce the temperature. Placing them in a lukewarm bath will have the same effect. BUT BEWARE – reducing the temperature too quickly can result in shock. For this reason some medical practitioners no longer recommend this action, but it may be effective as a last resort. It may be recommended for a child who has previously had a febrile convulsion. (see below)

Remember

1 **Never** give paracetamol to a baby of less than 3 months unless a doctor has prescribed the drug.
2 **Never** give any medicine to a child without the parent's consent.
3 **Never** give aspirin to a child under 14 years because of the danger of Reye's syndrome.

High temperature may be also associated with overheating which can be fairly easily resolved with cooling the child by:

- reducing the temperature of the body by removing clothing
- offering lots of cool fluids to drink
- staying in the shade or in a cool room.

Febrile convulsions

A febrile convulsion is a type of fit or seizure which occurs as a direct result of a raised body temperature. They usually occur in children between the ages of 6 months to 5 years at the beginning of an illness – children are vulnerable because the developing brain cannot cope with the sudden increase in temperature. A child who has had one febrile convulsion is more likely to have another one.

Signs

- Loss of consciousness.
- Rigidity (stiffness) of the body.
- Twitching movements of the body and/or face – eyes may roll back.
- May be incontinent of urine or faeces.

The child may regain consciousness briefly and then sleep or lapse straight into a deep sleep.

The child will probably be confused and irritable when they wake up.

Action by childcare worker/parent

1 Stay with the child throughout the convulsion and prevent them damaging themselves e.g. by falling out of bed. DO NOT INTERFERE with the process of the convulsion – allow it to take its course.

2   Ask a colleague to send for the doctor if possible.
3   Put the child into recovery position when movements have stopped and loosen tight garments.
4   Gently reassure the child if they regain consciousness before sleeping.
5   Call the doctor when the convulsion is over, if this has not been done already by a colleague.
6   Contact the parents to inform them of their child's condition.
7   Continue efforts to reduce the temperature i.e. by tepid sponging, etc.

The doctor may prescribe antibiotics to fight bacterial infections and may prescribe sedatives to be given if the temperature increases again to prevent future attacks.

✔ Progress check

1   Describe what signs and symptoms are.
2   How would you define a generalised sign and symptom?
3   What is a pyrexia?
4   What is the normal body temperature?
5   At what level is a temperature abnormal?
6   What different types of thermometers are available?
7   How would you take a child's temperature?
8   When would you contact the child's parents about a child's temperature?
9   How could the childcare worker try to reduce a child's temperature?
10   What are the possible dangers of tepid sponging?
11   How could you reduce the temperature of a child who was over-heating due to environmental conditions?
12   What is a febrile convulsion?
13   How would you recognise a febrile convulsion in a young child?

Case study

Andrea has enrolled on a first aid course for children at her local college. Now her son, Henry, was 9 months old, she thought she should be prepared for any accidents he may have in the future. Henry had seemed a little under the weather for the past few hours, he had refused his last evening feed and was crying and miserable. Although she had not taken his temperature she could tell he was hot, but now he had settled off to sleep she hoped he would be feeling better in the morning. A few hours later Henry started to cry, and as Andrea walked into the bedroom he began to shake violently and his feet and hands started to turn blue.

1   What do you think is happening to baby Henry?
2   What should Andrea do to help to relieve the situation?
3   What could Andrea have done earlier to try to prevent the febrile convulsion?

General malaise (feeling unwell)

When children feel generally unwell it is advisable to take their temperature and look for other signs of illness such as a rash, swellings, etc. Ask them if they have any pain or discomfort (such as a headache, earache, abdominal pain, etc.) and treat it accordingly.

Note whether there are any other signs of illness such as coughing, sore throat causing difficulty vocalising or eating, vomiting, diarrhoea, etc. It is useful to find out if the child has been in contact with any of the infectious childhood diseases because they could be incubating the condition themselves.

General malaise is usually the first sign of an infectious illness. Close observation is required because it could develop into something as straightforward as the common cold, or it could be a serious condition such as meningitis. However some children can feel unwell as the result of anxiety which can be caused by problems at school etc.

Signs

- Loss of appetite for food and drink.
- Tiredness, listlessness and lack of energy. Children may be uninterested in stimulating activity, preferring to sit quietly, perhaps gaining comfort from a familiar soft toy, comfort blanket or similar. Sleeping for longer than usual and drowsiness during the day are also signs of illness in young children.
- Change in skin tone. The skin may look pale or be flushed if the child has a high temperature. Lack of oxygen in the bloodstream may result in blueness (cyanosis) of the fingers, toes and sometimes of the lips. Yellowness of the skin may be caused by jaundice.
- Unhappy disposition. Babies and children may cry when they feel generally unwell. Older children may be able to tell adults about their discomfort, but not necessarily accurately. The clues are often picked up from non-verbal messages (such as holding or pulling on the ear), the posture of a child and the facial expression will give clues about the cause of the illness.

Remember

Always seek medical assistance if a child:
- is very drowsy and does not respond or communicate as NORMAL for them
- vomits for 12 hours or more
- refuses to drink for 6 hours
- has noisy and rapid breathing
- finds breathing difficult and laboured
- has a temperature of 39°C which does not respond to treatment
- has a flat rash of pink/purple spots which maintain their colour and do not change when pressed with the fingers – this could be meningitis and is usually accompanied by other signs.

FEELING GENERALLY UNWELL

If your child complains of feeling unwell, you should check his or her temperature and look for a rash. A symptom such as a headache may clear up with self-help measures, or it may be the first sign of an infection, such as influenza. If your child's condition worsens, consult your doctor.

DANGER SIGNS

Phone your doctor at once if your child has any of the following symptoms:

- Abnormal drowsiness or unresponsiveness.
- Temperature over 39° C (102° F).
- Vomiting for 12 hours.
- Fast or noisy breathing.
- Refusing to drink for 6 hours.
- Flat, pink or purple spots that do not disappear when pressed.

START HERE

Does your child have a fever – a temperature of 38° C (100° F) or above?

FEVER

NO FEVER

Does your child have any of the following symptoms?

VOMITING

DIARRHOEA

RASH

ABDOMINAL PAIN

NONE OF THE ABOVE

Go to chart
Rash with fever
(pp. 146-7)

POSSIBLE CAUSE

GASTRO-ENTERITIS (see p. 175 [babies]; p. 252 [older children])

ACTION NEEDED

MEDICAL HELP
Get medical advice within 24 hours.

SELF-HELP
See Good Practice: Preventing dehydration (p. 163).

Go to
Good Practice:
Helping to soothe abdominal pain (p. 155).

Does your child have a rash?

RASH

NO RASH

Go to chart
Rash with fever
(pp. 146-7)

Go to chart
Fever in Children
(pp. 138-9)

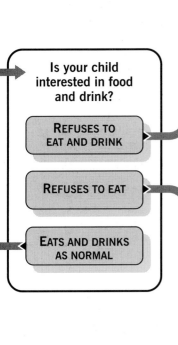

Is your child interested in food and drink?

- **REFUSES TO EAT AND DRINK**
- **REFUSES TO EAT**
- **EATS AND DRINKS AS NORMAL**

POSSIBLE CAUSE

Your child may be developing an infectious disease (see Chapter 8), particularly if he or she is listless or irritable or has other signs of illness.

ACTION NEEDED

MEDICAL HELP
If your child feels no better after 24 hours or develops other symptoms, make an appointment to see your doctor.

SELF-HELP
Try to make your child drink by offering his or her favourite liquid.

See Good Practice: Preventing dehydration (p. 163).

POSSIBLE CAUSE

Anxiety or problems at school can result in a child feeling unwell.

ACTION NEEDED

MEDICAL HELP
If your child feels no better after 24 hours or develops other symptoms, make an appointment to see your doctor.

Go to
Good Practice:
Comforting a sore throat (p. 294); Food and fluids (p. 334).

Might your child be anxious or worried about something?

- **POSSIBLY**
- **UNLIKELY**

In the past 3 weeks might your child have had contact with anyone who has an infectious disease?

- **NO CONTACT**
- **CONTACT**

POSSIBLE CAUSE

One of the childhood infectious diseases (see Chapter 8), in its incubation period, might be causing your child to feel unwell.

ACTION NEEDED

MEDICAL HELP
If your child feels no better after 24 hours or develops other symptoms, make an appointment to see your doctor.

If you cannot identify your child's problem from this chart, talk to your doctor within 48 hours.

Source: Valman, Bernard, *The British Medical Association Children's Symptoms*, Dorling Kindersley, 1997

RASH WITH FEVER

The combination of rash and fever – a temperature of 38° C (100° F) or over – is usually caused by an infectious disease. Most of these diseases are caused by viruses and generally clear up quickly without special treatment. You should, however, consult your doctor for a diagnosis.

DANGER SIGNS

Phone your doctor at once if your child has any of the following symptoms during, or after apparent recovery from, any of the common childhood infectious diseases:

- Abnormal drowsiness or floppiness.
- Seizures
- Temperature over 40° C (104° F) or above.
- Abnormally fast breathing.
- Noisy or difficult breathing.
- Severe headache.
- Refusing to drink for over 6 hours.

START HERE

What are the features of your child's rash?

- FLAT SPOTS THAT DO NOT DISAPPEAR WHEN PRESSED
- FINE RED RASH THAT TURNS WHITE WHEN PRESSED
- BLOTCHY, RAISED RED RASH
- CROPS OF ITCHY SPOTS THAT BLISTER AND DRY INTO SCABS
- FLAT, PINK SPOTS STARTING ON THE FACE OR TRUNK
- BRIGHT RED RASH CONFINED TO THE CHEEKS
- NONE OF THE ABOVE

If you cannot identify your child's problem from this chart, talk to your doctor within 48 hours.

POSSIBLE CAUSE

Blood infection with meningococcus, a bacteriun that causes MENINGITIS (see p. 208)

ACTION NEEDED

MEDICAL HELP
✚ **EMERGENCY!** Call an ambulance.

POSSIBLE CAUSES

CHICKENPOX (see p. 195)

ACTION NEEDED

MEDICAL HELP
If the spots become infected, make an appointment to see your doctor.

SELF-HELP
See Good Practice: *Reducing a raised temperature* (pp. 140-1).

POSSIBLE CAUSES

ERYTHEMA INFECTIOSUM (see p. 214)

ACTION NEEDED

MEDICAL HELP
If you are concerned about your child's condition or if your child has SICKLE-CELL ANAEMIA (see p. 325), make an appointment to see your doctor.

SELF-HELP
See Good Practice: *Reducing a raised temperature* (p. 140-1).

How high was your child's temperature during the 3 to 4 days before the rash appeared?

- 38.5° C (101° F) OR ABOVE
- BELOW 38.5° C (101° F)

POSSIBLE CAUSE

RUBELLA (see p. 207)

ACTION NEEDED

MEDICAL HELP
Make an appointment to see your doctor.

SELF-HELP
See Good Practice: *Reducing a raised temperature* (p. 140-1).

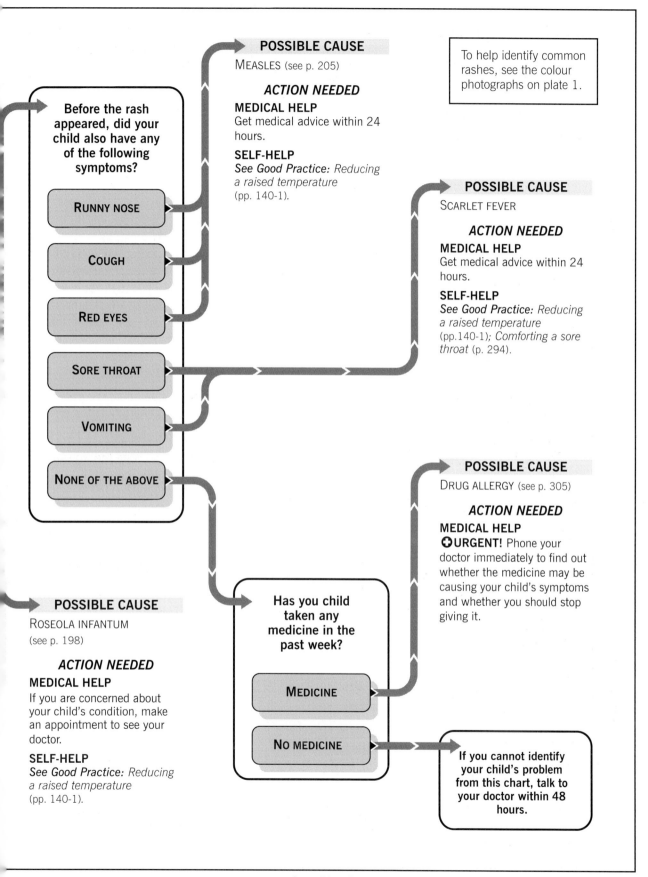

Before the rash appeared, did your child also have any of the following symptoms?

- RUNNY NOSE
- COUGH
- RED EYES
- SORE THROAT
- VOMITING
- NONE OF THE ABOVE

POSSIBLE CAUSE

MEASLES (see p. 205)

ACTION NEEDED

MEDICAL HELP
Get medical advice within 24 hours.

SELF-HELP
See *Good Practice: Reducing a raised temperature* (pp. 140-1).

To help identify common rashes, see the colour photographs on plate 1.

POSSIBLE CAUSE

SCARLET FEVER

ACTION NEEDED

MEDICAL HELP
Get medical advice within 24 hours.

SELF-HELP
See *Good Practice: Reducing a raised temperature* (pp.140-1); *Comforting a sore throat* (p. 294).

POSSIBLE CAUSE

DRUG ALLERGY (see p. 305)

ACTION NEEDED

MEDICAL HELP
⊕ **URGENT!** Phone your doctor immediately to find out whether the medicine may be causing your child's symptoms and whether you should stop giving it.

Has you child taken any medicine in the past week?

- MEDICINE
- NO MEDICINE

POSSIBLE CAUSE

ROSEOLA INFANTUM (see p. 198)

ACTION NEEDED

MEDICAL HELP
If you are concerned about your child's condition, make an appointment to see your doctor.

SELF-HELP
See *Good Practice: Reducing a raised temperature* (pp. 140-1).

If you cannot identify your child's problem from this chart, talk to your doctor within 48 hours.

Source: Valman, Bernard, *The British Medical Association Children's Symptoms*, Dorling Kindersley, 1997

Case study

Adil is 4 years old and attends the local state nursery school every afternoon. He is usually an energetic child who socialises well and is very popular with children and staff. One afternoon Adil was unhappy when his mother left, and cried briefly. He was unusually quiet and preferred to sit on a large cushion in the book corner instead of his more usual activities of building, creative play and outdoor pursuits. He looked pale and was obviously tired and withdrawn, refusing his milk and fruit at snack time. At story time he sat on the knee of the nursery assistant and she noticed that he felt hot. Adil later complained of a headache but pointed to his abdomen.

1 What signs of illness is Adil displaying?
2 Who should the nursery staff contact?
3 What important information should be conveyed to the parent and how?
4 What action could be taken by the staff in the nursery to comfort Adil?
5 What information should be recorded in the nursery records?

Swollen glands

The lymphatic system is part of the bodys immune system which creates lymphocytes – blood cells which destroy infection and make antibodies. It is made up of a network of lymphatic vessels and lymph nodes (glands) which circulate lymph. Lymph is a clear fluid which collects waste products and infection from the cells of the body. Lymph glands are filters which collect the pathogenic micro-organisms which are then destroyed by lymphocytes.

Lymph glands become enlarged and swollen as they try to fight infection and create antibodies.

The sites of lymph glands are shown in the diagram on page 149.

Swollen glands in the neck

Swollen neck glands are common in children with upper respiratory tract infections.

Characteristics

- The glands feel soft and smooth and are tender to touch.
- The glands may be swollen on one side of the neck only, as they drain infection from the site e.g. an ear infection in one ear.

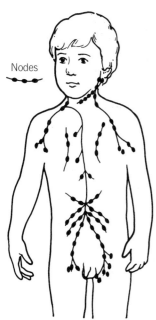

Nodes

The lymphatic system: areas of the body where glands that may swell are located

■ Glands may remain enlarged for 2–3 weeks or until the infection has gone.

Action

If a child is complaining of swollen, painful neck glands, it is advisable for a doctor or other adult to check other sites e.g. the glands under the armpits and in the groin and abdomen. If these are also enlarged it is a sign of a more widespread infection.

If the swollen glands are obviously associated with an infection which is getting better there is no necessity to call the doctor.

A child with swollen glands which are not improving in 2–3 weeks should be seen by a doctor.

If the gland(s) are swollen with no other signs of illness a doctor should be consulted.

Swollen glands in the groin

Lymph glands in the groin run along, just above and below, the crease between the top of the thigh and the base of the abdomen. In boys the term 'groin' also refers to the scrotum.

Small lumps in the groin can be felt when a child has a cough or cold and also when an infection near to the groin is present e.g. a cut or graze on the leg which has become infected.

A doctor should be consulted if a bacterial infection is suspected.

Generalised swollen glands

Swollen glands in the neck, groin and armpit may be a sign of infectious mononucleosis (glandular fever), but this is more common in adolescents and adults.

A doctor should be consulted.

 Progress check

1 What should the childcare worker do if a child seems to be generally unwell?
2 Why is close observation of the child necessary?
3 What are the signs of general malaise?
4 When should medical advice be sought for a child who is unwell?
5 Why do the lymph glands swell during an infection?
6 Where in the body are lymph glands situated?
7 What are the characteristics of swollen glands in the neck?
8 Where else in the body may the lymph glands be obviously swollen when the child has an infection?
9 When should the parents or doctor be called about swollen glands?

Coughing

Coughing is usually caused by a respiratory tract infection which is fairly common in young children. However there are several different types of cough associated with respiratory tract conditions.

- **Wheezy** – noisy breathing, usually on breathing out.
- **Productive** – the cough results in the movement of phlegm or mucus up the airways to the mouth. This is usually swallowed by the child.
- **Dry** – a rasping cough which does not result in any secretions from the respiratory tract.
- **Barking** – this croup-type cough sounds like a dog barking and is a hard, dry sound.
- **Whooping** – after a spasm of coughing the child 'whoops' when breathing in, before the coughing begins again.

Irritants to the respiratory tract

Coughs can be irritated by environmental conditions and as a result may be more severe at certain times of the day or night. Examples of factors which may affect coughs are as follows.

- **Smoking** –children in smoky atmospheres are more likely to develop coughs which will be irritated by the smoke.
- **Cold air** – inhaling cold air will increase the cough.
- **Allergens** – children may be allergic to a variety of substances and may develop a cough as a result.
- **Posture** – an upright position enables easy breathing and reduces coughing. Lying down in bed at night may increase the coughing spasms. Night-time coughs are associated with asthma (see page 300).

Remember

Call for an ambulance immediately if a child is:
- unable to talk or make any sounds
- blue around the mouth or tongue.

Soothing a cough

Good Practice

Soothing a cough
- Plenty of warm soothing liquids such as honey and lemon will help.
- Humidifying the atmosphere by putting a damp towel on a warm radiator may help to loosen phlegm and relieve the cough.
- Avoid overheating the room as this dries out the atmosphere and irritates the cough.
- Cough linctus may be prescribed by the GP and should be given according to the prescribed dosage.

✔ Progress check

1 What is the most common cause of coughing in childhood?
2 What do the different types of cough sound like?
3 List some of the environmental factors which may irritate the respiratory tract.
4 What are night-time coughs associated with?
5 How will humidifying the atmosphere help the cough?

Pain

Children may complain of pain in a specific part of the body or of a general hurting or aching all over. Young babies and children may not be able to tell you that they are in pain, so other clues will help to establish the cause such as crying, holding the affected part of the body such as the head, ear or tummy, difficulty with movement of legs, hands etc. The observant and experienced childcare worker should be able to identify the problem if he or she knows the child well.

Babies may experience pain caused by wind, colic, teething, nappy rash, etc. It is important to check the baby to find the cause of the crying.

Some possible sites and causes of pain in babies and children are the following.

Earache

Infection is the usual cause of earache. Children are particularly vulnerable to ear infections because of short passages (Eustachian tubes) connecting the nose and ear (see page 280).

Severe earache accompanied by a temperature and/or feeling poorly is usually the result of infection and a doctor should be seen.

Occasionally, earache can be caused by excessive wax production which may require removal by the GP or practice nurse.

Foreign bodies

Discharge from the ear and pain can be caused by a child pushing a small object into the outer ear canal. It is preferable to take the child to an accident and emergency department at a hospital so that the object can be removed. Trying to remove it yourself may result in it being pushed further into the ear.

Accidental injuries

Accidents may result in physical injuries which are painful and may need treatment to reduce the pain and prevent complications. Burns, scalds, grazes and cuts may occur at home or in a childcare establishment.

> **Remember**
> A child with earache should always be seen by a doctor.

Whenever a child is injured they will need a lot of comfort and reassurance. Minor injuries may be treated without requiring medical aid, but parents should always be informed of any incident involving their child. This can be done verbally when they come to collect the child but it is best practice to give them a written injury report as well.

All accidents should be recorded in an 'Accident Book' in all establishments including the date, time, details of the nature of the incident, who was involved, witnesses and first aid given.

INJURY	SIGNS	ACTION
Sprain	Child cannot put weight on the affected ankle May limp or hop Complains of pain	Remove the shoe and sock Raise and support the foot to reduce any swelling Apply a cold compress against it, wrap with cotton wool padding and a crêpe bandage. Rest, ice, compression, elevation (RICE) Keep the ankle elevated Call the doctor if the foot may be broken or take to the accident and emergency department at the local hospital
Fracture	Signs depend upon the site of the fracture: ■ pain ■ swelling ■ loss of use of a limb or inability to walk or stand ■ tenderness increased with movement	Call for the establishment's first-aider to administer first aid depending on the site of the injury Contact the parents Take the child to the accident and emergency department if a fracture is suspected
Swelling	May occur after a fall or knock when the injured area expands Compare the affected limb (arm or leg) with the other limb when a swelling will be apparent	Reduce swelling by holding a cold compress against it for 30 minutes Rest Ice Compression Elevation – raise and support the injured part
Splinter	Sharp pain in the hand Limping if in the foot Close inspection will reveal the site, and a small piece of the splinter may protrude through the skin	Wash the area with warm water and soap Use a pair of clean tweezers to remove the splinter Encourage a little bleeding by squeezing the area Inform parents if the splinter cannot be removed
Bruise	Purple-blue coloured areas on the skin – darker on black skin. They fade to yellow before disappearing 10-14 days later Common sites on children are forehead, elbows, knees, shins	Cold compress to prevent further bleeding underneath the skin Bruising in unusual and unexpected areas should be investigated e.g. armpits, back, abdomen, buttocks, inside the thighs, etc
Cuts and grazes	Bleeding	Sit the child down Wash the injured area with water and clean cotton wool or gauze – wipe away from the open wound Apply direct pressure if bleeding will not stop Remove any dirt and gravel carefully Cover the area with a gauze dressing

INJURY	SIGNS	ACTION
Poisoning	Child has swallowed poisonous berries or leaves, alcohol, drugs, chemicals or bleach Find out exactly what has been swallowed and how much Keep containers, berries or leaves to show to the doctor	Comfort and reassure DO NOT TRY TO MAKE THE CHILD VOMIT DO NOT GIVE THE CHILD ANYTHING TO DRINK Call the doctor or an accident and emergency (A & E) department Contact the parents. Put the child in recovery position if they are unconscious.
Bites	Irritation and pain at the site Puncture teeth marks in the skin after an animal bite	Rinse the wound under running water for 5 minutes Wash the area with soap and water Cover the wound with a dry dressing Check that the child is immunised against tetanus
Stings	Sudden cry when the sting occurs May see sting sticking out at the tip of a swollen area. Itching Irritation and pain at the site	Carers should remain calm as this will reassure a frightened child Sting may be removed carefully if possible, avoiding pressure on the poison sac Wasp sting – apply dilute vinegar Bee sting – apply bicarbonate of soda Apply cold compress followed by calamine Observe for signs of an allergic reaction
Burns and scalds	Pain Inflamed skin Blistering	Put affected area under cold, running water for 10–15 minutes to cool it. This will also help to reduce pain. Remove clothing when the area has been cooled (remove tight clothes before the area begins to swell) Cover with a clean, soft, non-fluffy cloth, cling film is adequate. These will keep the area cool and prevent infection Take to the A & E department if the burn is larger than a 10 pence piece

 Progress check

1 What are the possible causes of earache?
2 What information should be included in an accident report?
3 What are the signs of an ankle sprain?
4 How would you know that a child had fractured a limb?
5 How should a sprain be treated in a childcare establishment?
6 What action should be taken to treat a bruise and/or a swelling?
7 Describe the action you would take to treat a child with a severe burn to the arm.

Abdominal pain

Most children have tummy ache at some time and the cause is usually not serious. However the carer should notice the type, duration and location of the pain.

TYPE AND LOCATION OF PAIN	POSSIBLE CAUSE	ACTION
1 More severe when abdomen is pressed 2 Continuous (no relief with 'Good Practice' advice)	Appendicitis	Contact parents Call the doctor
Pain in the lower back and/or on one side of the abdomen	Urinary tract infection	Contact parents See the doctor
Generalised pain (all over the abdomen) with fever, vomiting/diarrhoea	Gastro-enteritis	Call the doctor for a baby under 1 year Offer clear fluids and rehydrating solutions to older children Call the doctor if condition persists for 24 hours with no improvement.
Recurrent attacks of abdominal pain with no other signs of illness	Anxiety Emotional problems Fear e.g. bullying	Try to soothe the pain – see below Discuss with parents and try to find the cause of the anxiety or fear The child should be seen by a doctor who may refer the child and family for specialist help

Remember

Call an ambulance if a child has:

- continuous abdominal pain for 4 hours or more
- greeny/yellow vomit
- pain in the groin or if the scrotum is swollen. This could be a serious complication of a hernia.

Good Practice

Helping to soothe abdominal pain

Always ask a child with abdominal pain if they have been to the toilet – having the bowels open can relieve some pains!

Contact parents and describe the child's symptoms.

Wrap a warm (not boiling hot) hot water bottle in a towel and encourage the child to lie with it on their abdomen to ease the discomfort.

Offer only water to drink while the pain lasts.

Case study

Oliver is $3\frac{1}{2}$ years old and is cared for at home by a live-in nanny because both his parents go out to work and live a long way from the nearest nursery. The large garden is very safe, secured by a high fence and security gate. Oliver is often allowed to explore and play on his slide and climbing frame outside. The nanny is vigilant and observes his play and activity closely. One day Oliver wants to give his soft toys a picnic, and together they collect leaves, seeds and berries to feed to the penguin, fox, squirrel and mouse. The picnic is great fun, but later that day Oliver complains of tummy ache and says he feels sick. He asks the nanny if the animals are sick too, because they had the same dinner. She wonders if he could possibly have eaten some of the seeds and berries.

1 What action should the nanny take now?
2 How could this accident have been prevented?

Skin conditions or allergies

Sunburn

This is severe burning of the skin by the sun and ultraviolet rays cause a serious inflammation. The skin is reddened in white races and black skin looks darker than usual and the skin is slightly swollen. The child will feel acute pain and discomfort and the skin is extremely tender and feels tight. Blistering, cracking or bleeding of the skin may occur.

Allergy

Allergy rashes are caused by something which has come into contact with the skin or by something a child has eaten, such as peanuts, shellfish, cheese, medicines, etc. The most common allergy rash is urticaria which is a very itchy, lumpy rash, common in the under-fives. It looks like swollen pale weals (lumps) on the skin surrounded by dark inflamed skin, and the rash may come and go. It may affect a small area of the body or be fairly widespread.

Good Practice

Soothing sore skin
- Keep the skin cool.
- Apply calamine lotion.
- Sodium bicarbonate in the bath water is soothing.

Antihistamine (anti-itch) cream and medicine are very effective. They can be purchased over the counter and the sedative quality of some of the medicines may induce sleep.

 Progress check

1 What observations should be made of a child with abdominal pain?
2 What is the difference between the symptoms for appendicitis and gastro-enteritis?
3 When should medical advice be sought for a child with abdominal pain?
4 How can abdominal pain be relieved by an adult?
5 Give three examples of allergens which may cause a skin rash.
6 What is urticaria?
7 How can sore skin be soothed?

Urinary tract infections (UTI)

Pain on passing urine is a sign of a UTI and the child should see the doctor as soon as possible. The child may also seem unwell, have a temperature and pass urine more often than usual. Frequent passing of urine without any other signs may be a sign of anxiety.

Drinking excessive amounts of fluid and passing large amounts of urine may be signs of diabetes mellitus and the doctor should be seen.

COLOUR OF URINE	POSSIBLE CAUSE	ACTION
Green or blue	Food colourings or medicines	None – try to find the food responsible
Dark yellow or orange	Concentrated because of low fluid intake, high temperature, diarrhoea/vomiting	Encourage the child to drink as much as possible
Dark brown	If stools are very pale or putty coloured – possible hepatitis	See doctor
Red/pink, blood-stained and cloudy	1. Urinary tract infection 2. Inflammation of the kidney (glomerulonephritis)	See doctor **See doctor urgently**

Remember

Always see the doctor if a child's headache is constant, happens regularly or is very severe. If a headache lasts more than 3 hours and does not respond to treatment at home or is accompanied by other symptoms of illness, call the doctor.

Call an ambulance immediately if you suspect meningitis.

Headache

Headaches often accompany infections but they may occur on their own or with a range of other symptoms. Observe the child for other signs of illness taking note of whether they are well, slightly off-colour or extremely poorly. One of the first symptoms of meningitis may be a headache so check for other signs – drowsiness, stiff neck, high temperature, vomiting, avoiding light and preferring the dark, or a flat rash of pink/purple spots which maintain their colour and do not change when pressed with the fingers. If any of these accompany the headache call for an ambulance.

Headaches can also be the result of:
■ worry or anxiety
■ eye strain
■ allergy to such foods as chocolate or citrus fruits.

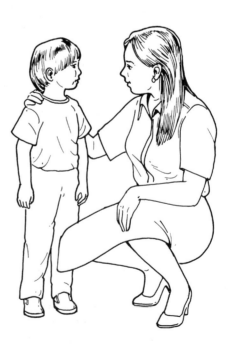

Is the child worried?

> ## Good Practice
>
> Headaches can be relieved by:
> 1 giving paracetamol elixir in the correct dosage – with the parents consent
> 2 encouraging a child to rest, preferably in a darkened room
> 3 (for headaches that occur as the result of low blood sugar levels) offering light food and/or a nutritious drink may relieve the symptom.

Painful joints and limbs

Painful joints and limbs require attention – they may be caused by a recent injury or infection. Carers may notice that a baby or child is not moving a part of the body at all, or that it is obviously painful for them to do so. Older children may tell adults that they have pain. Possible causes are:

- a fracture
- a dislocation
- sprains or strains
- a bone or joint infection
- cramp
- a generalised infection such as influenza which can result in aching limbs and joints
- juvenile arthritis which causes swollen, painful and reddened joints – this is quite rare.

> ### ✓ Progress check
>
> 1 How could you tell that a young child was experiencing pain?
> 2 List as many causes of pain as you can.
> 3 What are the signs of a urinary tract infection?
> 4 What action should the childcare worker take if he or she notices that a child's urine is a very dark colour?
> 5 What are the possible causes of a headache in a child?
> 6 How should the childcare worker respond to a child with a headache?
> 7 How can headaches be relieved?
> 8 What are some possible causes of painful joints and limbs?

Behaviour changes

Changes in behaviour are often the first sign of an illness developing. Children may be more clingy to their carers than usual and sometimes this is accompanied by apparently petty complaints.

Below are some behaviour changes which are characteristic early signs of illness:

- whining or crying child who does not want to play
- being quieter than usual
- attention-seeking behaviour

- sleeping more or less than usual
- lacking energy
- regression.

Crying

Babies cry for a variety of reasons – it is their only method of communicating a need. Some of these reasons are associated with illness, such as pain anywhere will cause in infant to cry. Crying in a very young baby which cannot be comforted by feeding or adult contact needs to be investigated. Ear infections, itchy skin and abdominal discomfort will all cause crying but may also provide other clues as to the cause of the crying such as temperatures, pulling the ears, rashes, diarrhoea, vomiting etc.

Children crying more than usual may be telling you that they feel unwell or that they are unhappy for another reason. Unexplained crying should not be ignored but should be investigated to find the cause of the discomfort or unhappiness. Other signs and symptoms may be seen as the child is supported and comforted.

Regression

Children who are unwell often experience regression in their development and/or behaviour. This means that they revert to a slightly earlier stage of development: they may wish to be carried instead of walking independently, may need to wear nappies, start to wet the bed again or want to play with familiar, undemanding toys which they have outgrown. This is perfectly normal and should be treated with understanding by their carers, however, it is also a sign that a child is not feeling as fit as usual and requires observation and attention.

Vomiting

Remember

Call an ambulance if a child has abdominal pain for 6 hours or more – this could be a sign of appendicitis.

Call an ambulance if a child who is vomiting has a flat rash of pink/purple spots which maintain their colour and do not change when pressed with the fingers.

Call an ambulance if a child produces greeny/yellow vomit.

All children vomit at some time! There are often signs to tell the difference between sickness as the result of too much excitement or party food, and more serious conditions. Although vomiting is often caused by an infection of the digestive system, it may be associated with infection in any part of the body, (urinary tract infections, hepatitis, appendicitis, meningitis, etc.) so it is important to observe the child carefully for any other signs of illness.

Noting how often the child is sick, what colour the vomit is, whether it contains blood, how long the illness has lasted, whether the child is drinking and managing to keep the fluids down without vomiting again, whether there is any pain associated with the illness, any diarrhoea, and the child's temperature will help to isolate the cause of the illness.

Greeny/yellow vomit can be a sign of a blockage (obstruction) in the bowel and the child should go to hospital immediately without having anything to eat or drink.

Good Practice

Helping a child who is vomiting

- Always reassure a child who is feeling or being sick. It is a very frightening experience for a young child.
- Support the head by putting your hand on the forehead – this is a practical help and also reassures the child of your presence.
- Wipe the child's face after vomiting and offer mouthwash or sips of water to freshen the mouth.
- Encourage small drinks often to prevent dehydration (about 30-60mls OR 1-2 fluid ounces every hour). Rehydrating powders can be purchased to replace the electrolytes lost during vomiting.
- Children who are feeling sick should be encouraged to rest with a bowl by the bed. It is preferable for an adult to stay with them until they have fallen asleep, or certainly nearby as they may vomit again.

✔ Progress check

1 What sort of behaviour changes might an ill child display?
2 How could a childcare worker establish the reasons for a child's crying?
3 What is regression?
4 List the possible reasons for vomiting in a child.
5 What observations should be made of a child who is or has vomited?
6 What might greeny/yellow vomit be a sign of?
7 What action should be taken by the childcare worker in this situation?
8 When should an ambulance be called?
9 What are the signs of dehydration in a child?
10 How could a sick child be comforted if he or she is vomiting?

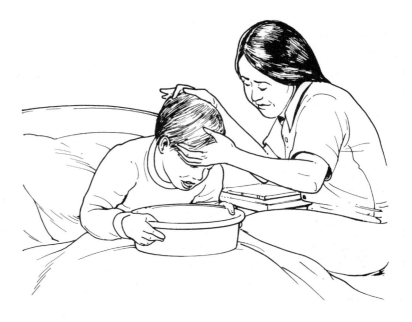

Helping a child who is vomiting

VOMITING IN CHILDREN

In children, an episode of vomiting without other symptoms is unlikely to indicate a serious disorder; it may be a result of overeating or excitement. Repeated vomiting is often caused by infection of the digestive tract, but infection anywhere else in the body can also be responsible.

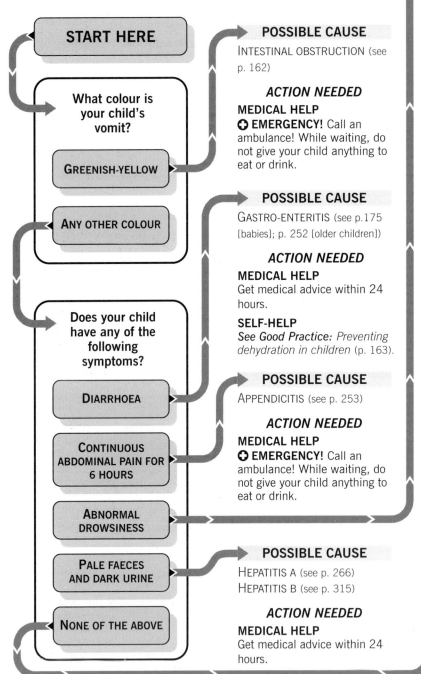

START HERE

What colour is your child's vomit?

- GREENISH-YELLOW
- ANY OTHER COLOUR

Does your child have any of the following symptoms?

- DIARRHOEA
- CONTINUOUS ABDOMINAL PAIN FOR 6 HOURS
- ABNORMAL DROWSINESS
- PALE FAECES AND DARK URINE
- NONE OF THE ABOVE

Has your child recently suffered a blow to the head?

- POSSIBLY
- UNLIKELY

Does your child have any of the following symptoms?

- FEVER
- PAIN ON PASSING URINE
- ABDOMINAL PAIN
- BEDWETTING

- ONE OR NONE
- TWO OR MORE

POSSIBLE CAUSE
INTESTINAL OBSTRUCTION (see p. 162)

ACTION NEEDED
MEDICAL HELP
✚ **EMERGENCY!** Call an ambulance! While waiting, do not give your child anything to eat or drink.

POSSIBLE CAUSE
GASTRO-ENTERITIS (see p.175 [babies]; p. 252 [older children])

ACTION NEEDED
MEDICAL HELP
Get medical advice within 24 hours.

SELF-HELP
See Good Practice: *Preventing dehydration in children* (p. 163).

POSSIBLE CAUSE
APPENDICITIS (see p. 253)

ACTION NEEDED
MEDICAL HELP
✚ **EMERGENCY!** Call an ambulance! While waiting, do not give your child anything to eat or drink.

POSSIBLE CAUSE
HEPATITIS A (see p. 266)
HEPATITIS B (see p. 315)

ACTION NEEDED
MEDICAL HELP
Get medical advice within 24 hours.

POSSIBLE CAUSE
URINARY TRACT INFECTION (see p. 156)

ACTION NEEDED
MEDICAL HELP
Get medical advice within 24 hours.

SELF-HELP
See Good Practice: *Reducing a raised temperature* (pp. 140-1).

POSSIBLE CAUSE

HEAD INJURY

ACTION NEEDED

MEDICAL HELP
✚ **EMERGENCY!** Call an ambulance! While waiting, do not give your child anything to eat or drink.

Does your child have any of the following symptoms?

- **HEADACHE**
- **STIFF NECK**
- **FLAT SPOTS THAT DO NOT DISAPPEAR WHEN PRESSED**
- **NONE OF THE ABOVE**

Did the vomiting occur in any of the following situations?

- **FOLLOWING A BOUT OF COUGHING**
- **BEFORE OR AFTER AN EXCITING OR STRESSFUL EVENT**
- **DURING A JOURNEY**
- **NONE OF THE ABOVE**

DANGER SIGNS

Call an ambulance at once if your child has any of the following symptoms:

- Greenish-yellow vomit.
- Abdominal pain for 6 hours.
- Flat, pink or purple spots that do not disappear when pressed.

Phone your doctor at once if your child has any of the following symptoms:

- Vomiting for 12 hours.
- Abnormal drowsiness.
- Refusing to drink for 6 hours.
- Sunken eyes.
- Dry tongue.
- Passing no urine for more than 6 hours during the day.

POSSIBLE CAUSE

MENINGITIS (see p. 208)

ACTION NEEDED

MEDICAL HELP
✚ **EMERGENCY!** Call an ambulance.

If you cannot identify your child's problem from this chart, talk to your doctor within 48 hours.

If you cannot identify your child's problem from this chart, talk to your doctor within 48 hours.

SELF-HELP

Dealing with vomiting

When your child vomits, the following measures may help.

- Support your child's head during vomiting. When the vomiting has stopped, sponge your child's face and give sips of water to rinse out his or her mouth.
- Reassure your child, who might be upset or frightened.
- Make your child take small drinks of water or rehydrating solution (30 mm/1 fl. oz) every hour to replace the fluids lost by vomiting.
- Encourage your child to lie down and rest, and provide a bowl by the bed in case he or she starts to vomit again.

POSSIBLE CAUSE

WHOOPING COUGH (see p. 202)

ACTION NEEDED

MEDICAL HELP
Get medical advice within 24 hours.

SELF-HELP *(see above)*
See Good Practice: *Helping a child who is vomiting* (p. 160); *Soothing a cough* (p. 298).

POSSIBLE CAUSE

Children often vomit in reaction to an exciting event or to stress.

ACTION NEEDED

MEDICAL HELP
If the vomiting persists, consult your doctor.

POSSIBLE CAUSE

TRAVEL SICKNESS

ACTION NEEDED

SELF-HELP
For any journey, you can give your child a travel sickness remedy obtainable over the counter. In a car, travelling at night or using motorways may lessen the problem.

Source: Valman, Bernard, *The British Medical Association Children's Symptoms*, Dorling Kindersley, 1997

Case study

Diana's dad has been in prison for more than a year and is due to be released soon. He has not allowed his daughter to visit him because he thought it would upset her to see him in prison.

Diana is 4 years old and complains of tummy ache in the reception class. The first time it happened the reception teacher phoned Diana's mum and asked her to come and collect the child, which she did. Diana was not sick and the doctor could not find anything wrong with her physically. Since then the tummy ache has occurred frequently. Diana's mum has asked to be informed if it happens again. The staff inform her when she comes to collect Diana from school at the end of the day.

1 Why do you think that this abdominal pain is occurring?
2 What observations should the nursery staff make of Diana?
3 How can they try to soothe her abdominal pain?
4 What support could be offered to this child?

Changes in bowel habits

Most children have an established pattern of bowel movements ranging from having their bowels open more than once a day to once every 5 to 7 days. This is normal but any changes in the frequency and consistency of the motions should be monitored.

Constipation

Constipation is passing hard, painful and infrequent stools. Infrequency alone is NOT constipation (see page 264).

It may be caused by generalised illness which results in a lack of fluid in the body.

Good Practice

Avoiding constipation
1 Offer lots of fluids, especially fruit juice.
2 Provide a diet rich in fruit and fresh vegetables.
3 Give roughage such as wholegrain bread and cereals, brown rice, salad, etc. at each meal.
4 Try to establish regular bowel habits by encouraging the child to have his or her bowels open regularly, such as after breakfast.

Stool changes

Changes in the colour, smell or consistency (whether stools are hard or runny) of the faeces may be due to changes in the diet. Parents should be informed of any stool changes noticed in a childcare establishment. The faeces should return to their usual state after a couple of days.

The doctor should be informed if:

■ any changes persist
■ there are any other signs of illness.

The table below shows possible changes to the appearance of the stools, possible causes and action to take.

APPEARANCE OF STOOL	POSSIBLE CAUSE	ACTION
Yellow	Breast feeding	None
Green – possibly runny	Gastro-enteritis if child is generally ill Bottle feeding formulas may cause green stools	Doctor None if child is well and gaining weight
Very pale, putty coloured, offensive smelling and floating	Food intolerance Coeliac disease	Doctor
Blood-stained	Gastro-enteritis Anal tear	Doctor
Pale, putty coloured with dark urine	Hepatitis	Doctor
Red and jelly-like	Intestinal obstruction	CALL AN AMBULANCE and contact parent

 Progress check

1 What is constipation?
2 How can this condition be avoided?
3 How would you define stool changes?
4 Which condition would you suspect if a child had green and runny stools?
5 What is the appearance of the stools in:
   ■ coeliac disease
   ■ hepatitis
   ■ food intolerance
   ■ intestinal obstruction
   ■ an anal tear

Remember

Call the doctor if a child:
- has sunken eyes – this is a sign of dehydration and the child may need fluids urgently
- has not passed urine for more than 6 hours or has consistently dry nappies
- vomits for 12 hours
- has abdominal pain constantly for 3 hours or more.

Diarrhoea

Diarrhoea is frequent, very loose stools usually accompanied by abdominal pain. It can result in dehydration if the excreted fluid is not replaced. Babies dehydrate very quickly and can become seriously ill as the result of diarrhoea.

Most children have diarrhoea at some time as the result of an infection of the gastro-intestinal tract. They should be given clear fluids only for 24 hours to rest the gut and prevent irritating the condition. This should allow the infection to resolve.

Diarrhoea may also be caused by:
- allergy
- reaction to drugs and medicines
- emotional factors e.g. excitement or worry.

Good Practice

Preventing dehydration
1 If a child has diarrhoea and/or vomiting it is important that the child has fluids to replace those that are being lost. Regular drinks of water or unsweetened fruit juice – 200mls every 2 hours – will help to prevent dehydration. Rehydrating solutions may also be given in place of the water. DO NOT offer milk for the first 24 hours as this may increase the diarrhoea.
2 Diarrhoea caused by infection is likely to spread in a childcare establishment unless there are stringent hygiene precautions (see Chapter 3). Children with diarrhoea should be sent home if possible.

Appetite loss

Children's appetites vary for a number of reasons – the appetite is dependent upon energy requirements and periods of growth and accelerated growth. If a child is generally well and gaining weight then a temporary loss of appetite is not a cause for concern. Appetite loss is associated with many illnesses. Look for the following signs in the child to decide whether or not it is a sign of illness:
- temperature
- sore throat
- rash
- swollen glands.

If any of these signs are apparent further investigation is needed to find the cause. It is best to see the doctor to be sure of the correct treatment.

Is the child:

■ passing urine frequently or finding it painful to urinate?
■ bedwetting?

If so the child may have a urinary tract infection which will need medical treatment.

Is the child:

■ gaining weight normally?
■ passing urine and faeces normally?

If the answer to the above is 'yes' and the child is otherwise well, they may just need tempting to eat or be too busy playing to take time out for a meal or a snack!

See page 334 for suggestions for offering food and drinks to a sick child.

Good Practice

Encouraging a child to eat

Tempting a reluctant child to eat should not include pressurising them to eat – gentle encouragement combined with providing attractive and appetising food in small quantities is enough (see page 334). The following list provides some tips.

1 Remember that children do not eat as much at one mealtime as an adult – they need smaller helpings at 5–6 meals or snacks.
2 Make mealtimes social occasions which incorporate fun – food faces or games may encourage eating.
3 Sick children may not want to eat at all, but plenty of nutritious drinks and yoghurt/ice cream to soothe sore throats will provide some nutrients.

 Progress check

1 What is a serious complication of frequent diarrhoea?
2 How should diarrhoea be treated in the first instance?
3 Apart from infection, give three other causes of diarrhoea.
4 What factors influence a child's appetite?
5 What other signs and symptoms should a childcare worker look for in a child with loss of appetite?
6 How can a reluctant child be gently tempted to eat?

When to call the doctor

The following lists are a guide to when the doctor should be consulted. They cannot replace the common sense of parents/carers or their thorough knowledge of the child(ren) they care for.

Remember

Always seek immediate medical help from a doctor for a baby under 6 months with a raised temperature

The doctor should always be consulted if there is any concern about a child's condition. It is always preferable to make an appointment with the doctor – it could be serious.

Babies under one year with any of the following symptoms should be seen by a doctor IMMEDIATELY:

■ temperature over 38.5° C
■ rapid, difficult or noisy breathing
■ persistent drowsiness – a floppy baby is always worrying
■ irritable behaviour accompanied by persistent crying (sometimes high pitched)
■ refusal to feed and/or not drinking for 6 hours or more
■ vomiting and/or loss of appetite
■ a sunken anterior fontanelle can be a symptom of dehydration (see page 176).
■ a bulging anterior fontanelle feels hard and can be clearly seen pulsating as the heart beats. It is a symptom of raised pressure inside the skull. A doctor should be seen urgently.

Children should be seen by a doctor immediately if they have any of the following signs and symptoms:

■ a pyrexia of over 39°C
■ signs of meningitis such as headache, photophobia or a stiff neck
■ hypothermia
■ convulsion
■ drowsy and difficult to wake up
■ breathing difficulties e.g. gasping for breath or cannot talk due to difficult breathing, pain when breathing, coughing foul sputum or blood, or noisy breathing
■ very drowsy and irritable
■ vomiting for more than 24 hours OR if associated with pain.
■ loss of appetite for more than 24 hours.
■ pain in any part of the body.

Remember

Call the parents and the doctor for advice if there is any doubt about a child's condition.

✔ Progress check

1 When should a doctor be consulted about a baby who is ill?
2 Which signs and symptoms in an older child would make you realise that medical advice should be obtained?

Key terms

You need to know what these words and phrases mean. Go back through the chapter and find out.

axillary temperature	sign
diarrhoea	symptom
earache	tepid sponging
febrile convulsion	urinary tract infection
malaise	vomiting
pyrexia	

Chapter 7 Conditions in babies

This chapter includes:

- Nappy rash
- Milk spots
- Heat rash
- Mongolian blue spots
- Seborrhoeic dermatitis
- Colic
- Gastro-enteritis
- Cows' milk intolerance
- Lactose intolerance
- Umbilical hernia
- Pyloric stenosis
- Thrush
- Blocked tear ducts
- Sticky eyes
- Squint
- Croup
- Bronchiolitis
- Failure to thrive
- Sudden infant death syndrome (SIDS)
- Hypothermia

This chapter aims to provide information about illnesses and conditions which occur in babies. Where further information is available in other chapters, the location is given.

There are several conditions which are far more common in babies, or only occur during the first year of life. Childcare workers who care for young babies must be aware of these conditions so that appropriate care and reassurance can be offered. Knowledge of the signs and symptoms, knowing what to do when an abnormality is suspected and when to seek medical advice is vital.

Babies are very vulnerable to infection because of their immature immune systems although they have some protection from their mother (see page 75). Their good health depends upon high standards of hygiene and care to prevent infection and observational skills to note any deviation from the norm.

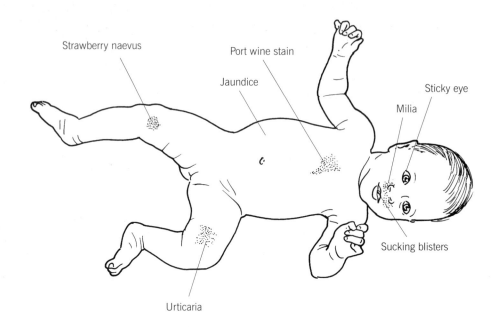

Strawberry naevus

Port wine stain

Jaundice

Sticky eye

Milia

Sucking blisters

Urticaria

Common skin problems in the new baby

NAPPY RASH

What Is Nappy Rash? Nappy rash is red, sore skin in the nappy area – the bottom, genital area and/or groin. It may spread to the lower abdomen and back. Most babies get a mild form of nappy rash at some time. It need not be seen as the result of poor care – although this will create the condition – and prompt treatment should cure it.

What Causes Nappy Rash? Nappy rash may be caused by:
- infection by bacteria or fungal infection, usually thrush
- reaction or allergy to medicines, food, washing powders (especially biological brands), creams, baby-wipes etc.
- concentrated urine as a result of illness or insufficient fluids
- irregular changing of nappies resulting in wet or dirty nappies being left on too long. Ammonia in the urine irritates the skin. Diarrhoea may cause nappy rash if the nappies are not changed very frequently
- inadequate cleaning of the nappy area
- babies with eczema or dermatitis are more likely to develop nappy rash.

How To Recognise Nappy Rash Gradual reddening of the skin in the nappy area which may proceed to spots, blistering and raw areas which may bleed. The baby will cry in pain especially when the nappy is changed.

Immediate Action	<ul><li>Remove the nappy.</li><li>Clean the area carefully with unperfumed baby soap and warm water and dry carefully.</li><li>Expose the bottom to warm air for as long as possible.</li><li>Lie the baby on a nappy but do not replace until the area is completely dry</li><li>If creams are used, ensure that the skin is completely dry before applying. Creams on damp skin will cause the rash to worsen.</li><li>Establish the cause of the rash and treat, for example provide more fluids, change nappies more often, change brand of washing powder or disposable nappies.</li><li>If there is no improvement in 48 hours see the health visitor for advice – the doctor will be able to prescribe treatment for an infection.</li></ul>

Ongoing Care

To prevent nappy rash, stringent hygiene routines are required which include the following.

- Regular nappy changing.
- Thorough cleaning of the nappy area.
- Leaving the nappy area exposed to the air as often as possible.

Remember

Regular nappy changing, thorough cleansing of the skin and frequent exposure of the nappy area to the air are the most effective ways to prevent nappy rash.

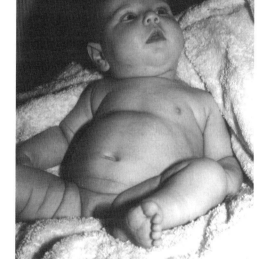

Leave the nappy area exposed to the air as often as possible

Creams may be used but are not essential – they can sometimes cause rashes! A baby in disposable nappies should not need barrier creams.

Possible Complications

Severe skin infection e.g. impetigo (see page 227) can spread to other areas of the body.

MILK SPOTS

What Are Milk Spots?	Milk spots (milia) are tiny white-headed spots on the face of a new baby – usually around the nose and cheeks. They are not itchy and do not irritate the baby at all.
What Causes Milk Spots?	Milk spots are caused when fluid blocks the immature sebaceous glands in the skin.
Immediate Action and Ongoing Care	None – these are quite normal and eventually disappear.
Possible Complications	Very occasionally milia may become infected and require treatment from the GP.

 Progress check

1 What are common causes of nappy rash?
2 What would you do if you found a baby had a nappy rash in your childcare establishment?
3 How can nappy rashes be prevented?
4 What complication may occur if a rash is left untreated?
5 Describe what milk spots are and what they look like.

HEAT RASH

What Is Heat Rash?	Heat rash is faint, red rash on the skin.
What Causes Heat Rash?	Heat rash is caused by overheating – such as wearing too many clothes on a warm day or in a warm room.

| How To Recognise Heat Rash | Lots of tiny, itchy red spots which join to form a faint, red rash in areas of the body where there are many sweat glands such as the face, neck, shoulders, chest and skin creases. |

| Immediate Action | ■ Cool the baby by removing clothing and bathing.
■ Dress in weather-appropriate clothes made of natural fibres e.g. cotton.
■ Calamine lotion will relieve the itching and increase comfort.
■ The rash should disappear in a few hours. |

| Ongoing Care | Dress the baby appropriately for the weather and room temperature. Using layers of light clothing which can be removed or increased is beneficial. |

| Possible Complications | If the rash persists it is best to consult a doctor to rule out any other cause. |

| Further Information | Intertrigo is an inflammation of the skin caused by wet surfaces rubbing together. This may be confused with heat rash. |

MONGOLIAN BLUE SPOTS

| What Are Mongolian Blue Spots? | Mongolian blue spots are areas of changed pigmentation of the skin usually found at the base of the spine or on the buttocks, although they can be anywhere on the body (see plate 4). |

| What Causes Mongolian Blue Spots? | Mongolian blue spots are caused by genetic information. They usually affect babies of Asian, African-Caribbean or Mediterranean descent and are especially common in babies of mixed parentage. |

| How To Recognise Mongolian Blue Spots | They are flat bluish/grey/purple areas present at birth which resemble bruising. |

| Immediate Action | Because they can be confused with bruising they should be measured and plotted on a body diagram to prevent later allegations of child abuse. |

| Ongoing Care | None – they disappear naturally by the age of 5 years. |

| Possible Complications | None. |

| Further Information | Child protection procedures may be implemented if inadequate recordings have been made by the midwife or health visitor. Children attending casualty departments for other conditions have been investigated for suspected child abuse by hospital staff who are unfamiliar with mongolian blue spots. |

SEBORRHOEIC DERMATITIS

What Is Seborrhoeic Dermatitis? Seborrhoeic dermatitis is a skin rash which can be mistaken for eczema. Cradle cap seen in babies is an example.

What Causes Seborrhoeic Dermatitis? There is no known cause of seborrhoeic dermatitis. It usually appears in the first few months of life and clears completely before the age of 2 years.

How To Recognise Seborrhoeic Dermatitis Cradle cap results in the front of the child's head being covered in a yellowish crust which at times extends to the eyebrows. The underlying skin is red and inflamed.

The rash does not usually itch.

Other parts of the body may be affected (such as the armpits, groin and areas where plump skin rubs, for example the neck in babies) with a scaly, blotchy rash.

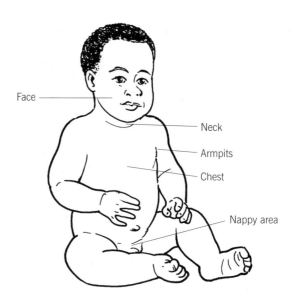

Face — Neck — Armpits — Chest — Nappy area

Areas of the body affected by seborrhoeic dermatitis in babies

Immediate Action *Cradle cap*
Rub olive oil or baby oil into the area and allow it to soak in, preferably overnight, to soften the crusts. The following morning gently comb the hair to loosen the crusts, and then shampoo the area rubbing the crusts gently to assist their removal. Special preparations can be purchased in a pharmacy to treat cradle cap.

Other areas
Affected areas should be cleaned with emulsifying ointment rather than soap.

Ongoing Care Consult the doctor if the rash does not improve or becomes inflamed or infected. In very severe cases an antibiotic or steroid cream may be prescribed. These will help to clear the rash within a few days.

Possible Complications Impetigo (see p. 227) may result if the skin becomes infected.

Further Information Seborrhoeic dermatitis may recur in puberty and throughout life.

Good Practice

Parents and carers should not be afraid to rub the baby's head when bathing and washing the hair. Firm massaging helps to remove dead skin cells and thorough rinsing removes all traces of shampoo.

 Progress check

1 What may cause a baby to have a heat rash?
2 What other rash may this be confused with?
3 What immediate action would you take for a baby with a heat rash?
4 How is heat rash prevented?
5 What are mongolian blue spots and in which races are they most commonly found?
6 What may a mongolian blue spot be confused with?
7 What is seborrhoeic dermatitis?
8 Which parts of the body does it commonly affect in babies?
9 How can cradle cap be treated successfully?
10 When should the doctor be consulted in cases of seborrhoeic dermatitis?

Activity

Make a chart to include all the skin conditions which may affect a baby in the first year of life. Include the following information.
- Name of condition
- Appearance
- Cause(s)
- Treatment
- Prevention.

COLIC

What Is Colic? Colic is pain resulting in inconsolable crying which is very distressing for parents and carers. It usually occurs between 2 weeks and 3 months of age and it is commonly known as '3 month colic' because that is the typical duration.

What Causes Colic?   Wind taken in during feeding or crying passes through the stomach and becomes trapped in the small intestines. This results in contractions of the intestines which causes quite extreme pain.

How To Recognise Colic
- Crying, reddened face, drawing knees up and appearing to be in pain.
- Common in the evenings in breast-fed babies.
- Some babies are affected by colic in the day and night as well.

Immediate Action
- Comfort the baby – pick her up and rub the back to dislodge any trapped wind.
- Lying on the tummy on the carer's lap and rubbing the back may help.
- Rocking movements such as those created by car journeys, baby slings and walks in the pram may help.

Ongoing Care   Some doctors advise breast-feeding mothers to monitor their diet to avoid foods which may exacerbate colic.

Bottle-fed babies should be winded regularly, with teats checked for hole size and flow of milk. A small hole which does not allow much milk to flow will increase the amount of swallowed air.

Homeopathic remedies are available from registered homeopathists. The GP may prescribe medicinal drops to be taken before a feed.

Possible Complications   Lactose intolerance may result after a bout of gastro-enteritis if milk is reintroduced into the diet too quickly and this will result in colic.

Further Information   It is unsafe to assume that colic is to blame for all crying, so exclude other possible causes. Any concerns should be discussed with the health visitor or doctor.

Remember

Many breast-fed babies experience 'evening colic', a period of restlessness and crying in the early and/or late evening. This is very common and quite normal. It is generally resolved by regular feeding, thorough winding and rocking the baby.

 Progress check

1 What is colic in babies?
2 What is the typical picture of an infant with colic?
3 How can the baby be comforted?
4 What are the possible complications of colic?

Case study

Hayley was discharged from hospital with her mother when she was 12 hours old. She was fully breast fed and woke every 2 to 3 hours for a feed. After 2 weeks at home she began to get unsettled in the evenings – she would cry a lot and refused to be comforted. She would not bring up any wind and drew her knees up as though she was in pain. Her mother thought it was because she was hungry, probably because her milk supply was inadequate at the end of the day. She started to express her milk after every feed to give to Hayley in the evening. This made no difference and the crying increased, occurring at other times of the day as well.

1 What remedies would you advise to try to relieve this colic?
2 How could you reassure this mother about her baby's condition?

GASTRO-ENTERITIS

What Is Gastro-enteritis? Gastro-enteritis is inflammation or infection of the stomach and intestines.

What Causes Gastro-enteritis?

Gastro-enteritis can be caused by:
- bacteria in food and drinks or on feeding equipment. Rotaviruses are responsible for most cases of gastro-enteritis in children under 2 years of age.
- airborne viruses/bacteria
- contact with infected faeces

How To Recognise Gastro-enteritis

- Vomiting.
- Diarrhoea.
- Reluctance to feed.
- High temperature.
- Generally unwell and lethargic.

Immediate Action

Preventing dehydration
- Call the doctor if the baby is under 3 months or if there are signs of dehydration. Vomiting and diarrhoea in a young baby is potentially very serious.
- For the first 24 hours offer clear fluids – cooled, previously boiled water – or rehydrating solution to drink. Breast-fed babies should be given clear fluids or rehydrating solution before their breast feed.

If there is no improvement in this time seek medical help.

Ongoing Care

- Gradually introduce the usual diet.
- Scrupulous attention to hygiene, including sterilising feeding equipment, personal hygiene, etc.

Possible Complications

Dehydration which, if not treated, can lead to death.

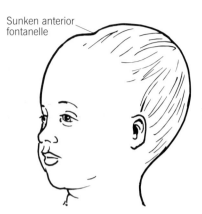

Sunken anterior fontanelle

Good Practice

Rigorous attention to hygiene in making feeds and storing them is essential to prevent gastro-enteritis. Carers should wash their hands before making feeds and before feeding an infant. All bottles and teats should be sterilised according to the manufacturers instructions. Feeds should be refrigerated until required. All remaining milk left in the bottle after a feed should be discarded.

COWS' MILK INTOLERANCE

What Is Cows' Milk Intolerance?	Cows' milk intolerance is an inability to digest the protein content of cows' milk. It generally begins in the first year of life but has usually resolved by 3 years of age.
What Causes Cows' Milk Intolerance?	The cause is uncertain. Most infant formula milks are based on cows' milk with the animal fat removed. It is the protein in the milk which is difficult to digest and results in intolerance in some children.
How To Recognise Cows' Milk Intolerance	Diarrhoea (the baby may also vomit) which begins after cows' milk is introduced into the diet and clears up when cows' milk is withdrawn. The condition recurs if cows' milk is offered again.
Immediate Action	<ul><li>A baby should be seen within 24 hours of the symptoms occurring.</li><li>Under medical supervision cows' milk is withdrawn for 2 weeks. Soya milk may be given to replace cows' milk. If the condition clears up then a small trial amount of cows' milk is offered. The diagnosis is confirmed if the symptoms recur.</li></ul>
Ongoing Care	<ul><li>The baby may need to take soya-based formula milk.</li><li>If breast feeding, mothers can reduce or exclude dairy products from their diet.</li></ul>

- A dietician will advise and support the family.
- The cows' milk trial can be repeated every 3 months.

Possible Complications Failure to thrive (see page 188).

LACTOSE INTOLERANCE

What Is Lactose Intolerance?	Lactose intolerance is an intolerance to lactose which is a sugar found in milk.

What Causes Lactose Intolerance?
- Lack of the required enzyme (in the small intestine) which digests lactose.
- Genetically inherited lactose intolerance is common in people of Asian and African-Caribbean descent.
- May occur as the result of gastro-enteritis (see page 252) or coeliac disease (see page 254).

How To Recognise Lactose Intolerance
Diarrhoea.
Vomiting.

Immediate Action See the doctor. A test dose of lactose may be given to the child and a stool specimen taken for examination to see if an excessive amount of sugar has been excreted.

Ongoing Care A dietician will plan a lactose-free diet, which does not contain milk but may contain some milk products.

Possible Complications Failure to thrive may result if the condition is not treated.

Further Information Some children with cows' milk intolerance are also lactose intolerant.

Case study

Ida Kennedy was concerned about her son Jacob, aged 5 months. Ida had recently started to wean Jacob off the breast, and was giving him bottles of formula milk in preparation for when she was due to return to work a month later. Although she was a vegan she did not intend to bring up her children with the same diet, thinking that they would make up their own minds as they matured. Jacob had been grizzly and unsettled for several days, vomiting back some of the feeds and then wanting more. His stools had become very runny and his bottom was sore. At the last visit to the child health clinic he had not gained any weight at all. The health visitor thought he may have a mild dose of gastro-enteritis and advised Ida to give him clear fluids only, for 24 hours. This was the longest 24 hours she had spent, because Jacob cried with hunger and would not sleep. She gave him some more milk feeds and although he was not sick, the diarrhoea increased and his nappy rash worsened. Ida wondered if he could have an allergy.

- What signs of an allergy is Jacob displaying?
- Why are these signs only apparent now, when Jacob is 5 months old?
- What sort of diet will Jacob need if the allergy is confirmed?

✔ Progress check

1 What are the most common causes of gastro-enteritis in young babies?
2 What are the signs of dehydration in a baby?
3 What immediate action should be taken if a baby has a high temperature and vomits?
4 Describe the hygiene precautions which should be taken in a baby nursery to prevent the spread of gastroenteritis.
5 Why are babies vulnerable to cows' milk intolerance?
6 How would you recognise cows' milk intolerance?
7 What is a possible complication of cows' milk intolerance?
8 What is lactose intolerance?
9 Which other conditions may be associated with lactose intolerance?

UMBILICAL HERNIA

What Is An Umbilical Hernia?   An umbilical hernia is a small loop of intestine which protrudes through the abdominal wall and causes a small lump around, or just above, the umbilicus.

What Causes An Umbilical Hernia?   A weakness in the muscles of the abdominal wall.

How To Recognise An Umbilical Hernia

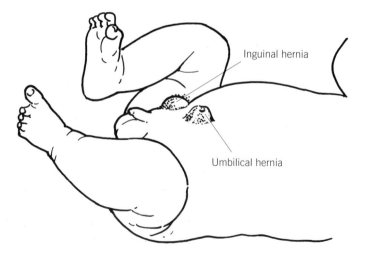

Typical sites of umbilical and inguinal hernias

A small swelling usually appears around the navel a few weeks after birth which:

- may not be present in the morning, but appear gradually through the day
- is more noticeable when the baby cries or tenses the abdomen
- is soft and completely painless.

Immediate Action	This is not uncommon and no immediate treatment is required. It usually resolves as the child develops strength in the abdominal muscles, for example in sitting up and crawling. It usually disappears by the first birthday.
Ongoing Care	An operation may be required if the hernia has not disappeared by the age of 5 years. This is more usual if the hernia is above the navel.
Possible Complications	If the lump becomes painful and hard and cannot be pushed back inside the abdomen, URGENT medical attention is required. This is a very rare strangulated hernia.
Further Information	An old remedy for an umbilical hernia was to bandage an old penny on top of the umbilical lump. This was intended to push the loop of intestine back through the abdominal wall. There is no evidence to suggest that this was any more successful than leaving it alone !

PYLORIC STENOSIS

What Is Pyloric Stenosis?	Pyloric stenosis is a thickening of the muscle around the pylorus, (the outlet from the stomach to the small intestine) which causes the pylorus to narrow. As the baby feeds, the stomach fills with milk which cannot pass through into the small intestine. The pressure in the stomach increases causing the baby to vomit.
What Causes Pyloric Stenosis?	The cause is not known but the condition is: - five times more common in boys - occurs between 3 to 6 weeks of age – typically at 5 weeks
How To Recognise Pyloric Stenosis	- Projectile vomiting. Increased pressure in the stomach results in the feed being forcefully ejected – several metres across the room. This is a distinctive sign of pyloric stenosis. - The hungry baby is impossible to satisfy. After vomiting the child will be hungry and want to feed again. - There is failure to thrive. Weight gain is poor because of recurrent vomiting. - Dehydration may result from a lack of fluid being absorbed. - Constipation. Food is not reaching the intestines.

| Immediate Action | ■ Contact the doctor.
■ Feed small amounts often to prevent over-filling the stomach. |

| Ongoing Care | After an ultrasound scan to confirm the diagnosis minor surgery may be required to widen the pylorus. |
| Possible Complications | If treated surgically there are no permanent ill-effects. |

> **Remember**
> All babies who experience projectile vomiting on more than one occasion should be examined by a doctor. Pyloric stenosis is much more common in boys between 3 and 6 weeks of age.

THRUSH

| What Is Thrush? | Thrush is a fungal infection, usually in the mouth (oral thrush) although it can affect the bowel and the nappy area as well. |

| What Causes Thrush? | Candida albicans is the infecting organism. It is present in small quantities naturally in the mouth, but abnormal growth can be caused by general illness, a course of antibiotics or poor hygiene. |
| How To Recognise Thrush | Raised white or cream coloured spots inside the mouth, on the cheeks, gums, and roof of the mouth (see plate 3). They look like milk deposits seen after feeding but they cannot be rubbed off. The mouth looks red and sore. |

| Immediate Action | ■ If you think a baby has thrush, report to the parents so that they can arrange to see the doctor within the next day or two.
■ The doctor will prescribe some anti-fungal treatment. If the baby has nappy rash too, then the treatment will probably be drops to cure the condition in the mouth, and anti-fungal cream for the nappy area. |

| Ongoing Care | ■ Ensure scrupulous hygiene in sterilising equipment and preparing feeds.
■ Do not use dummies until the infection has cleared up. |
| Possible Complications | None, if treated. |

Case study

The baby unit at Cedars Day Nursery is always busy, usually full to capacity with nine babies and four members of staff. The nursery was registered with social services to take babies from 6 weeks of age and the youngest baby is usually about 3 months old. During one week in July, two babies of 7 weeks and 9 weeks were enrolled at the nursery for full-time care. Over the next few days they both developed a similar nappy rash around the anus and buttocks. Despite the thorough procedures adopted by the staff the rashes would not improve. Both sets of parents were informed and supplied extra quantities of barrier creams. The conditions got worse over the next 24 hours and red, inflamed spots developed in the nappy areas. One of the babies began to refuse their bottle feeds and the nursery nurse noticed white spots which looked like milk curds inside the baby's mouth. She reported this to the officer-in-charge who thought the spots looked like thrush. She continued to try to feed the baby, encouraging her to take milk off a spoon to prevent the irritation of her sore mouth. The officer-in-charge looked at the other baby and was not surprised to see that he, too, had a raised white rash in his mouth.

1 What action should now be taken by the officer-in-charge?
2 How is the nappy rash associated with the oral thrush?
3 Do you think it was a coincidence that both babies were affected at the same time? Give reasons for your answer.
4 How could the nursery organise its hygiene procedures to prevent the further spread of the condition?

Progress check

1 What is an umbilical hernia?
2 How would you recognise the condition?
3 Why do you think that many parents would be very concerned about the condition?
4 In what circumstances would urgent medical attention be required for an umbilical hernia?
5 Explain how pyloric stenosis occurs.
6 What are the characteristic signs of pyloric stenosis?
7 What action should be taken if the condition is suspected?
8 What is the usual treatment for oral thrush?

BLOCKED TEAR DUCTS

What Are Blocked Tear Ducts? The tear ducts in one or both eyes may be blocked preventing tears from being drained away from the eye/s into the nose.

What Causes Blocked
Tear Ducts?

Dead cells at birth may block the duct/s.

How To Recognise
Blocked Tear Ducts

■ The eyes constantly water even if the baby is not crying.
■ Infection of the eyes is common.

Immediate Action

Consult the doctor.
If there is no infection treatment includes:
■ keeping the eyes clean by regular bathing
■ massaging the affected tear duct/s. With a very clean finger massage the inner corner of the eye to remove the blockage. This should be done 3-4 times a day and is often successful.

Ongoing Care

Continue to massage the eye/s. If there is no improvement by the first birthday an ophthalmic doctor may clear the blockage under general anaesthetic using a thin probe.

Possible Complications

■ Recurrence may happen even after surgical treatment.
■ Infection in the eyes may occur as a result of this condition.

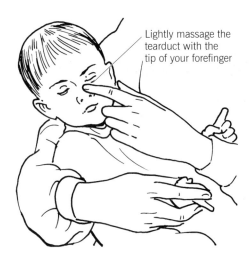

Lightly massage the
tearduct with the
tip of your forefinger

Unblocking a tear duct

STICKY EYES

What Is Sticky Eyes?

Sticky eyes is a common condition in new-born infants – an infection of one or both eyes.

What Causes Sticky
Eyes?

Sticky eyes is caused when narrow tear ducts cannot drain tears from the eye, resulting in a warm, moist area where bacteria can multiply. The bacteria in the birth canal may infect the eye/s.

How To Recognise
Sticky Eyes

The eye/s are affected with a yellowy/green discharge which can cause the lids to stick together and prevent the baby from opening its eye/s.

The area around the eye may become red as the infection spreads.

Immediate Action

- Bathe the eye/s with warm water and cotton swabs, wiping from the inner eye to the outer corner and using a fresh swab for each eye. This helps to prevent infection spreading to the other eye.
- Contact the doctor who may prescribe some antibiotic cream.

Ongoing Care

As the baby grows, the tear ducts get larger. There is usually no recurrence unless the tear duct is blocked (see page 181).

Good Practice

Regular bathing of the eyes in the early days and weeks helps to prevent infection. Using a separate swab for each eye, bathe the eye/s with warm water and cotton swabs. Wipe from the inner eye to the outer corner, away from the tear duct.

SQUINT

What Is a Squint?

A squint is when the eyes do not look in the same direction at the same time. This is very common in young babies who are co-ordinating the movement of their eyes – all babies squint before 3 to 4 months of age.

For more detailed information see page 274.

What Causes a Squint?

In babies the mechanism which controls the movement of the eyes is not fully developed.

There is also a tendency to inherit a squint from either parent.

How To Recognise a
Squint

One eye turns too far in or out, or up or down, when looking straight ahead. Babies are more likely to squint when they are tired or when they have just woken up.

A wide bridge to the nose can give the appearance of a squint an 'apparent squint' or 'pseudo squint'.

Look at the baby when a bright, distant object is reflected in the eyes – when a squint is present it will not be in the same place in both eyes.

Immediate Action

If a squint appears to continue after 4 to 6 months of age, seek a medical opinion.

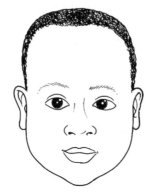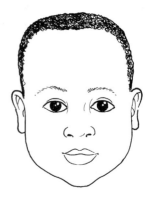

A wide bridge to the nose can give the appearance of a squint

Ongoing Care

Treatment by expert ophthalmologists (eye doctors) may include:
- patching the unaffected eye to encourage use of the squinting (lazy) eye
- eye exercises
- surgical correction of the squint.

Possible Complications

Poor vision in the affected eye will result if the squint is not treated. The brain eventually ignores the distorted image from the lazy eye.

 Progress check

1 Why do you think that babies' tear ducts are vulnerable to infection?
2 How would you recognise an eye infection?
3 What causes blocked tear ducts?
4 How can the condition be recognised?
5 How can blocked tear ducts be treated?
6 What immediate action should be taken to deal with sticky eyes?
7 How would you recognise a squint in a baby?
8 When is a squint considered to be normal?
9 When should a squint be investigated by a doctor?
10 What sorts of treatment may be given to a baby with a squint when the condition has been diagnosed?

CROUP

What Is Croup?

Croup is an inflammation and narrowing of the airway. It usually affects children between 6 months and 3 years of age. A doctor should see children with croup to exclude **epiglottitis** (see page 292) which is potentially fatal.

What Causes Croup?

Croup is caused by a viral infection or less often, an allergy.

How To Recognise Croup
- Signs of a cold – runny nose and sneezing.
- Hoarse breathing.
- Characteristic cough which sounds like a dog barking.
- Some children may have a severe attack which makes breathing difficult or abnormally fast.
- Blueness (cyanosis) of the tongue and mouth, extending to the skin are serious signs – the doctor should be called.

Croup attacks usually occur in the early morning hours.

Immediate Action
- When the baby is having a croup attack, create a humid, warm atmosphere. Taking the child into the bathroom and running the hot taps, or continuing to boil kettles in their room will provide the required moist, steamy air. There should be an improvement within about 20 minutes.
- Close physical contact with the parent/carer will reassure the baby.
- Offer liquid paracetamol and lots of warm drinks.
- A baby with croup should be seen by a doctor.
- Croup lasts for about 5 days.

Ongoing Care

Croup does recur in babies and children who have had one attack. When they show the first signs of a cold, vaporise the air in their room while they sleep. Try to keep the atmosphere moist – putting a wet towel on a warm radiator to achieve this is much safer than steaming kettles.

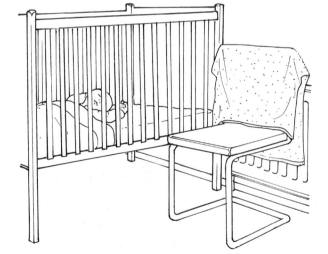

Damp towels drying near a radiator will humidify the air

Remember

If a baby is cyanosed at any time due to breathing difficulties, call an ambulance immediately.

Possible Complications

Children with asthma are prone to attacks of croup.

Case study

Ryan was 3 months old when he had his first attack of croup in the middle of the night. His mother is a trained nurse, so she recognised the barking cough and hoarse breathing. It terrified her to hear such a small and young baby making such a dreadful sound and it seemed much worse in the early hours of the morning. She picked up the baby and took him into the bathroom and turned on the hot taps but there was no hot water.

1 What would you do next in this situation?
2 What other action would relieve Ryan's symptoms?
3 If this was not an attack of croup, what could it have been?
4 What steps should be taken when Ryan shows signs of a cold in the future?

Good Practice

When a baby seems to be developing a cold or snuffles, a few drops from a Karvol capsule on the baby's bib or cot sheet will help to clear the airways and improve breathing.

BRONCHIOLITIS

What Is Bronchiolitis? Bronchiolitis is an acute lung infection of the smaller airways (the bronchioles) which affects babies under 1 year of age.

What Causes Bronchiolitis? A syncitial viral infection is the cause of bronchiolitis.

How To Recognise Bronchiolitis
- Symptoms of the common cold after 2 to 3 days developing into this serious condition.
- Reluctance to feed.
- High temperature.
- A dry, rasping cough.
- Breathing varies between:
  – rapid panting breathing at up to 60 breaths a minute and
  – difficult, wheezy breathing – sometimes with more than 10 seconds between each breath.
- There is obvious distress in the baby.
- Drowsiness may occur.

Immediate Action	■ Call an ambulance immediately if the baby finds breathing difficult.
	■ The baby may need hospital treatment and severe cases will be ventilated
	■ Send for the doctor if there is wheezing and a cough.
	■ Hold the baby in an upright position to help the breathing – propped against a shoulder is ideal.
	■ A paracetamol elixir such as Calpol will help to reduce the temperature.

Ongoing Care

Offer lots of fluids and small, regular feeds. Babies often prefer to suck at the breast or on a bottle and refuse their weaning foods and any solids.

Mild cases last about a week, by which time the baby should be feeding normally again.

The cough may continue for up to six weeks.

Possible Complications

Bronchiolitis does not usually cause serious lung damage, but children who have had this illness as babies will wheeze when they have a cold.

Further Information

Bronchiolitis occurs in epidemics during the winter months.

Good Practice

Easing a cough in a baby

Put the baby across your knee, facing downwards. Pat the back firmly to loosen any mucus and this will help him to cough it up.

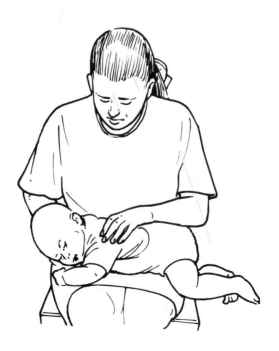

Placing the baby across your knee, face downwards, will help the baby to cough

> ✅ **Progress check**
> 1 What is croup?
> 2 Why is it a frightening condition for the baby and the parents?
> 3 How would you recognise bronchiolitis?
> 4 What immediate action should be taken if the condition is suspected?
> 5 When is bronchiolitis most common?

FAILURE TO THRIVE

What Is Failure To Thrive?

A baby who does not gain weight as expected according to the centile charts for growth may be described as failing to thrive.
Older children can also fail to thrive for similar reasons.

What Causes Failure To Thrive?

Genetic
Small parents generally have small babies who grow into small children.

Low birth weight
Babies who weigh less than the average for their gestation may remain small.

Underfeeding
Not taking in enough calories will prevent the required weight gain. Here are some reasons why babies may be underfed.

- It may be assumed that premature babies, because they are small, do not require as many calories as full-term neonates. In fact they need more (to replace the constant supply of nutrients which was available inside the womb) to enable rapid growth.
- Babies do not always cry when they are hungry. Inexperienced parents who are demand feeding their baby, may mistake a quiet baby for a satisfied baby.
- Babies need 150mls of milk per kilogram of their body weight every day. If this is not supplied via breast or bottle there will be weight loss or static weight.
- *Malabsorption:* a digestive problem which prevents the nutrients from food being absorbed. Diseases which may cause this are cystic fibrosis (see page 308), coeliac disease (see page 254), cows' milk intolerance (see page 176).
- *Illness:* early illness may prevent growth from accelerating.
- *Physical disorders*: pyloric stenosis (see page 179), infections of the kidney and disorders of the heart are rare but possible causes of failure to thrive.
- *Emotional difficulties*: neglect of care by parents and/or carers may include failure to feed the baby – this may be intentional or unintentional, due to ignorance. Sometimes parents feel unsupported themselves and as a

result find it difficult to meet the needs of another individual. They may be depressed or suffering from stress, for example experiencing social or financial difficulties which reduce their ability to cope. Failure to thrive may be due to a poor quality of care and in older children may occur as a result of unhappiness, insecurity and separation.

How To Recognise Failure To Thrive

Failure to gain weight adequately will probably be noticed at the child health clinic if the baby is a regular attender.

Immediate Action

Investigation of the cause.

Is the baby active with good muscle tone and achieving his or her developmental milestones?

- Was the baby premature? What was the birth weight? How big are the parents?
- Is the baby getting enough nutrients. How much milk is taken and how often?
- Is there an underlying illness?
- What is the appearance of the stools?
- How does the relationship with the parents seem? Is there an established bond?

Ongoing Care

The treatment offered to the child will depend upon the cause of the condition as will the ongoing care provided by parents and carers. Babies will be weighed regularly to check that they are making satisfactory progress. Their diet will be monitored closely to ensure that they are taking the required amount of nutrients each day, and to make sure that the diet is the right one for them. For example a baby with coeliac disease will have a gluten-free diet.

Children with no medical cause for their failure to thrive, or family history of small stature, will need regular monitoring to check their growth and development. This may be performed by the health visitor. Families who need extra support may also be monitored by social services.

Possible Complications

If the failure to thrive is caused by a medical condition, the complications of that condition may occur. If it is caused by inadequate care at home, the child may become the subject of child protection proceedings.

Remember

Children and babies who are happy and physically small but have lots of energy, are usually quite normal. Their small size is usually inherited from their parents or grandparents.

 Progress check

- What is failure to thrive?
- Describe the possible causes of the condition.
- How much milk should young babies be offered?
- How can the condition be recognised?
- What sort of questions will be asked to identify the cause of the failure to thrive?
- Which professionals may be able to help and support families and children as a result of this condition being diagnosed?

SUDDEN INFANT DEATH SYNDROME (SIDS)

What Is Sudden Infant Death Syndrome?

Sudden infant death syndrome is the unexpected and usually unexplained death of an infant. It was previously called 'cot death syndrome' because the baby is usually found in the cot after failing to wake for a feed. This may occur between 1 week and 2 years of age, but 3 months is the most common age. Estimates suggest that 1 in 700 babies are affected, but this figure is falling as parents adopt the recommended practices for cot death prevention.

What Causes Sudden Infant Death Syndrome?

A lot of research has not isolated a particular cause, but has established that there are some risk factors linked to SIDS.

■ Over-heating.

■ Smoking.

■ Being generally unwell in the few days prior to the death – possibly off feeds and/or snuffly.

SIDS is commoner in:

■ winter months

■ boys

■ premature babies

■ low birth-weight babies.

How To Prevent Sudden Infant Death Syndrome

There are 4 basic guidelines which, when adopted, reduce the risks of a cot death.

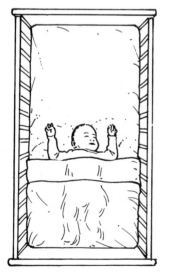

✔ Put the baby to sleep on their back with the feet touching the end of the cot.

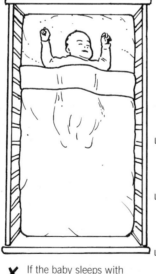

✗ If the baby sleeps with their head at the top of the cot, they may move down under the blankets and either overheat or suffocate.

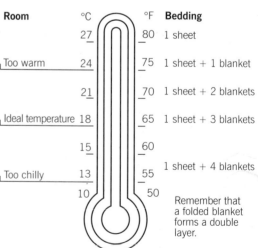

Temperature and bedding
How much bedding is required depends on the temperature of the sleeping area.
This illustration shows how to keep the baby's temperature at a healthy level.

Room	°C	°F	Bedding
	27	80	1 sheet
Too warm	24	75	1 sheet + 1 blanket
	21	70	1 sheet + 2 blankets
Ideal temperature	18	65	1 sheet + 3 blankets
	15	60	
	13	55	1 sheet + 4 blankets
Too chilly	10	50	

Remember that a folded blanket forms a double layer.

Prevention of SIDS

1 *Put the baby to sleep on their back* in the cot, pram or buggy to prevent them from rolling over onto the tummy.
2 *Do not allow the baby to over-heat.*
   ■ Place 'feet to foot' in the cot. Place the baby at the foot of the cot, with their feet touching the end. This prevents the baby from wriggling down under the covers and overheating, or suffocating.
   ■ Do not use duvets. Use a sheet and layers of blankets instead because these can be adjusted to suit the temperature of the room. The ideal temperature for the baby to sleep in is 18°C.
3 Keep the baby out of smoky atmospheres. It is preferable that people do not smoke in the rooms which the baby uses. Parents should stop smoking during the pregnancy.
4 The baby should be examined by a doctor if it is unwell in any way. If there is any concern it is better to be safe than sorry.

Ongoing Care

Support for parents

Parents will go through the stages of grieving. Initially they will feel shocked and numb, unable to accept what has happened. Confusion, anger, guilt and despair will follow. They may want to talk and should be given every opportunity to do so.

A support network of families who have experienced the same trauma may be available via local voluntary groups.

Professional counselling may be required and should always be offered.

Possible Complications

There is a slightly increased risk that a second baby may also suffer IDS (see CONI below) and parents will be naturally anxious for the safety of their future children.

Further Information

> **Remember**
> SIDS may occur in a childcare establishment (see page 386: 'Dealing with SIDS in a childcare establishment').

■ The Foundation For The Study Of Infant Deaths (FSIDS) can give advice.
■ Care of the Next Infant (CONI) is a programme set up to support parents who have lost an infant – to offer advice, practical help and reassurance.
■ Each cultural group has their method of child rearing. In the UK the rate of SIDS is lower amongst Asians. This may be because most Asian parents keep the baby in the parental bedroom through the night.
■ FSIDS recommend that parents keep their baby in their bedroom, in a separate cot, for at least the first 6 months.

HYPOTHERMIA

What Is Hypothermia?

■ Hypothermia is low body temperature sometimes called *neonatal cold injury.*
■ Premature babies are more vulnerable.
■ It is more usual in the first few months of life.

What Causes Hypothermia?

Babies cannot control their temperature because the thermostat in the brain is not yet fully developed.

The following will cause a baby to lose body heat very quickly:

- a cold room
- a bath in a cool room
- going outside with too few clothes for warmth
- not wearing a hat in cool temperatures because babies lose a lot of body heat through the head.

How To Recognise Hypothermia

- Healthy skin colour – BUT
- Skin feels cold. Feet and fingers are often cooler than the rest of the baby, but in hypothermia the tummy and limbs feel cold to the touch.
- Refuses to feed.
- Tired and lethargic.
- Feet and hands may be swollen.

Immediate Action

For baby

- Call the doctor.
- *Warm the baby gradually BUT DO NOT APPLY DIRECT HEAT.*
- Put a hat on the baby's head.
- Cuddle the baby against your warm body – skin-to-skin contact is best.
- Wrap the baby loosely in warm blankets.
- Encourage the baby to feed.

Immediate Action

For older child

- Call the doctor.
- Put the child in a warm bath until the skin colour has returned to normal
- Dry quickly and wrap in warm blankets – put the child to bed dressed warmly (with a hat on) and give warm glucose drinks and high energy food such as chocolate.
- An adult should stay with the child until the temperature has returned to normal.

Ongoing care

Prevention

- Keep room temperature constant 18-20°C.
- Dress the baby in appropriate clothes for the weather and room temperature.
- Bath in a warm room.

Possible complications

Babies and children whose temperatures drop can lapse into a coma and if they do not receive urgent medical attention, death may be the outcome.

Further information

Hypothermia in an older child may occur after playing outside in very cold weather or falling into cold water. They will be:

- shivering
- cold to the touch
- pale
- confused or lethargic
- breathing shallowly
- with a weak pulse.

Remember

Always warm babies and children very gradually. Never put a hot water bottle or similar hot objects next to the skin.

✔ Progress check

1 When is SIDS most common?
2 Between which ages can it occur?
3 What are the risk factors for SIDS?
4 What steps can be taken to reduce the risks of SIDS?
5 What support is available for parents who have experienced a cot death?
6 What is hypothermia?
7 What circumstances may result in a baby losing body heat?
8 What are the signs of hypothermia in a baby?
9 What action would you take for a baby with a low temperature?
10 How can hypothermia be prevented?
11 What are the signs of hypothermia in an older child?
12 Why should babies and children be warmed very slowly?

Chapter 8 Infectious diseases

This chapter includes:

- Chickenpox
- Hand, foot and mouth disease
- Roseola infantum (3-day fever)
- Mumps
- Tetanus
- Whooping cough (Pertussis)
- Measles
- Rubella (German measles)
- Meningitis
- Diphtheria
- Polio (Poliomyelitis)
- TB (Tuberculosis)
- Erythema infectiosum (Slapped cheek syndrome)
- Kawasaki disease

This chapter aims to describe the above diseases and offers the specific action and care required for each. A general approach to caring for ill children and meeting their needs is given in Chapter 15.

Childcare workers will inevitably see a range of infectious childhood illnesses during their careers, because children's immature immune systems make them more susceptible to these infectious diseases than adults.

It is important to recognise the signs and symptoms of various conditions so that appropriate treatment can be offered and urgent medical attention sought if necessary. Knowledge of incubation periods will help childcarers to identify any children who may have been in contact with the illness before it was recognised, and during the period when it was infectious, and to seek appropriate medical help (especially in the case of contact with meningitis). It will also enable carers to be alert to early signs and symptoms in vulnerable children. Awareness of immunisation schedules and individual records of children's immunisation status will enable them to provide reassurance to parents. For example, children who have been immunised against whooping cough are unlikely to contract the illness. It is possible for children who have been immunised to develop a mild form of any disease, but the symptoms are slight compared to those in an unimmunised child.

Many of these diseases are accompanied by a specific rash. Identifying rashes can be difficult – there are many different types of rashes and they look different on different types of skin. The main causes are infection and allergy. The descriptions given here, and the colour photographs on plate 1 will enable fairly accurate identification – but even doctors can sometimes find it difficult to identify particular rashes. The colour of spots may vary and on black skin may be difficult to identify.

One of the most important aspects of any rash is the signs and symptoms which accompany it. In childhood illnesses the rashes are usually not irritating or itchy – with the exception of the chickenpox rash – and the child will be generally unwell with a raised temperature. This does not happen if the rash is caused by an allergy.

Seek medical advice if a child has a rash and is showing other signs of illness or if there is any doubt about the cause of a rash.

CHICKENPOX

What Is Chickenpox? Also known as varicella, chickenpox is a highly infectious, common childhood illness which is not immunised against in the UK. It is most common in the late winter and spring. Most seriously affected are :
- very young babies
- children who are immunosuppressed (taking drugs to suppress their immune system) to treat another condition e.g. leukaemia
- children who are HIV positive or have AIDS.

For these children chickenpox can be life threatening.
Incubation period: 11–21 days.

What Causes Chickenpox? Chickenpox is caused by viral infection: herpes zoster, and spread by droplet infection. This virus is also responsible for shingles which usually affects older people. Children can catch chickenpox from older people who are suffering from shingles.

How To Recognise Chickenpox
- Mild fever and headache.
- Red spots on the back and chest appearing in 'batches' or 'crops' of spots occurring in an area at the same time (see plate 1).
- Spots quickly become fluid-filled blisters (vesicles) with red bases. They are very itchy (see plate 1).
- The fluid in the blisters becomes cloudy or yellowish.
- Rash spreads to all areas of the body, with new batches appearing over a period of days.
- After 2–3 days the blisters dry to form scabs.
- Spots at various stages are present at the same time.

Immediate Action
- Reassure the child.
- Contact parents.
- Call the doctor if the child is under 1 year of age.
- Offer paracetamol to reduce the temperature (See pages 140–1) 'Reducing a raised temperature').
- Discourage the child from scratching as this can cause permanent scarring. Apply calamine or caladryl lotion to the skin.
- If at home, a warm bath with a handful of bicarbonate of soda added will reduce the irritation.

Ongoing Care
- Offer plenty of fluids to drink.
- Treat a raised temperature with paracetamol and tepid sponging.
- Continue with calamine lotion, comforting baths etc. to reduce the itching. The doctor may prescribe some antihistamine (anti-itch) cream or medicine if necessary. These can be purchased in the pharmacy over the counter.
- Dress child in loose cotton clothing.
- Keep fingernails short and explain to the child why they must try not to scratch the spots – cotton mittens in very young children can help.
- If the spots become weepy or are very deep, the doctor may prescribe antibiotics to avoid infection.

Possible Complications
- Scarring from scratched spots.
- Secondary infection from scratched spots. Impetigo may develop which requires antibiotic treatment.
- Encephalitis – inflammation of the brain.
- Pneumonia – inflammation of the lungs.

Further Information

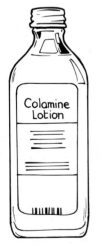

Calamine lotion and mittens help to prevent scratching

An affected child is infectious for 2 to 3 days before the rash appears and until all the scabs have dried. If the child is well he can then return to playgroup, nursery, infant school etc. It is not necessary to wait until all the spots have disappeared completely. The most important consideration is that the child feels well before returning to a childcare establishment.

Having the disease should give life-long immunity, but the virus does remain in the body and can develop into shingles in later life.

Immunisation for immunosuppressed and other ill children is being developed.

> ### *Remember*
> Chickenpox in a childcare establishment is not a cause for panic! Many children will have become infected before the first case is confirmed. For most children it is a fairly mild illness and they can return after all the scabs are dry when they are generally well. All children need some 'TLC' at home to encourage their full recovery.

Good Practice

Call the doctor immediately if a child with chickenpox shows signs of developing complications. Coughing, abnormally rapid breathing, seizures, drowsiness and an unsteady gait are signs of serious complications.

 Progress check

1 Which children will be most seriously affected by chickenpox?
2 How is the virus spread?
3 What are the first signs of chickenpox?
4 What are the stages the spots progress through during the infection?
5 How can the irritation from the rash be controlled?
6 What are the possible complications of chickenpox?

Case study

Bob was a regular at Fairview Infant School. After his retirement, every Wednesday afternoon he played the piano for all the infant children while they sang and danced. One week he complained of a severe pain in his back and ribs and had to go home, he did not look at all well. The next day three children were sent home from school in the morning complaining of headaches and feeling poorly. In the afternoon two others were changing for PE when the teacher noticed a red rash on their chests. Bob's wife telephoned the headteacher on Friday to say that, unfortunately, Bob would not be able to come to the school for a few weeks, because the doctor had diagnosed shingles. That day, six mothers rang to say that their children had got chickenpox.

1 What is the connection between shingles and chickenpox?
2 What is the incubation period for chickenpox?
3 Why do you think so many children were affected at the same time?
4 What are the risks of other children contracting chickenpox?
5 When could the school assume that the small epidemic is over?

HAND, FOOT AND MOUTH DISEASE

What Is Hand, Foot and Mouth Disease?

Hand, foot and mouth disease is a mild viral infection which is common in children from 1 to 4 years. It is highly infectious and usually occurs in epidemics in the summer and early autumn. The condition was first recognised in Canada in 1957 and there is no connection with foot and mouth disease in cows.

What Causes Hand, Foot and Mouth Disease?

Hand, foot and mouth disease is caused by the coxsackie virus. The incubation period is unknown.

How To Recognise Hand, Foot and Mouth Disease

- A slight fever may be present.
- Tiny blisters appear on the inside of the cheeks and the tongue which may develop into ulcers.
- Loss of appetite if sore mouth ulcers are present – babies will refuse feeds and older children will be unwilling to eat.
- 1–2 days after the mouth blisters, flat, greyish white blistery spots with a red halo surrounding them develop on the hands and feet, usually on the fingers and backs of the hands, and the top surfaces of the feet.
- These blisters do not usually cause any itching or discomfort.

Immediate Action

- Relieve the symptoms of the disease.
- Give paracetamol elixir for raised temperature and headache.
- Soft foods and bland fluids for mouth soreness.

Ongoing Care

Blisters will usually have disappeared within 3 to 5 days. If mouth ulcers have developed these will take longer – the doctor may prescribe treatment for these.

Children should stay away from school until the blisters have disappeared.

Possible Complications

In rare cases the rash can extend to cover the body, but will disappear within 3–5 days.

There are no long-term effects.

Further Information

One infection will give a child natural active immunity.

Good Practice

How to relieve soreness in the mouth
1 Offer soft foods such as soup, pureed foods, bland yoghurts etc.
2 Give the child plenty of non-acidic liquids to drink, such as milk – (fruit juices may irritate the mouth). Using a straw avoids contact with the sore areas.
3 Liquid paracetamol can be offered if the child is in pain.
4 Anaesthetic gels applied directly to the sore areas/ulcers will reduce the discomfort.
5 Mouthwashes can reduce the soreness.

ROSEOLA INFANTUM (3-DAY FEVER)

What Is Roseola Infantum?

Roseola infantum is a common infection in early childhood, most prevalent between the ages of 6 months and 2 years.

What Causes Roseola Infantum?

Roseola infantum is caused by the herpes virus.

How To Recognise Roseola Infantum

Roseola infantum has two distinct phases.

Phase 1
- irritable and feverish – the temperature increases rapidly
- sore throat
- enlarged glands in the neck
- earache
- diarrhoea
- cough.

Phase 2
After 4 to 5 days the fever disappears and a rash of tiny pink spots appears – firstly on the front and back – spreading to the arms and legs and face. The rash lasts for about 5 days.

Immediate Action

- Temperature control is essential, in this condition the temperature can rise to 40°C.
- Call the doctor if the temperature does not respond to paracetamol and sponging or if the child has a febrile convulsion.

Ongoing Care

- The child recovers quickly as the rash subsides.
- Antibiotics are not usually necessary.

Possible Complications

- Febrile convulsion as a result of the rapid increase in temperature.
- Other complications are rare.

Further Information

- Some children appear well apart from the high temperature.
- Having the disease provides natural active immunity.

Remember

Roseola and meningitis have similar symptoms. Remember that in meningitis the temperature continues to rise with the appearance of the rash. Call the doctor or send for an ambulance if you suspect that a child has meningitis.

 Progress check

1 What is hand, foot and mouth disease?
2 How would you recognise the symptoms?
3 How long will the blisters last?
4 How long is the child infectious for?
5 How can an adult relieve soreness in the mouth for a child?
6 When is roseola infantum most prevalent?
7 Describe the two phases of the disease.
8 What care should be taken to prevent the temperature increasing to dangerous levels?

MUMPS

What Is Mumps? Also known as epidemic parotitis, mumps was a common childhood infection until the introduction of the MMR vaccine. It involves inflammation and painful enlargement of the salivary glands (parotid glands) which are just in front of, and slightly below, the ear. Other salivary glands beneath the chin and tongue, may also be affected.
Incubation period: 14–21 days.

What Causes Mumps? Mumps is caused by the parotitis virus and is spread by droplet infection. Children continue to be infectious for several days after the symptoms appear.

How To Recognise Mumps
- Generally unwell for 2–3 days before mumps is recognised.
- Raised temperature.
- Extreme tenderness and swelling of one or both sides of the face lasting 5–7 days.

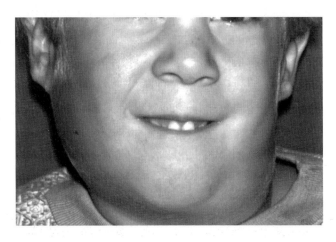

In mumps, the glands in the cheeks and the angle of the jaw swell

- May complain of earache.
- Loss of appetite because of pain when moving the jaw.
- Dry mouth caused by the reduction in saliva produced by the salivary glands.

Immediate Action
- Offer paracetamol to reduce the temperature and relieve the pain.
- Offer plenty of fluids through a straw.
- Children with mumps should be seen by a doctor to confirm the diagnosis.
- Call the doctor if the child has a severe headache or complains of abdominal pain

Ongoing Care
- Give paracetamol half an hour before a meal to reduce the intense discomfort of eating.
- Offer soft foods and fluids such as soups, jellies and liquidised food.

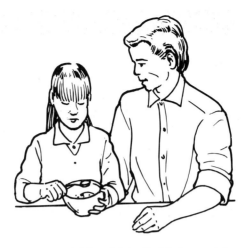

Soft foods are easier to eat when the mouth is sore

Children usually recover quickly within 7–10 days with no ill effects. They can return to their childcare establishment when they feel well.

Possible Complications

- Meningitis. Inflammation of the meninges (covering of the brain) can occur up to 10 days after the first symptoms of mumps. Children usually make a full recovery from mumps meningitis.
- Pancreatitis. Inflammation of the pancreas can occur, causing acute abdominal pain. Although there is usually no permanent damage to the pancreas, in rare cases, diabetes can result.
- Orchitis. Inflamed testes can develop about a week after mumps has started. This is rare before puberty.
- Deafness in one or both ears. A hearing test must be conducted on any child whose hearing seems to have deteriorated after an attack of mumps.

Further Information

Having the disease provides natural active immunity.

TETANUS

What Is Tetanus?

Tetanus is an illness affecting the central nervous system (CNS) – the brain, spinal cord and nerves. It is not often seen in the UK because of the immunisation programme.
Incubation period: 3–21 days.

What Causes Tetanus?

Tetanus is caused through infection by the bacteria, tetanus bacillus. Spores live in the soil and in animal manure and can enter the body through a wound.

How To Recognise Tetanus

- Lockjaw, or difficulty in opening the mouth.
- Difficulty swallowing.
- Tightening of the facial muscles, giving the appearance of a fixed smile.
- Muscle spasms in the back, neck, abdomen, arms and legs.

Immediate Action	**CALL AN AMBULANCE. This is a medical emergency.**

Ongoing Care — The child will be admitted to hospital. Mild cases will be sedated and given small helpings of easily digested food. Severe cases may require help to breath – some may be put on a life-support machine.

Possible Complications — Tetanus can cause death, however the few children who do contract the disease usually recover in about 3 weeks.

Remember

Tetanus is effectively prevented with a course of immunisations offered to babies at 2, 3 and 4 months, followed by a pre-school booster at 4 or 5 years. Boosters every 10 years will continue the protection for life.

✔ **Progress check**

1 Why are mumps and tetanus rarely seen these days?
2 What are the characteristic signs of mumps?
3 How can children with mumps be helped to feel more comfortable?
4 What are the possible complications of mumps?
5 How is the tetanus bacillus spread?
6 What are the recognisable signs of tetanus?
7 Why is tetanus possibly life-threatening?
8 How often should boosters of the tetanus vaccine be given?

WHOOPING COUGH (PERTUSSIS)

What Is Whooping Cough? — Whooping cough is a serious infection of the lungs causing a characteristic 'whoop' on breathing in, after a bout of coughing.
Most seriously at risk are:
■ babies under 6 months of age.
■ children who have not been immunised.
The disease kills 50,000 children each year worldwide, but the incidence in the UK has been reduced with the childhood immunisation programme. Epidemics continue to occur every 3–4 years and were most noticeable when immunisation rates fell in the 1970s – serious epidemics occurred in 1978–9 and 1982–3.
Incubation period: 7–10 days.

What Causes Whooping Cough? — Whooping cough is caused by the bacteria, bordetella pertussis influenzae, which is spread by droplet infection. The bacteria attacks the respiratory tract, producing the early symptoms, and then the bacteria produces toxins which attack other cells throughout the body. Antibiotics have no effect on the later toxins.

How To Recognise Whooping Cough — *Stage 1: The catarrhal stage (lasts 7–10 days)*
■ Dry cough mainly at night.
■ Symptoms of a cold.
■ Mild fever.

Plate 1

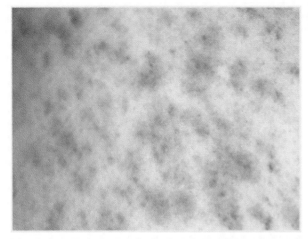

Measles rash

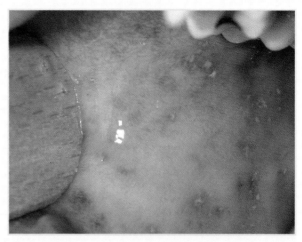

Koplik's spots, which appear on the inside of the cheek, are characteristic of measles

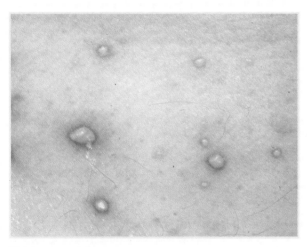

Chickenpox rash

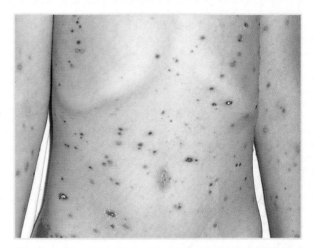

Chickenpox spots appear in batches on the chest and back

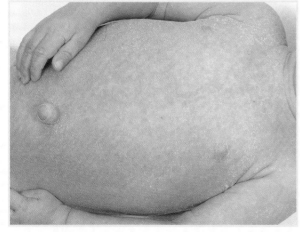

Rubella rash

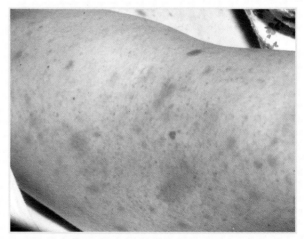

Meningococcal rash

Plate 2

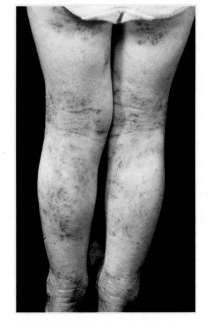

Eczema

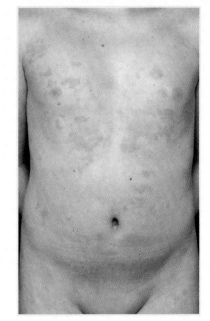

Urticaria

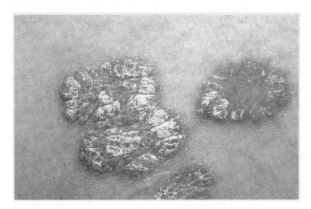

Psoriasis

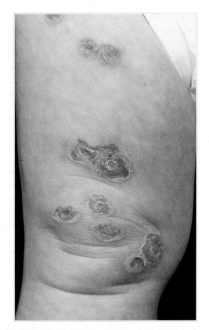

Impetigo

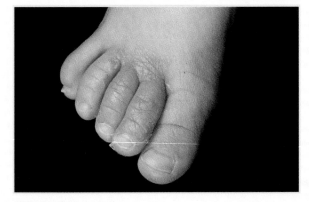

Athlete's foot

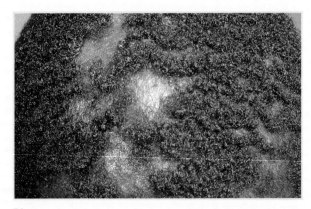

Ringworm

Plate 3

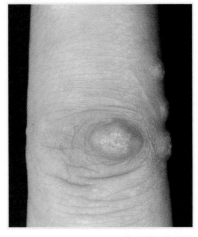
Warts

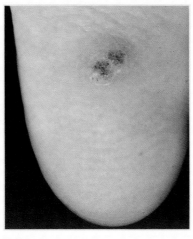
Verruca

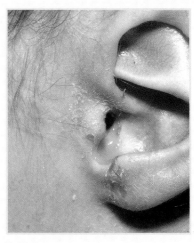
Otitis externa

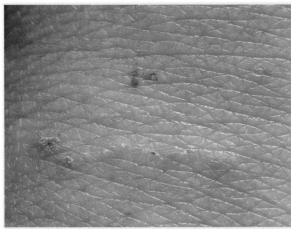
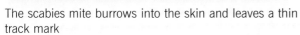
The scabies mite burrows into the skin and leaves a thin track mark

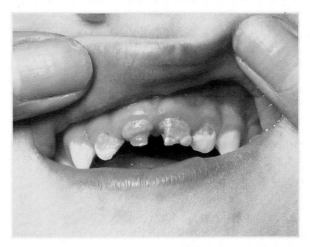
Dental caries

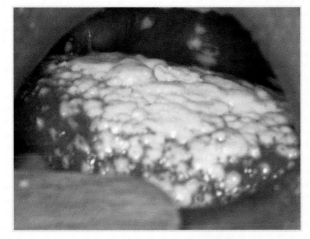
Oral thrush

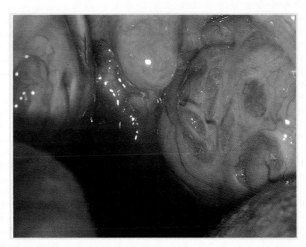
Tonsillitis

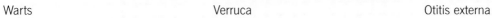

Plate 4

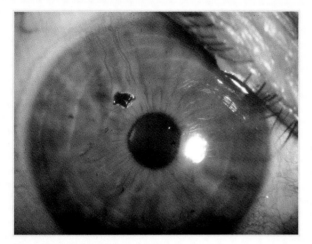

Foreign body in cornea

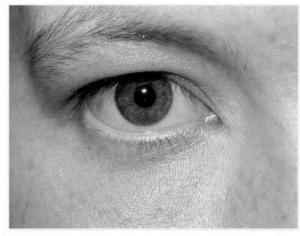

Hepatitis A causes jaundice, a yellowing of the skin and whites of the eyes

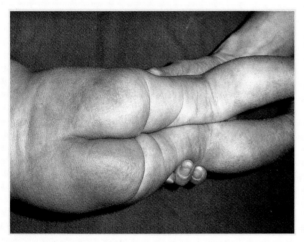

Mongolian blue spot

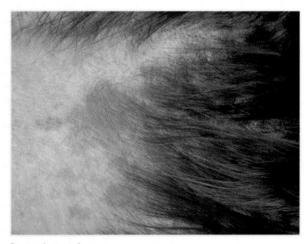

Port wine stain

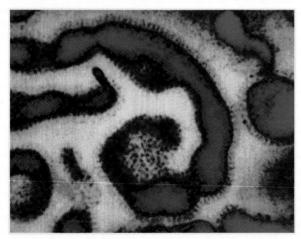

A false-colour electron micrograph of the influenza A virus

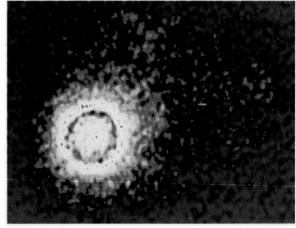

A false-colour electron micrograph of the rhinovirus – one of some 200 viruses that cause the common cold

Stage 2: The paroxysmal stage (lasts 8–12 weeks)
- Bouts of short, dry coughs occurring day and night.
- Prolonged coughing (paroxysmal attacks)with the characteristic whoop when breathing in. Babies may not whoop.
- Vomiting as a result of coughing.
- Occasionally the child may have a convulsion.

Lack of oxygen during the coughing attacks can produce haemorrhages – bleeding – in some parts of the body e.g. the eyes, nose and the skin.

Immediate Action	CALL THE DOCTOR IF YOU SUSPECT WHOOPING COUGH. Reassure the child.

Ongoing Care
- Whooping cough is an extremely distressing illness for the child and for the carers.
- Antibiotics will be given (usually erythromycin) but are only really effective if they are given in the very early stages before the toxins have been produced.
- Some children – especially babies – will be admitted to hospital for treatment.

Relieving the cough
- Ensure the child sits upright when coughing – pat the back firmly to help them to bring up any mucus.
- Encourage them to expectorate – cough the mucus out of their airways
- Hold a baby and gently rub and pat their back as they cough.
- No smoking in the same house.
- Remain calm and comfort and reassure the child.
- Physiotherapy may be required to help the cough.
- Parent and child should share a room for the duration of the illness so that care can be offered quickly at night.

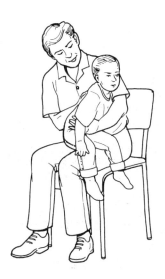

Relieving a cough

General Care

- Avoid changes of temperature which can cause a coughing attack.
- Give plenty of fluids to drink. Give nutritious drinks if possible as the child may not feel like eating.
- Provide soft and attractive meals. Avoid crumbly food as this may stimulate the cough.
- The child will be exhausted with coughing and will need plenty of rest.
- Nights will be disturbed for several weeks – parents/relatives could alternate caring duties so that one parent sleeps and is not over-tired.
- Call a doctor if the child's lips turn blue during a coughing attack, or if they have a convulsion.

Possible Complications

Permanent lung damage is rare, but collapse of part of the lung does sometimes occur because of the violent coughing attacks. Most children who have had whooping cough are affected with the same type of cough if they have a viral infection within the next year to eighteen months.

- Bronchopneumonia can occur with an attack of whooping cough. It is treated with antibiotics.
- Otitis media, infection of the middle ear, will result in earache and fever.
- Hernia may occur, usually in the groin in boys, as the result of strenuous coughing.
- Haemorrhages (bleeding) can occur as a result of the violent coughing spasms causing bleeding under the skin, nose bleeds, coughing up blood and bleeding in the conjunctiva of the eyes. They usually improve as the disease gets better.

Further Information

The child is infectious from about 7 days after they contacted the disease until 21 days after the symptoms appear.

The child should only return to school when they feel well enough to do so – this can take several weeks. Teachers and carers should know that the child is not infectious during the convalescent stage, after antibiotics have been given.

Brothers and sisters should be given antibiotics to prevent a serious infection.

Having the disease provides natural active immunity.

Remember

An effective immunisation programme exists for many childhood diseases – encourage families to have their children immunised to protect them from serious illness.

Good Practice

Call a doctor if:
- a child under 6 months is coughing
- coughing results in vomiting
- a cough does not improve after a week.

✅ Progress check

1 What causes whooping cough and how is it spread?
2 Describe the two stages of whooping cough.
3 Find out why the immunisation rate for pertussis fell in the late 70s.
4 What is the medical treatment for pertussis?
5 How can children with this condition be cared for at home?
6 How long are children with pertussis infectious for?

Case study

Sian, aged 7 years was the eldest of five children aged 5, 3, 18 months and 8 weeks. Her parents did not believe in immunisations because they thought that a natural diet and healthy lifestyle were all the protection that their children required. They did not like seeing the doctor and regularly went to a homeopathist. Despite the lack of immunisations, none of the children had been ill except for the usual childhood coughs and colds. Soon after Christmas, Sian caught a cold which made her cough at night. The cough got worse and worse and the homeopathic treatment did not seem to help. Sian could not eat because it made her cough, and the cough was so violent that her nose bled profusely. She was completely exhausted and had to fight for breath when she coughed. In desperation her parents took her to the GP who immediately diagnosed whooping cough. He prescribed antibiotics, but explained that for them to be fully effective against the bacteria Sian should have been given them several days before. He thought that Sian should be admitted to hospital.

1 How can the infection be prevented in Sian's brothers and sisters?
2 Which of the other children are most at risk and why?
3 How could Sian's parents be persuaded to allow their children to participate in the immunisation programme?
4 What are the possible complications of whooping cough for Sian?

MEASLES

What is Measles? Also known as rubeola, measles is a highly infectious disease with a characteristic rash. It is now uncommon due to the successful MMR immunisation, but before the immunisation 800,000 children a year contracted the disease in the UK. In developing countries without immunisation, 25 per cent of deaths in the first 5 years of life are due to measles.

Incubation period: 8–14 days.

What Causes Measles?   Measles is caused by a virus and is spread by droplet infection. It is a highly infectious condition.

How To Recognise Measles

- Generally unwell for about 4 days before the rash appears, with a runny nose and a harsh, dry cough.
- Raised temperature which sometimes results in a febrile convulsion.
- Sore, red eyes – the child may avoid bright light because the eyes are painful (photophobia).
- Koplik's spots on the inside of the cheeks (see plate 1). These small white spots with a red base, are characteristic of measles and appear a day before the rash on the body. They look like grains of salt.
- Rash first appears behind the ears and along the hairline spreading to the face and neck. It then spreads over the whole body and limbs.

Appearance of the rash
Tiny separate spots which merge together to give a blotchy appearance. The rash is flat and a deep and dusky reddy/brown colour. After 3–4 days the surface skin begins to shed.

- A high fever occurs as the rash appears, which improves as the rash disappears (see plate 1).

Immediate Action

- Call the doctor if measles is suspected – the child should be examined within 24 hours.
- Control the temperature with paracetamol and fluids.
- Care for the child in a darkened room to protect the sensitive eyes, and comfort the child.

Ongoing Care

- Antibiotics will be prescribed by the doctor to prevent secondary infection caused by bacteria.
- Eye-drops will help to soothe the eyes.
- Offer plenty of fluids and continue to control the temperature.
- Ensure that the child rests during the early stages. Quiet play as recovery begins will help.
- The child will begin to feel better as the rash disappears after about 3–4 days.

Possible Complications

- Conjunctivitis, which is an infection of the eye.
- Infection of the middle ear (otitis media). Hearing should be checked about a month after the illness if the ears have been affected.
- Bronchitis can be treated with antibiotics.
- Pneumonia can be treated with antibiotics.
- Encephalitis (inflammation of the brain) in 1 in 1,000 cases because the infection spreads to the brain. This occurs 7 to 10 days after the original illness began.

Because of these possible complications the doctor should be called at once if a child has any of the following symptoms: earache, rapid breathing, drowsiness, convulsions, severe headache or vomiting.

Further Information	■ A child is infectious from 1 day before symptoms appear until about 4 days later.
	■ Having the disease provides natural active immunity.

> ## Remember
> Measles will continue to occur until 90 per cent of children have been immunised.

RUBELLA (GERMAN MEASLES)

What Is Rubella?	Rubella is a mild infection which can affect the fetus if contracted by a woman in early pregnancy. These effects of the disease were not detected until as recently as the 1960s. Rubella is chiefly a disease of childhood, being most common in children between the ages of 5 and 12 years. It has been a notifiable disease since 1988. **Incubation period: 14–21 days.**

What Causes Rubella?	Rubella is caused by a virus.

How To Recognise Rubella	■ Mild fever and generally unwell for 2–3 days before the rash appears. ■ Enlarged lymph nodes (glands) behind the ears. ■ Non-irritating rash appears on the face. ■ Joint pain may affect some children.

Appearance of the rash
Tiny, flat pink spots. Starts on the face and spreads to the chest, back and limbs. The spots may merge together but the rash remains quite pale compared to the measles rash (see plate 1).

Immediate Action	■ Call the doctor to confirm the diagnosis – do not take the child to the health centre or surgery because of the risk of infecting pregnant women. A blood sample may be taken to confirm that the rash is due to rubella. ■ Offer fluids and paracetamol.

Ongoing Care	Avoid contact with pregnant women and women who may be pregnant. Children usually recover quickly from this infection with paracetamol to treat any pain and reduce the temperature.

Possible Complications	Fetal development is affected and can result in: ■ deafness ■ blindness ■ heart deformities ■ delayed intellectual development.

Further Information A child is infectious from 5 to 7 days before the rash appears until about 4 days later.

Remember

MMR (mumps, measles and rubella) immunisation is offered to boys and girls at 12 to 15 months. It is still offered to girls at 10 to 14 years if they have not had the MMR as babies.

 ### Progress check

1 What causes measles and how is it spread?
2 Why do you think an immunisation for measles is necessary?
3 What are Koplik's spots?
4 How would you be able to recognise a measles infection in a child?
5 What does the measles rash look like?
6 What treatment and care will the child require?
7 What are the possible complications to a measles infection?
8 Why is rubella immunisation important?
9 What are the signs of rubella infection?
10 How long is a child infectious with rubella?
11 What are the potential effects of rubella infection on the fetus?

Remember

If you think that a rash may be due to meningitis – send for an ambulance.

MENINGITIS

What is Meningitis? An inflammation of the meninges – the meninges are a protective covering of the brain and the spinal cord.
Incubation period: 2–10 days.

What Causes Meningitis? A virus or bacteria (usually meningococcus, pneumococcus or haemophilus influenzae) can cause this disease. The HIB immunisation protects against the haemophilus influenzae strain of the disease.

The bacterial form is most common in children under 5 years of age and tends to occur in isolated cases.

The viral form is less severe and tends to occur in epidemics in the winter.

How To Recognise Meningitis A child with meningitis will become seriously ill very quickly.

The symptoms of the bacterial and viral form of meningitis are similar in the early stages, but the bacterial type is more severe and can develop in a few hours.

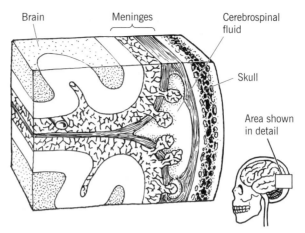

Brain   Meninges   Cerebrospinal fluid

Skull

Area shown in detail

The meninges cover the brain and spinal cord

Signs in a baby:
- very drowsy and irritable
- high temperature
- vomiting
- loss of appetite
- crying (sometimes high pitched)
- restlessness
- a very young baby may have bulging fontanelles caused by the increased pressure inside the skull.

Signs in children:
- headache
- photophobia – avoidance of light. May close the eyes and prefer to be in the dark
- stiff neck – the neck muscles become very rigid and it is too painful for a child to try to put their chin on their chest.

Bacterial meningitis
The above signs will progress very quickly and the child will become more and more drowsy. Older children may become incoherent (it is difficult to understand their speech and actions).

A bacterial rash may develop (see plate 1). The rash is the result of septicaemia (infection of the blood). The rash:
- is flat with purple or pink spots
- can look like bruising
- does not disappear or fade when pressed.

This is a very serious sign and the child will need urgent medical aid.

Immediate Action
- CALL AN AMBULANCE IMMEDIATELY or take the child to the nearest accident and emergency department at a hospital if this is quicker.
- If you call a doctor, while you are waiting, care for the child in a darkened room and try to reduce the temperature. Reassure the child and provide comfort. The doctor will give penicillin at home before arranging for the child to be admitted to hospital.

Ongoing Care

Children will be admitted to hospital where they will be given intravenous antibiotics and a lumbar puncture to:

1 confirm that it is meningitis
2 find out which pathogenic organism is causing the disease, so that the correct treatment can be given.

Possible Complications

Viral meningitis usually has no complications.

Bacterial meningitis can result in damage to the brain, epilepsy, deafness and learning difficulties. If it is not treated promptly it can be fatal.

Further Information

Short-term protection to meningococcal meningitis may be given during local outbreaks by immunisation.

Remember

Children who have been in contact with meningitis can be given antibiotics to prevent the spread of the disease.

✔ Progress check

1 What is meningitis?
2 Why is it considered to be such a serious condition?
3 Why is the bacterial disease more serious than the viral disease?
4 What are the signs of meningitis in a baby?
5 How can the diagnosis be confirmed?
6 What immediate treatment will the child require?
7 What are the possible complications of the condition?

Activity

Prepare a large poster/display for your establishment to inform parents of the signs and symptoms of meningitis. Include:

■ the immediate action they should take if they suspect that their child may have the disease
■ immunisation information
■ possible effects and complications of meningitis.

Case study

Ian had been playing in the garden in the sunshine for most of the afternoon, splashing in the water and chasing his new kitten, laughing with glee. He was 3 years old and loved to play with his dad after nursery, while mum was at work. He started to feel ill quite quickly and told his dad that he had a 'headache in his tummy' before he vomited. His dad comforted him, gave him a drink, washed him quickly and put him to bed. Ian groaned as his dad undressed him and put his pyjama top over his head. His neck hurt, and the bedroom light was too bright – it hurt his eyes. An hour later his dad went into the bedroom to check on his son's condition. To his dismay he saw that Ian was sweating, he had a very high temperature and when he changed his wet pyjamas there was a flat purple rash all over his tummy.

- What action should his dad take now?
- If bacterial meningitis is confirmed, what treatment will Ian be given in hospital?
- What protection can be offered to the children Ian contacted at nursery?
- What were the early signs of illness that Ian was displaying?

DIPHTHERIA

What Is Diphtheria?

Diphtheria is a severe throat infection which is very rare due to the effective immunisation programme. The infection produces toxins which may attack the heart and central nervous system (CNS). **Incubation period: 2–6 days.**

What Causes Diphtheria?

Diphtheria is caused by bacteria and spread by droplet infection.

How To Recognise Diphtheria

Three strains of bacteria causing diphtheria produce symptoms of varying degrees, but the following are the characteristic signs:

- generally unwell
- headache
- sore throat
- white/grey membrane forming in the back if the throat which restricts the airway (the diphtheretic membrane)
- breathing difficulties
- fever.

Immediate Action

Call the doctor if you suspect diphtheria.

Ongoing Care

Child will be admitted to hospital and given an anti-toxin to prevent further damage and antibiotics to fight the infection. Tracheotomy may be necessary to assist breathing.

- As the disease progresses the heart may be involved causing a weak and irregular pulse and reduced blood pressure.

Possible Complications

Diphtheria toxins may produce the following side-effects.

- Heart failure.
- Respiration may be affected resulting in further infections e.g. bronchopneumonia.
- Central nervous system complications such as paralysis of the arms and/or legs, and squint.

Further Information   Children who have been in contact with diphtheria should be given a further vaccine and close family should also be given antibiotics to prevent them developing into 'carriers'.

POLIO (POLIOMYELITIS)

What Is Polio?   Polio is an infection which attacks the central nervous system and causes paralysis.
Incubation period: 5–21 days.

What Causes Polio?   Polio is caused by a virus.

How To Recognise Polio
- Suddenly unwell.
- Headache.
- Stiff neck and back.
- Loss of movement and paralysis.
- Breathing difficulties.

Immediate Action   Call the doctor.

Ongoing Care   Hospital treatment is essential.
Physiotherapy.

Possible Complications   Permanent paralysis often in the legs.

Further Information   Rarely seen but odd cases do still occur.

Good Practice

Carers who change babies' nappies should be particularly careful to keep their polio boosters up to date as they may be vulnerable to this infection.

TB (TUBERCULOSIS)

What Is Tuberculosis?   TB is a chronic infection which usually affects the lungs, but can also affect the kidneys, bones and brain.
Incubation period: 28–42 days

What Causes Tuberculosis?   TB is caused by the bacteria – tubercle bacillus.

How To Recognise
Tuberculosis
- Persistent cough.
- Tiredness.
- Loss of appetite.
- Weight loss.
- May have a raised temperature.

Immediate Action
Contact the doctor if a cough lasts more than a week without improvement.

Ongoing Care
- Child will have a chest X-ray (CXR) which will show the affected patch in the lung(s).
- Antibiotics will be given for up to a year to combat the bacteria.
- High quality diet to help the child regain strength and be able to recover.
- Lots of rest.
- Other members of the family will be examined to try to find out where the infection originated

Possible Complications
Tuberculous meningitis

Further Information
TB is increasing in the UK, partly because of people travelling to areas of the world where the disease is prevalent. Also, visitors to the UK may not have been immunised and pass the disease to family and social contacts.

BCG immunisation for TB is offered to all children at secondary school after a HEAF test to detect antibodies. Children who have already been exposed to the disease and have a positive HEAF test will be examined to see if the disease is still in its active stages.

TB contact tracers are employed within health authorities to find all the people that a confirmed case has had contact with, to ensure that they are treated if necessary.

Good Practice

BCG vaccine should be given to high risk babies and children – some ethnic groups in certain geographical areas are most vulnerable e.g. babies born to parents from India, parts of Africa, Central and South America should be given a BCG immunisation soon after birth.

 Progress check

1 What part of the body does diphtheria affect?
2 How could you recognise the condition in a child?
3 What are the possible complications of diphtheria?

4   When are children usually immunised against diphtheria and polio?
5   What are the effects of polio?
6   How would you recognise polio?
7   Which parts of the body may be affected by tuberculosis?
8   What are the signs of tuberculosis?
9   To whom is BCG vaccine given and why?
10 Why is the incidence of TB increasing in the UK?

ERYTHEMA INFECTIOSUM (SLAPPED CHEEK SYNDROME)

What Is Erythema Infectiosum?
Also called 'fifth disease' it is a mild infection which usually occurs in small epidemics and affects children over 2 years of age.
Incubation period: 4–14 days

What Causes Erythema Infectiosum?
Erythema infectiosum is caused by a virus.

How To Recognise Erythema Infectiosum
The child will have:
- bright red cheeks and a pale area around the mouth
- raised temperature
- rash coming 1–4 days after the reddened cheeks. It appears on the trunk and limbs with a blotchy appearance. It is far more obvious after a warm bath. It lasts for 7–10 days
- occasional joint pain.

Immediate Action
Call the doctor if the child has sickle cell anaemia or thalassaemia. Otherwise comfort the child and reassure. Ensure that they drink well and offer paracetamol for a raised temperature.

Ongoing Care
No specific treatment is required.

Possible Complications
The rash may recur over a period of months and may be more severe after exposure to sunlight.

Further Information
The child is infectious for 2 days before the rash and 2 days after the rash appears.

Remember

Having the disease provides natural active immunity and gives life-long protection.

KAWASAKI DISEASE

What Is Kawasaki Disease? Kawasaki disease is an inflammatory condition which affects the small arteries all over the body.

An illness which affects children only before puberty and is most common under the age of 5 years.

What causes Kawasaki Disease? Possible infection by bacteria or virus – the exact cause has not been identified. There have been few reports of the illness being passed from child to child.

How To Recognise Kawasaki Disease
- High temperature lasting about 5 days.
- Cracked and swollen lips.
- Sore throat.
- Conjunctivitis – the whites of the eyes will be red.
- Swollen glands in the neck.
- Swelling of the hands and feet.
- Reddening of the palms of the hands and soles of the feet.
- Red, blotchy rash over the whole body.
- Skin peeling off the hands during the second week of the illness.

Immediate Action The doctor should be called immediately.

Admission to hospital may be recommended for treatment with:
1 injections of gammaglobulin which reduces the risk of damage to the coronary arteries. It must be given within 10 days of the start of the illness
2 aspirin tablets to reduce the risks of heart complications. Aspirin acts by reducing the inflammation in the walls of the blood vessels.

Ongoing Care A child will be acutely ill for about 10 days and full recovery takes 3 to 8 weeks.

Possible Complications *Heart disease*
- Inflammation of the heart muscle (myocarditis).
- Heart attack (myocardial infarction).
- Coronary artery disease.

Heart disease may persist in about 1 to 2 per cent of cases, but many children may have complications which can last for up to a year. Twenty per cent of children who have had Kawasaki disease will suffer from coronary artery disease later in life.

Arthritis

This inflammation of the joints may last for 6 to 8 weeks before improving. There are not usually any long-term effects on the joints.

Further Information

Kawasaki Disease was first described in Japan in the 1960s and the first cases in Britain were diagnosed in the 1970s.

Case study

Sophia, aged 3 years, woke up feeling awful – her mouth was so sore that it hurt to swallow and she could hardly gather the strength to call for her mother. When her mum came in and turned on the light she was amazed to see Sophia's red eyes and sore, red lips. When she touched her it was obvious that Sophia had a high temperature, so she gave her daughter some Calpol to reduce the temperature and soothe her sore mouth. Eventually the child went back to sleep. The next day Sophia would not eat or drink because it hurt her mouth. The high temperature continued, despite doses of paracetamol, and her hands and feet reddened and began to swell. The GP was contacted and when he saw the extent of Sophia's symptoms he diagnosed Kawasaki disease. Mother and child were sent to the local hospital for immediate treatment and care.

1 What were the signs of illness that Sophia was displaying?
2 What specific treatment will she be given and why?
3 How would you care for a child with these symptoms?

Progress check

1 What is fifth disease and who does it most commonly affect?
2 How could you recognise the infection?
3 What care should be offered to treat the condition?
4 What is Kawasaki disease?
5 What are the possible complications of Kawasaki disease?

Chapter 9

Conditions affecting the skin and hair

This chapter includes:
- The skin
- Eczema
- Urticaria
- Psoriasis
- Impetigo
- Cold sores
- Athlete's foot
- Ringworm
- Alopecia
- Warts
- Verrucae
- Sunburn

All children need adult help and supervision in their personal hygiene requirements. This chapter explains the structure and functions of the skin to raise the awareness of childcare workers of the importance of the organ. This will also reinforce the value of hygiene in maintaining good health. The chapter continues to explain the many conditions which affect the skin including the specific care of each.

Good standards of hygiene in childhood are important because they:
- help to prevent disease
- increase self-esteem and social acceptance
- prepare children for life by teaching them how to care for themselves.

The skin

The structure of the skin
The skin is a very complex organ which is composed of several layers (see the diagram on page 218).

Functions of the skin
The functions of the skin include the following.

Protection

The skin provides protection:

- of underlying organs
- against germs entering the body.

Sensation

The skin is the organ of touch and contains specialised skin cells which detect pressure, pain and temperature, conveying sensations of hot, cold, soft, hard, etc.

Secretion of sebum

Sebum is an oily substance, which:

- lubricates the hair
- keeps the skin supple and waterproof
- protects the skin from moisture and heat.

The manufacture of vitamin D

Vitamin D is manufactured by exposure of the skin to ultra violet rays from the sun. It is necessary for healthy bone growth. Black children may need a supplement in the winter as their skin does not easily make vitamin D.

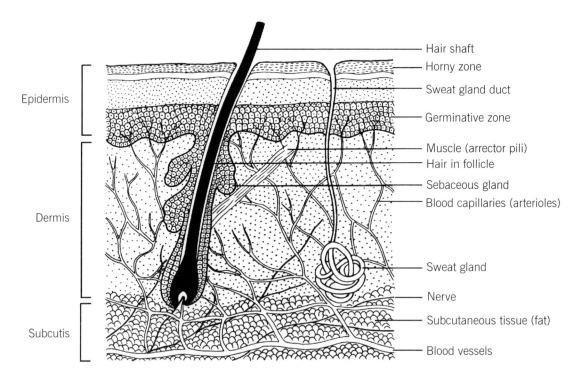

The structure of the skin

Sweating

The skin excretes sweat which:

- gets rid of some waste products
- helps to regulate the temperature when the body is hot.

Care of the skin

Because the skin has so many important functions and because it is the first part of the body to come into contact with the environment, it must be well cared for. This does not mean obsessive cleaning of the skin: too much cleaning can be as harmful as too little because it may make the skin dry and sore and also wash away protective sebum. However, clean skin is important because washing reduces the number of bacteria living on the skin and helps to prevent skin infections such as abscesses and impetigo. Bacteria thrive on damp, sweaty skin especially in the skin creases, for example the nappy area in babies. However, conditions that affect only the skin are usually quite mild and with the correct treatment they improve quickly.

Skin conditions are usually due to the following.

Irritation

Young skin is delicate and sensitive to many environmental factors, for example different soaps, washing powders and plants can result in rashes and soreness. This is the commonest cause of widespread, itchy rashes.

Infection

- Breaks in the skin such as cuts, grazes and abrasions allow the entry of pathogens which can cause skin infections and sometimes more serious generalised infections.
- Rashes on the skin are often a sign of other diseases, for example chickenpox or measles and are accompanied by other signs of illness.

Allergy

Allergies can be potentially serious because there are usually other effects as well as an itchy skin rash. They are caused by a direct irritant (something which has come into contact with the skin) or by something a child has eaten such as peanuts, shellfish, cheese or medicines.

Parents and carers must be observant so that they are aware of what a child has come into contact with or eaten for the first time, and to note any changes in the skin and/or hair which indicates a possible allergic reaction.

The skin provides many clues about the general health and well being of babies and children. Healthy skin is clear with shiny hair. Good blood flow produces glowing colour, fine texture, suppleness and elasticity. Spots, blemishes and dryness all indicate the need for further investigation of the cause of the skin problem.

ECZEMA

What Is Eczema? Other names are atopic dermatitis and infantile eczema. It is a common skin condition affecting about 1 in 30 children. Atopic eczema is the usual type affecting children. See plate 2.

Eczema takes its name from the Greek word meaning 'to boil out' which effectively describes the red and boiling nature of the rash.

What Causes Eczema? There is an inherited tendency to develop eczema which is triggered by an environmental condition such as:
- infection
- direct irritants on the skin e.g. perfume, soap, washing powder
- specific foods e.g. dairy products
- heat and humidity
- inhaled irritants e.g. smoke, pollen
- drugs
- emotional triggers such as stress and excitement.

Seventy per cent of children with eczema have family members who suffer from allergic conditions, such as hay-fever, asthma or eczema.

How To Recognise Eczema The rash of atopic eczema usually develops before 18 months of age, but is unusual before 3 months.

Under 4 years
- Dry skin
- Itchy rash of inflamed pimples – may be moist or weepy.
- Face, scalp, trunk, fronts of legs and forearms are the usual sites of the rash.
- Lack of sleep due to itching

4–10 years
- Dry, scaly rash with cracked skin. It is very itchy.
- Red, sore skin where it has been scratched – the skin may weep and as it dries a crusty, yellow layer is left on the skin.
- Thickened, leathery skin in affected areas which may look pale due to the loss of pigmentation.
- Sites: face, neck, backs of knees, inside elbows, ankles i.e. inside surface of joints.

Immediate Action
- A doctor should be consulted if a child has sore and itchy skin. If eczema is diagnosed there are many ways of trying to reduce the child's discomfort. The doctor may prescribe drug treatment if the condition is severe.
- Some children will experience a worsening of their rash in cold weather and others will have a more severe reaction during hot and humid weather. Each child must be treated individually according to their specific condition.

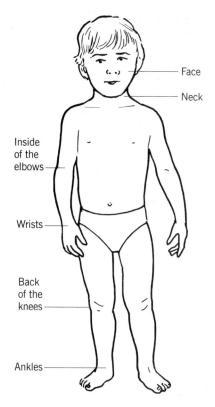

Face

Neck

Inside of the elbows

Wrists

Back of the knees

Ankles

Sites of atropic eczema in children aged 4 years and over

Ongoing Care

Preventing dry skin

- Trying to keep the skin soft and supple is fundamental in the treatment of eczema. When the skin is dry it itches and becomes inflamed.
- Moisturise the skin regularly with emollient cream – as many times a day as possible and especially after a bath. Wrapping cling film loosely around the affected areas, after the cream has been applied, will increase the absorption of the emollient.
- Use aqueous cream in place of soap.
- Put an oil such as oilatum in the bath water. Daily baths are not necessary and can make the skin even drier.
- Dress the child with loose, cotton clothes next to the skin.
- Keep the child's nails clean and short to prevent infection caused by scratching. A young child may benefit from wearing cotton mittens at night to prevent damage to the skin.
- Avoid overwarm rooms, especially at night, as heat can irritate the condition.
- Excluding possible irritants from the diet may help the condition, but should only be done with the help of a doctor and dietician.

Prescribed drugs

It may be necessary to use medicines prescribed by a doctor.

- Steroids. Corticosteroid cream or ointment to reduce itching and inflammation during a severe episode of eczema.
- Antihistamines. These are anti-itch creams and may help the child to sleep when the condition is severe.

Remember
Always follow medical advice when applying steroid creams or ointments. Carers should wear gloves during application.

- Antibiotics. Used to treat infections of the skin which may occur as a result of scratching, they may be in the form of creams or taken internally as medicine.

Possible Complications

There may be infection as a result of scratching, e.g. impetigo (see page 227).

Children can be cruel – an affected child with visible rashes may be subject to taunting and teasing at school. Childcare workers must deal promptly and vigorously with this.

Good Practice

Encourage a child who is scratching to rub the skin in a circular movement and apply pressure instead – this avoids the possibility of damaging the skin with the nails. Keep the nails short.

Further Information

By the teenage years most children (about 90 per cent) are no longer affected by eczema.

About 50 per cent of children affected by eczema develop other allergic conditions such as asthma.

Complementary therapy
Chinese herbal medicine (a mixture of many plants) has been used by many children with impressive results – some have improved dramatically. The medicine should be given under a doctor's supervision but is not yet available in all NHS hospitals.

Seborrhoeic dermatitis
This condition can be mistaken for eczema. Cradle cap seen in babies is an example (see page 172).

Self-help group
National Eczema Society
4 Tavistock Place
London
WC1H 9RA

Remember

Always wear gloves when applying creams to broken or inflamed skin. This protects the child from the risk of further infection and protects the carer from absorbing the cream into their body.

Good Practice

Use non-biological washing powders and avoid using fabric softeners especially if a child has any type of skin condition. The chemicals in biological washing products can irritate healthy young skin and are best avoided.

Supporting a child with eczema in the childcare establishment

AREA OF DIFFICULTY	EFFECT ON THE CHILD	COPING STRATEGY
Over-heating in the playroom/classroom	Irritates eczema and causes scratching	Allow child to be away from radiators and sunny areas Use emollient creams Avoid tights and wool next to the skin Soothe with a cool, damp flannel Distract child from scratching with activities
Classroom pet	Increases the irritation	Encourage the child to be interested in other creatures e.g. goldfish
Contact with paints, dough, clay, sand in the classroom. Chlorinated water in the swimming pool	Creates rashes on the hands and other contact points	Provide plastic or cotton gloves for the child to use. Use lots of emollients before the child goes into the water Shower well after swim and re-apply creams Ensure that the child has the opportunity to participate in all activities
Writing, drawing, painting,	Difficulties in developing fine motor control with painful hands and greasy creams on the fingers.	Offer other activities when the hands are sore and reintroduce when they are improved
Using a knife and fork	Child is frustrated and self-confidence is affected	Food can be cut up so the child can use a fork to eat
Paper towels and soap	Irritate the skin	Encourage the parents to bring in aqueous solution and flannel towel

Case study

Jake has eczema. He is due to start school soon and his mother is concerned about all the possible irritants there, which may worsen his condition and prevent him from enjoying school. She is also keen to stress to the staff that his eczema is not catching and is not a reflection of poor hygiene. Jake has had eczema since he was a baby and his skin is very sensitive to environmental factors, especially heat, paint and perfume. When he is anxious or upset the condition rapidly deteriorates. When Jake visits the school with his mother he is very excited about all the activities and meeting the other children.

1 How can the staff prepare the other children and avoid unnecessary negative reactions?
2 What information would the school require to make sure that Jake received the correct care during the school day?
3 How could the childcare worker reassure this parent about Jake's entry to school?
4 How could Jake be made to feel secure in the school environment?

Activity

You are a nanny who is responsible for the care of two young children at home – Sam aged 3 years and his sister Beth, aged 18 months. Both children have eczema which is treated with steroid creams from the doctor when severe. Write a routine for their care over a 24-hour period aiming to meet their individual needs.

 Progress check

1 What are the probable causes of eczema?
2 How can eczema be recognised in a young child?
3 Which parts of the body are most commonly affected?
4 What can a parent/carer do to keep the skin as soft and supple as possible?
5 What type of drugs may be used in the treatment of eczema?

URTICARIA

What Is Urticaria? Urticaria is also known as nettle rash or hives. It is a very itchy, lumpy rash which is common in the under-fives. See plate 2.

What Causes Urticaria? Usually, urticaria is an allergy to an environmental factor which has irritated the skin, for example clothing such as wool or nylon, washing powders, metal in zips, food the child has eaten such as dairy products or medicine such as penicillin etc.

How To Recognise Urticaria
- The child is generally well although itching may cause grumpiness.
- Swollen, pale weals (lumps) on the skin are surrounded by dark inflamed skin.
- It may affect a small area of the body or be fairly widespread.
- The rash may come and go.
- Acute attacks can last for as little as half an hour, but a chronic case can last several months.

Immediate Action
- Keep the skin cool.
- Apply calamine lotion.
- Sodium bicarbonate in the bath water is soothing.
- Antihistamine (anti-itch) cream and medicine are very effective. They can be purchased over the counter and the sedative quality of some of the medicines may induce sleep.

Ongoing Care   Establish the cause of the rash. This can be very simple or almost impossible!

   If the cause is found then all measures should be taken to eliminate contact of the allergen with the child.

Possible Complications   *Anaphylactic Shock*
Allergies can lead to anaphylactic shock in extreme cases. This is a generalised reaction to an allergen and it is very dangerous because the mouth and face will swell, breathing and swallowing become difficult as the airways swell. It can be fatal. Call the doctor or take the child to the Accident and Emergency Department of the nearest hospital if this will be quicker. Support the child in a semi sitting position to ease the breathing. Children who have had this type of allergic response should wear a bracelet indicating their allergy, and parents and teachers may have adrenaline to inject in case of an emergency.

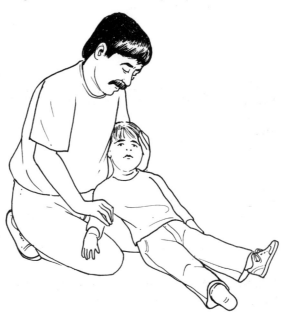

Support child in a semi-sitting position to ease breathing

✔ *Progress check*

1 What causes urticaria?
2 What is the difference between an eczema rash and a nettle rash?
3 How can urticaria be treated?
4 How would you know that a child had gone into anaphylactic shock?
5 What would you do if this was the case?

PSORIASIS

What Is Psoriasis?   Psoriasis is a severe skin condition which is most common in children over 10 years of age, but it can occur in younger children with a family history of the condition. See plate 2.

What Causes Psoriasis?

The cause is unknown, but it is thought to be dominantly an inherited disorder. It sometimes appears for the first time after an acute infection such as tonsillitis or a stressful event, for example an accident or emotional trauma such as bereavement. The rash develops as new skin cells are created more quickly than the dead cells are shed. The new cells form thicker areas of skin and are covered with flaking skin.

How To Recognise Psoriasis

In children the psoriasis rash is often preceded by an upper respiratory tract infection caused by streptococcal bacteria.

- Red and scaly patches appear on the arms, legs, body and head – typically on the knees and elbows.
- The rash is not itchy but it can be uncomfortable and feel 'tight'.
- The rash is more severe during times of stress and worry.
- The skin may crack and become sore.
- Thickened nails

Immediate Action

The doctor will usually refer a child to a dermatologist (skin doctor) for specialist treatment.

Ongoing Care

- The doctor will prescribe treatment, probably coal tar cream or corticosteroid creams. Avoid and prevent dry skin by using an emollient cream.
- Coal tar formulations may help, especially if added to the bath water.
- Exposure to moderate amounts of sunshine can help, but care must be taken to avoid sunburn.

Possible Complications

- Infections of the skin.
- Psychological effects and isolation if the rash results in unsympathetic responses from peers.

Further Information

Long-term follow-up should be provided by the same doctor who knows the child's skin condition. Reassurance and encouragement is important.

Psoriasis cannot be cured but the effects can be controlled with care and preventive treatment such as avoiding dry skin, controlling stress and treating the first signs of a rash.

Some careers are best avoided by children with this condition, for example chemistry, beauty therapy, hairdressing and any jobs which involve contact with possible irritants.

Self-help group
The Psoriasis Association
7 Milton St
Northampton NN2 7JG

<table>
<tr><td>

Remember

Although some exposure to sunshine can be beneficial to the skin, sensible precautions must be taken to prevent sunburn. It is essential for a child in the sun to wear a hat, a tee-shirt and high factor suncream or sun block.

</td><td>

Good Practice

Children with skin conditions can be affected by bullying at school. Cruel remarks from other children and social isolation from peers are not uncommon. Childcare workers must be alert to these possible reactions from other children and be vigilant in supporting children with skin conditions.

</td></tr>
</table>

IMPETIGO

What Is Impetigo? This is a highly contagious skin infection. It usually affects the mouth and nose areas in children and can also affect the nappy area in babies. See plate 2.

What Causes Impetigo? Impetigo is caused by bacteria – usually streptococcal or staphylococcal – which enter through a break in the skin as the result of a cut, graze, insect bite, scratching, atopic eczema etc.

How To Recognise Impetigo
- Reddened skin with small blisters usually around the mouth and nose.
- Raw, weeping areas appear as the blisters burst. The affected area rapidly gets larger as the infection spreads.
- Yellow/straw-coloured crusts form over the sores.

Immediate Action
- See the doctor immediately.
- If the child is away from home and with other children, contact the parents immediately. The child should be cared for at home, away from other children.
- Make sure that the child uses only their own face flannel and towel to prevent the spread to others.

Ongoing Care The doctor will prescribe some antibiotic cream which should be applied as directed, probably several times a day. Carers should wear gloves when removing crusts and applying the cream.

Discourage the child from touching the affected area(s).

Hygiene precautions include washing of bedding, face flannels and towels and ensuring that each member of the family is careful to only use their own bedding and washing equipment.

As it takes about 5 days for the infection to clear up the child should stay at home for this period. Impetigo can spread like wildfire through a group of children.

Possible Complications
- Generalised infection can occur if impetigo is not treated – without treatment it can last for months.

- Scarring of the skin may occur after repeated scratching.
- Impetigo caused by streptococcal bacteria can cause kidney complications. Observe the child for any swelling of the tissues, especially around the face, and look for blood in the urine.

Further Information

If a child has a cold, put Vaseline around the nose to prevent the skin being broken as the nose is wiped.

> ## Remember
> Keep children's nails short and clean to prevent bacteria growing under the nails which may enter the skin if it is scratched and broken.

Case study

Amelia was just recovering from a cold which had made her feel tired and miserable, her skin was red and looked sore around her nose. She had not been to nursery for 3 days and now she was beginning to feel better she wanted to see her friends again. Her mother thought that, as it was Friday, a morning at nursery would not overtire her and she could regain her full energy over the weekend. The nursery staff and children were happy to see her back again, and Amelia joined in with all the activities. She began to get tired at story time and sucked her thumb and fingers as she sat and listened.

That afternoon her mother noticed small blisters appearing around her nose and mouth which were itching. By the evening they were bursting and Amelia was crying with the discomfort. Her mother comforted her and applied some antiseptic cream before she went to bed.

In the morning yellow scabs had formed over the burst blisters. The GP diagnosed impetigo and prescribed antibiotic cream.

1 How do you think Amelia caught impetigo?
2 Could anything have been done to prevent the infection?
3 What hygiene precautions should Amelia's mother take to prevent the rest of the family being affected?

COLD SORES

What Are Cold Sores?

Cold sores are small blisters that appear around the lips. They are very common between 1 and 4 years of age.

What Causes Cold Sores?

Cold sores are caused by the herpes simplex virus. Triggers for cold sores may be:
- cold weather
- dry winds
- sunlight
- raised temperature.

How To Recognise Cold Sores

- A tingling, pricking sensation around the mouth a few hours before the cold sore appears.

- Small, clear blisters appear around the mouth forming crusts as they burst. Cold sores have a more regular shape than impetigo.
- Reddened skin surrounds the cold sore. It is itchy and sore.

Immediate Action
- For many children no treatment is necessary from the doctor – but if the sores are causing discomfort the doctor may prescribe an anti-viral cream.
- Cold drinks and ice will relieve the itchiness.
- Use lipsalve for dry lips.

Ongoing Care
Cold sores should have healed within 2 weeks.

Using a cold sore remedy containing acyclovir (an antiviral drug found in most over-the-counter cold-sore creams) as soon as the tingling starts will reduce the severity of an attack.

Possible Complications
Touching the cold sore can spread the virus to other parts of the body.

Further Information
There are no cures for cold sores but as the child gets older they tend to get fewer outbreaks.

Remember

Frequent hand washing reduces the risk of skin infections and avoids spreading them to other areas of the body and to other people.

 Progress check

1 How would you recognise psoriasis?
2 What type of treatment will a child with psoriasis require?
3 How could a childcare worker help to prevent the child experiencing social isolation because of their skin condition?
4 What is impetigo?
5 How is impetigo spread from person to person?
6 What are the signs and symptoms of the condition?
7 What immediate action should a childcare worker take if they suspect impetigo?
8 How could you tell the difference between a cold sore and impetigo?
9 What hygiene precautions should be taken if a child has a cold sore?

ATHLETE'S FOOT

What Is Athlete's Foot?
Athlete's foot is a fungal infection between the toes which is more common in children who wear trainers all the time, especially during the summer. Fungal infections can affect the hair, skin and nails. Fungi like warm moist areas in which to grow and multiply – in childhood the two most common infections of this sort are athlete's foot and ringworm. See plate 2.

What Causes Athlete's Foot? The fungus is usually caught from the floors of changing rooms and showers at swimming pools, leisure centres and gyms.

How To Recognise Athlete's Foot
- Itchy areas between the toes.
- Sore and cracked skin between the toes – the skin is flaky and may bleed.
- Toenails may be thick and easily broken.

Immediate Action
- Remove shoes and socks. Wash the feet carefully to examine the extent of the rash.
- Over-the-counter remedies are available for treatment or a doctor can prescribe anti-fungal sprays and powders.

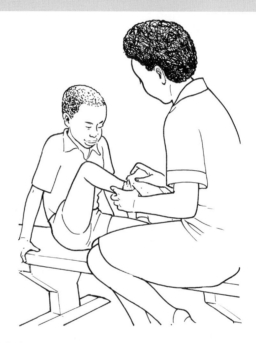

Dry the feet carefully, especially between the toes

Ongoing Care
- Wash and dry feet twice daily, taking care to dry carefully between the toes. Ensure that the child uses their own towel to prevent cross-infection.
- Cotton socks and shoes made of natural fibres, for example leather or canvas, are preferable when the feet must be covered.
- Sprinkle athlete's foot powder in the socks and shoes.
- The condition should have cleared up in 1–2 weeks. If it has not improved or if the nails seem infected, consult a doctor.

Further Information To prevent a recurrence leave the feet open to the air – going bare foot is ideal if possible, or use open-toed sandals. Avoid constant use of trainers which do not let the feet breath.

Good Practice

Feet should be washed daily and dried between the toes.

RINGWORM

What Is Ringworm? Ringworm is a common rash in school children which can affect the scalp, the face and the body. See plate 2.

What Causes Ringworm? Ringworm is a fungal infection usually caught by direct contact with infected children, animals or soil. It can also be passed by sharing hats, combs and clothing. Fungal infections can affect the hair, skin and nails. Fungi like warm moist areas in which to grow and multiply – in childhood the two most common infections of this sort are athlete's foot and ringworm.

How To Recognise Ringworm

Scalp
- Hair breaking close to the scalp resulting in bald patches.
- Large flakes of skin in the hair.
- Severe itching.

Skin
- Rash is a red/pink ring or oval.
- Raised, inflamed edges.
- Severe itching.

Immediate Action A doctor must be seen, who will prescribe the appropriate anti-fungal cream or lotion. If the scalp is affected or if the condition is widespread an antifungal medicine may be prescribed.

Ongoing Care
- If the cause is an animal, treatment should be given by a vet.
- Separate towels and flannels.
- No sharing of combs or other personal equipment.
- Regular hand washing.

Possible Complications A kerion, which is a pus-filled area of inflammation, may result. This will need treatment with antibiotics from a doctor.

 Progress check
1 What sort of conditions do fungi thrive in?
2 How can children catch athlete's foot and how is it encouraged to reproduce?
3 What would the child complain of if they had athlete's foot?
4 How can the condition be treated and its recurrence prevented?
5 How would you recognise ringworm on the scalp and on the skin?
6 What treatment and ongoing care is recommended?

ALOPECIA

What Is Alopecia?	Alopecia means baldness.

What Causes Alopecia?

Alopecia can be a symptom of another condition, for example ringworm. In babies bald patches are increasingly common, especially on the back of the head because of current recommendations to put babies to sleep on their backs – fine hair can be rubbed off.

In children alopecia can be the result of worry and anxiety – children may pull and twiddle with their hair as they concentrate and pull the hair out resulting in bald patches.

Tight braids, plaits and pony tails can put stress on the hair root and pull the hair out.

Alopecia areata is caused by a simple illness or emotional upset and results in scattered bald patches anywhere on the head.

Chemotherapy used to treat malignant conditions usually results in severe hair loss.

How To Recognise Alopecia

- Hair loss.
- Hair coming out in large quantities when combing or brushing the hair.
- Bald patches on the scalp.

Immediate Action

- Examine the scalp – ringworm will result in reddened, scaly patches and itching (see page 231).
- Remove braids and hair styles that may be the cause of the hair loss.
- Consult a doctor if there is no obvious cause or if you suspect ringworm.
- Hair will usually grow back slowly.

Ongoing Care

- Reassure the child.
- Children should be discouraged from pulling their hair.
- Hairstyles must not put strain in the hair root.
- Causes of anxiety should be dealt with sympathetically.

Possible Complications

Psychological problems associated with excessive teasing and even bullying about their appearance.

Remember

Hair loss in children is usually only temporary. Children will require gentle support and understanding from their carers to enable them to cope with this short-term situation.

Case study

Cassandra had lots of thick, black, curly hair which her mother braided for her. Because the hair quickly escaped from the plaits her mother braided them more tightly, sometimes using beads and ribbons. It took several hours to complete but lasted for several weeks and her hair could be washed with the braids still in. Cassie loved the beads and enjoyed the admiring looks and comments from her friends at primary school. When the hair began to grow out and her mother undid the plaits, she was amazed to see some bald patches. These were especially noticeable at the front and on the top of Cassie's head. When she noticed lots of hair loose in her hands her mother fainted.

1 Why had Cassie developed bald patches?
2 What could be done to prevent the hair loss?
3 How could a childcare worker support this child at school?

WARTS

What Are Warts?
Warts are small, hard growths on the skin surface which occur individually or in clusters. They are very common in children, usually on the fingers, feet, knees and face. See plate 3.

What Causes Warts?
Papillomavirus, a virus which invades the outer skin cells causing them to overgrow, is the cause of warts. They are passed by direct contact with an infected person but are not highly contagious. The immune system takes time to recognise the virus but when it does, the wart disappears within days.

How To Recognise Warts
There are three different types of warts:

Common wart
A hard, raised growth with a rough surface. They are not usually painful.

Plane wart
A smooth growth very slightly raised from the skin surface, generally on the hands and face. They may be slightly itchy.

Plantar wart
A verruca (see page 234).

Immediate Action
- Check for other warts – if there are none it is probably best to wait for the wart to disappear without interfering, especially if the wart is painless and not causing any distress.
- If pain is present it is because the surrounding skin has become infected, so a doctor should be consulted.

Immediate Action (cont)	■ There may be many warts. If so over-the-counter remedies can be purchased, but great care must be taken when they are applied not to damage the surrounding skin. The instructions should be followed carefully.
	■ Warts on the face can be treated by a dermatologist who may use cryotherapy (freezing).
Ongoing Care	Treatment usually takes several weeks. Most warts eventually disappear. Children should be advised not to pick or scratch them as this can spread the infection.
Possible Complications	■ Skin infections.
	■ Burns to healthy skin if treatment solutions are not applied correctly.

Remember
Always consult a doctor if a lump on the skin is causing concern.

VERRUCAE

What Are Verrucae?	Verrucae are warts on the soles of the feet (plantar warts), which are flat due to the pressure on them when walking. See plate 3.
What Causes Verrucae?	Papillomavirus – usually caught on the feet from the floors of changing rooms and showers at schools, swimming pools, leisure centres and gyms – is the cause of verrucae.
How To Recognise Verrucae	■ Small, hard, gritty area(s) on the sole of the foot.
	■ The surface is usually speckled with black spots (very small blood clots).
	■ Pain and discomfort when walking if the verruca is on the ball of the foot or the heel.
Immediate Action	■ Verrucae are difficult to eradicate without medical treatment and should be examined by a doctor or chiropodist.
	■ They are best treated with cryotherapy (freezing) with liquid nitrogen if they persist.
Ongoing Care	Prevent spread by ensuring the child wears a plastic sock when using communal changing rooms and swimming pools.
Possible Complications	Skin infections.

Further Information   School nurses used to conduct regular verrucae clinics to try to eliminate the problem. However these had limited success so now most health authorities have discontinued them. Verrucae are not as highly infectious as they were once believed to be.

 Progress check

1 What are the possible causes of alopecia in children?
2 How could you find out why a child was losing their hair?
3 How could you help them to cope with this situation?
4 What are the three different types of warts?
5 What causes them?
6 Explain the different types of treatment for warts.
7 What are the possible complications?
8 How would you recognise a verruca?

Case study

The Year 2 Infants at Rosewood Primary School go swimming once a week at the local leisure centre. Several of the children have learnt to swim there and they all enjoy their time in the water. One of the parents insists that her son wears plastic socks when he goes swimming to avoid the risk of getting a verruca. Some of the other children laugh at him because they think he looks silly with socks on in the swimming pool.

1 Do you think that this is a sensible precaution to avoid verrucae? Explain your answer.
2 How could a childcare worker or teacher reassure this parent?

Activity

Prepare an information leaflet for parents to explain about verrucae and palmar warts.
Include the following.

- How the conditions are spread.
- Risk areas for transmission.
- Appearance.
- Treatment and prevention.

SUNBURN

What Is Sunburn?   Sunburn is intense burning of the skin by the sun.

What Causes Sunburn?   Over exposure to sunlight. Ultraviolet rays cause a serious inflammation of the skin.

How To Recognise Sunburn
- Reddened skin in white races. Black skin looks darker than usual.
- Area affected is slightly swollen.
- Acute pain and discomfort. The skin is extremely tender and feels tight.
- Blistering, cracking or bleeding of the skin may occur.

Immediate Action
- Take the child indoors.
- Apply calamine lotion or a cold compress to the affected areas.
- Leave clothing off when indoors – cover the body with loose cotton clothing if it is necessary to go outside.
- Provide plenty of drinks to prevent dehydration.
- Give liquid paracetamol to ease the pain.
- If the child develops a temperature, tepid sponging of the face will increase comfort.

Ongoing Care   Keep the child away from sunshine for at least three days. Continue to soothe the burns with calamine.

Prevention
Most cases of sunburn are the result of less than vigilant care. Children are not aware of the dangers of sunshine – they simply want to enjoy their outdoor play. Parents and carers must take responsible precautions when children are outside. A high factor suncream or sunblock is essential on all skin types and colours, black skin can burn as easily as pale skin. This should be reapplied frequently, especially after swimming. Shoulders and face are vulnerable in the water, so swimming in a tee-shirt is advisable. A wide-brimmed hat helps to protect the face. Gradual exposure to the sun is sensible.

Water, sun and sand reflect the ultra violet rays and children can burn even when the sun is not shining directly on them.

Possible Complications   Children with severe blistering or feverishness should be seen by a doctor.

Heatstroke
This can be serious and results in dehydration and problems with circulation. The child will be feverish, lose their appetite and be generally unwell. They may develop drowsiness and confusion – if this is the case a doctor should be seen urgently.

Malignancy in later years
Over exposure to the sun in childhood has been proven to cause skin cancer in some people. This is becoming more common with the thinning of the ozone layer.

Remember
'Slip, slap, slop': tee-shirt, hat and high-factor sun-cream. This is the best protection against sunburn and heat stroke.

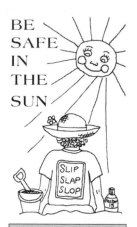

BE SAFE IN THE SUN

Follow the simple
SLIP, SLAP, SLOP
guide.

Slip on a shirt, slap on
a hat, slop on some
sun-cream

 Progress check

1 How can you recognise sunburn?
2 What steps should be taken to prevent it from occurring?
3 How could you recognise heatstroke?

Case study

Leroy, aged 4 years is an energetic child who loves to play outside in all weathers. In the summer his child-minder often takes the children to a local outdoor paddling pool where they have a picnic on the grass next to the water – there is a playground nearby where the children also play. She always makes sure that the children are protected by using creams, hats and tee-shirts when the sun is shining. One warm but overcast day in May, she takes them to the park for a picnic, not expecting them to use the pool. Leroy insists on stripping down to his underpants for a paddle and proceeds to spend two and a half hours playing in the water. On arriving home, he complains that his shoulders and back hurt. When she looks at them, the child-minder sees that Leroy's black skin is dark and swollen.

1 What is the cause of Leroy's discomfort?
2 How could this have been prevented?
3 What treatment should the child-minder give to Leroy immediately?
4 What signs should she be aware of that may indicate more serious effects?
5 What is the possible long-term damage to Leroy's skin?

Chapter 10 Infestations

This chapter includes:

- Head lice
- Scabies
- Fleas
- Threadworms
- Toxocara

Infestations are common in childhood and also occur amongst childcare workers. The main defence against these parasites is stringent hygiene safeguards in childcare establishments and at home. Constant vigilance, armed with the knowledge of how to recognise specific infestations, is crucial.

Parents and carers must also be involved in the prevention, detection and treatment of infestations and be provided with relevant and topical health education.

Epidemics of some parasites are fairly common because those which are spread by direct contact usually involve touching hands and heads. Children work and play very close to each other so the parasites can spread easily. Early detection and treatment is the only way to control their transmission, so childcare workers have an important role to play. Because they work with children they are in a position to notice the first signs and take active steps to control the spread by informing parents and suggesting relevant and appropriate treatments.

Remember

Human parasites are not aware of social class and so an infestation is no reflection on a child or their carer. Head lice, for instance, are thought to prefer clean hair and are just as prevalent in private establishments as they are in state schools.

HEAD LICE

What Are Head Lice?	Small, wingless insects which infest the scalp and suck blood.

What Causes Head Lice?

Head lice are transmitted from head to head via close contact. They are not particular about which head they infest and they like clean hair and skin.

Children are most vulnerable because they work and play together with heads in close proximity.

Most children are infested with head lice at some time in their school career!

How To Recognise Head Lice

- Intense itching because head lice bite the skin to suck blood. Any child scratching their head repeatedly should be checked.
- Nits can be seen cemented onto the hair shaft, near to the scalp. These

are eggs which look like dandruff, but are impossible to brush off as they remain firmly attached to the hair.

■ The eggs hatch leaving an empty shell, still cemented to the hair. These look like small white specks near the base of the hair. Children who have been infested for some time will have a series of nits in varying stages of development down the hair shaft towards the root.

■ Long-term infestations can cause lack of sleep, reduction in energy and vitality – the phrase 'feeling lousy' resulted from the effects of the louse.

Immediate Action

■ If the child has asthma or a history of allergies, or is under 2 years of age, a doctor should be consulted for advice about treatment.

■ Inform the childcare establishment so that other parents can be advised to check their children's heads.

■ Wet the hair and comb it with a fine tooth comb over a piece of white paper. It may be easier to comb after conditioner is applied. Lice will fall out of the hair and can be seen crawling on the paper.

■ Fine tooth combing is the preferred method of treatment and should be performed every 3–4 days for 2 weeks.

■ There are a range of insecticides available to treat head lice but some species are becoming resistant to particular treatments. It is therefore preferable to check with the doctor or health visitor about which brand to use before commencing treatment.

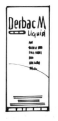
Derbac M Liquid – used for treating head lice, crab lice, scabies mites and their eggs

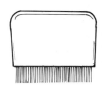
Nit comb – used for removing nits from the hair after treatment

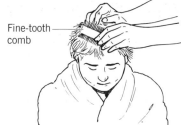
Fine-tooth comb

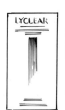
Lyclear Creme Rinse – used for treating head lice and their eggs

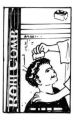
Robi Comb – electronic comb used for detecting and killing lice

Useful remedies for hair lice

Homeopathic remedies

Media scares about the dangers of organophosphates in insecticides have resulted in some alternative therapies being used to treat head lice. However, overuse of essential oils in unskilled hands can be hazardous, so a qualified aromatherapist should be consulted.

Tea-tree oil and eucalyptus oil are effective in dealing with head lice and are not harmful to children.

Recipe

Mix together:

15 drops of tea-tree oil

15 drops of eucalyptus oil

5 drops of oil of rosemary

5 drops of oil of geranium

30mls of olive oil or vegetable oil.

Rub into the child's hair, allow the solution to soak in for several hours and comb with a fine tooth comb to remove dead lice and nits. Apply tea-tree oil shampoo to wash out the oil. Check the hair regularly and reapply 2–3 times a week.

Ongoing Care

All combs and brushes should be washed and scrubbed in hot, soapy water to remove any eggs.

Insecticides should not be used to prevent infestation. The best prevention is regular combing or brushing of the hair, preferably straight after school or nursery as well as morning and evening. This breaks the legs of the louse and makes it incapable of laying eggs. Regular inspections of the head by parents and carers will spot infestations early – the hair behind the ears and at the back of the head/neck are the most likely areas.

Possible Complications

Infected scalp.

> **Remember**
>
> Daily combing of the hair (especially after a playgroup, nursery or school session) is an effective way of preventing infestations. This breaks the legs of the louse and prevents them from laying any eggs.

Good Practice

Head lice infestation is not a cause for excluding a child from any childcare establishment or activity. The child should not be made to feel uncomfortable or dirty.

The procedure to implement if a child is seen to have head lice is as follows.

1 Inform the parent sensitively in private when the child is collected. Some parents will be horrified and require reassurance that head lice are very common and that they prefer clean heads.

2 Offer an explanatory leaflet to support your comments – the local health centre will have current literature.

3 Discuss possible treatments.

4 Suggest the parent contacts their health visitor for advice, especially if they are anxious.

5 Remind the parent about the policy of the establishment which should include the following points.
- All parents will be informed when head lice have been detected and their co-operation will be required to deal with a possible outbreak.
- Apply treatment solutions of preference.
- Inform the establishment if lice or nits are found.
- Regularly comb and brush the hair, especially after a session in any childcare establishment.
- Regular head checks at home.
- Parents who refuse to deal with the problem and repeatedly send affected children will require special consideration.

 Progress check

1 Why are children vulnerable to head lice infestations?
2 What is the best means of preventing head lice infestations?
3 How can infestations be treated?

Case study

Geoffrey is an only child. His parents had wanted to have a family since they got married and had tried almost every kind of fertility treatment. When they had given up trying Geoffrey arrived. His parents are obviously devoted to him. A few weeks after he started at infant school an outbreak of head lice occurred. All the parents were informed and asked to check their children's heads for lice and nits and advised about the current treatment. The next day Geoffrey's mother stormed into the infant school exclaiming that her child had caught nits from a dirty child. She said that unless the staff could prevent her son from playing with this child again she would not be bringing him back.

1 Why do you think that this parent reacted in this way ?
2 How can she be reassured by:
- the staff
- other parents
- the school nurse?

SCABIES

What Are Scabies? External animal parasites which infest the skin, they are also known as itch mites. The itch mite burrows into the skin to lay eggs. See plate 3.

What Causes Scabies? Scabies are passed from person to person by skin-to-skin physical contact. They are also transmitted via clothing, bedding and towels. Anyone can catch scabies – it is not only associated with poor personal hygiene.

How To Recognise Scabies

- Itchy skin which is worse at night.
- Thin track marks (where the mite has burrowed) in areas where the skin is thin, such as between the fingers and toes, the inner wrist and arm, genitals etc. These may be difficult to see if the child has been scratching furiously.
- Sore rash and scabs caused by scratching.
- Scabies can be mistaken for eczema.

Immediate Action

- The doctor should be seen within 24 hours. Scabies will not clear up without treatment with lotions and emulsions prescribed by a doctor.
- The whole family should be treated as should all bedding and clothing.
- The lotion should be applied to the whole body and washed off after 24 hours.

Ongoing Care All clothing and bedding should be washed and ironed to kill the parasites and prevent re-infestation.

Mites usually die within 3 weeks of treatment, but itching can continue for a few weeks. This itchiness can be treated with an antihistamine cream.

Possible Complications Impetigo (see page 227). Intense scratching can damage the skin, allowing other pathogenic organisms to enter. This secondary infection is common.

Good Practice

People who have been in contact with the affected child(ren) should be told about the infection so that they can be examined and get treatment if necessary.

 Progress check

1 What are scabies and how would you recognise an infection?
2 What may a scabies rash be mistaken for?
3 What are the possible complications of scabies infection?

Remember

In scabies infestations, thin track marks can usually be clearly seen in areas where the skin is thin, such as between the fingers and toes, the inner wrist and arm.

Case study

The Baker family and the Wilson family decided to celebrate New Year's Eve together – they would have a party and all of their friends could bring their children because baby-sitters would be impossible to find. The children could sleep together – boys in one room and girls in another. It was exciting to be allowed to stay up late and then go to sleep with your friends. David Wilson had been scratching his arms for the past few days and the itching had kept him awake at night at home. He fell asleep easily that night as they all snuggled into the same bed for warmth and company. The next morning the children were up and about, encouraging their parents to do likewise. A few days later Mrs Baker noticed that her two sons were scratching – they both suffered from eczema so she applied some E45 cream to moisten their skin. That night they were both crying because the itching was much worse. Mrs Wilson called in the next day and in the course of their conversation she commented on the rash that David had developed on his arms and hands, and the itching that had kept him awake recently. Both mothers decided to take their children to the doctor.

1 What is a possible cause of this itchy rash?
2 What other signs could the parents have observed?
3 How could all the children have been infested?
4 What hygiene precautions should be taken now?
5 Should the other parents be contacted and if so, how could they be told about the infestation?

FLEAS

What Are Fleas? Fleas are small insects which are able to bite through skin and suck blood. The human flea is virtually extinct in Britain.

What Causes Fleas? Children may be bitten by fleas which usually infest cats and/or dogs. These fleas also live in parts of the house where the animal sleeps or plays, for example carpets, sofas and soft furnishings, and can live for a long time without contact with the animal. They will bite humans if they cannot get back to their host cat or dog.

How To Recognise Fleas
- Fleas cannot fly but they can jump from person to person and, although very small, can be clearly seen with the human eye.
- Bites may be painful, itchy and swell.
- Severe cases can result in painful lumps and swellings.

Immediate Action	■ Wash the bite with unperfumed soap and water.
	■ Calamine lotion will soothe the itching.

If there is no improvement the doctor may prescribe:

■ antihistamines to control itching and/or
■ antibiotics if the bite is infected

Ongoing Care	Fleas can be controlled by applying insecticide powder to animals and their bedding and to carpets, floors and furnishings.
Possible Complications	■ Severe allergic reaction.
	■ Impetigo if bacteria enters through broken skin.
	■ Fleas can transmit typhus, bubonic plaque and anthrax. Some fleas may carry other germs which they pass from person to person as the fleas feed.

 Progress check

1 Where may fleas live?
2 How could you recognise a flea bite?
3 What treatment should be started as soon as possible after a diagnosis is made?
4 What are the possible complications associated with fleas?

THREADWORMS

What Are Threadworms?	Parasitic worms which live in the intestines and most commonly affect children, although several members of the family may also be affected. They are most common in children between 5 and 9 years of age. Children living in urban areas are most vulnerable – it is estimated that up to 50 per cent of children living in London are affected at any one time.
What Causes Threadworms?	Threadworms are transmitted via unwashed vegetables, soil, towels, bedding and less than scrupulous hygiene. Children catch threadworms by sucking contaminated objects or eating foods which contain worm eggs. The swallowed eggs develop into adult worms in the intestines. The female worms come out of the anus at night, when the child is quiet and still, to lay their eggs on the skin around the bottom. It causes severe itching around the bottom and when the child scratches her/his bottom the eggs are caught under the finger nails. If the fingers are then put in the mouth the fresh eggs are ingested to develop into more threadworms.

The nails will contaminate all that the child touches, and so worms can spread quickly and easily around any childcare establishment.

The eggs can survive at room temperature in dust for 2–3 weeks.

How To Recognise Threadworms

- Itching around the anus especially at night, when the female lays her eggs.
- Girls may also have an itchy vulva.
- Constant scratching may cause an inflamed anus and very sore bottom.
- Sleep may be disturbed.
- Some children may begin to wet the bed although enuresis is not a definite sign of threadworms.
- Threadworms look like small, white threads and may be seen in freshly passed stools.
- Occasionally abdominal pain may result from a heavy infestation of threadworms.

Immediate Action

- See the doctor who will prescribe an oral anti-worm medicine. This is usually repeated 10–14 days later.
- The doctor may ask for a sample of the eggs for examination – these can be collected by pressing some sellotape onto the child's anus first thing in the morning before the child washes or uses the toilet. The tape will collect any eggs.
- The whole family should be treated as many may be affected without symptoms.

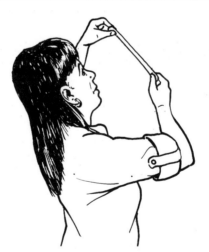

Eggs can be collected on a piece of sticky tape

Ongoing Care The drug treatment combined with thorough hand washing, nail scrubbing and scrupulous attention to hygiene including separate towels, flannels, bedding etc. is generally effective.

Keep fingernails short and clean – worms depend on long, dirty nails to pass from person to person.

Children should be encouraged to maintain careful handwashing and nail scrubbing first thing in the morning and after having the bowels open.

Remember
Children who complain of an itchy or sore bottom, especially at night, should be investigated for threadworm infestation.

Hand washing before all meals and after going to the toilet should be reinforced.

Ensure that fresh food is washed well before eating.

Further Information

Stringent hygiene precautions should be maintained to prevent the spread of threadworms. Children are especially vulnerable in their childcare establishment if there has been an occurrence of threadworms. Carers must pay strict attention to the cleanliness of toys and objects which children may put in their mouths – as well as maintaining routine food hygiene.

> ## Good Practice
>
> Childcare workers should reassure parents that this infestation is not a reflection on their parenting skills. Threadworm are very common in childhood and children do not suffer from permanent harm.

 Progress check

1 What are threadworms?
2 How can they get into the human digestive system?
3 How would you recognise a threadworm infection?
4 How can a sample of eggs be collected?
5 What hygiene precautions must be taken to prevent the spread of the threadworm?

Activity

Prepare an information leaflet for parents about threadworms. Include the following.
- How threadworms are spread.
- Signs and symptoms of threadworm infestation.
- Treatment.
- Prevention.

Case study

Juliet, aged 7, enjoyed helping her uncle and aunt on their allotment; they grew carrots, potatoes, beans and cabbages, and she loved to dig and try to pull up the root vegetables. She was always careful to wash her muddy hands before meals but enjoyed eating her weekly sweet allowance while she was digging. She had been finding it difficult to get off to sleep for the past week because her younger brother Jason kept calling for their father and complaining that he could not sleep because his bottom hurt. She began to think it could be catching, because now her bottom was itchy and if she scratched it, it got very sore. She called her parents.

1 What is causing these itchy bottoms?
2 How could both children have been affected by this infection?
3 What precautions can the family take to prevent any further infestations?

TOXOCARA

What Is Toxocara?

Toxocara is a type of roundworm which is active in young dogs and foxes. Older dogs gain immunity by about 6 months of age.

In the human the larvae – which result from the eggs – find it difficult to locate the intestines. They move around the body resulting in inflammation of organs, for example lungs, brain, eyes, kidneys and muscles.

The toxocara affecting cats can cause similar symptoms.

What Causes Toxocara?

Very young children are the most commonly affected and they swallow the tiny toxocara eggs as a result of contact with:

- the tongues of puppies as they lick their faces
- crawling or falling on carpets, grass or other areas where eggs may be deposited.

How To Recognise Toxocara

There may be a combination of several vague and non-specific symptoms which makes diagnosis difficult. However, affected children have usually had a new puppy in the family and are aged between 1 and 7 years.

Signs and symptoms may include some or all of the following depending upon the site(s) of the larvae:

- failure to thrive with associated poor weight gain
- pica – an urge to eat unusual substances such as coal, soil or strange combinations of food
- cough
- anaemia – pale skin, tiredness and general lethargy
- convulsions
- blurred vision if the eyes are infected.

Immediate Action

- The doctor may take some blood samples to check for toxocara antibodies and anaemia.
- Specific signs and symptoms will be treated, for example anaemia can be treated with iron supplements and an increased amount of iron in the diet. Antibiotics will resolve any infections.
- Treatment for toxocara may take several weeks with specific drugs.

Ongoing Care   If the condition is left untreated, the body's immune system and defence mechanisms will usually overcome the infection within about 18 months.

Possible Complications   Blindness can result if the larvae affect the eyes.

Good Practice

To reduce the risk of toxocara infection to young children to a minimum, the following precautions can be implemented.

- Puppies should be wormed regularly.
- Children should be discouraged from allowing dogs to lick their faces.
- Children should wash their hands after playing with pets and especially before eating.
- Dog owners should not allow their animals to foul public areas such as parks and pavements.
- Communities can ensure the safety of playing fields, sandpits and playgrounds by erecting fencing and inspecting the areas regularly.

 Progress check

1 What is toxocara?
2 How is toxocara spread?
3 How would you recognise the signs and symptoms?
4 What is a possible complication of toxocara?
5 How can the risk of toxocara infection be reduced?

Chapter 11 Digestive and dietary disorders

This chapter includes:

- The digestive system
- Gastro-enteritis
- Appendicitis
- The coeliac condition
- Diabetes mellitus
- Obesity
- Anorexia nervosa
- Constipation
- Hepatitis A
- Food refusal
- Toddlers' diarrhoea
- Rickets

A well-balanced diet is essential in childhood to ensure healthy growth and development. Childcarers must be familiar with the components of a healthy diet so that they can provide the essential nutrients to the children in their care. However, even with a well balanced diet, illnesses involving the digestive system are extremely common in childhood; only coughs and colds are more prevalent. Childcare workers will certainly be present when a child is showing the first signs of digestive problems and will be responsible for recognising symptoms and caring for the child in the early stages of illness. To do this effectively, they require insight into the possible childhood conditions so that safe care of the child can be maintained and medical assistance sought when it is necessary.

They may also care for a child with a chronic – long-term – digestive condition and will need knowledge and understanding of that illness in order to provide competent and empathetic care.

The digestive system

Digestion is the process which breaks down food into smaller components that the body can absorb and use. Each part of the digestive tract has a specialised function in breaking down the foods and liquids swallowed.

Dietary needs

Good nutrition is essential for general health and well-being.

Food is essential for four reasons:
- to enable growth, repair and replacement of tissues
- to help fight disease
- to maintain the proper functioning of body systems
- to provide energy and warmth.

The food eaten should contain the *nutrients* children need. Before these nutrients can be used the food must be digested by the body.

Inadequate dietary intake is still the most common cause of failure to thrive. Good eating habits begin at an early age and childcare workers need to ensure that children establish healthy eating patterns which will promote normal growth and development.

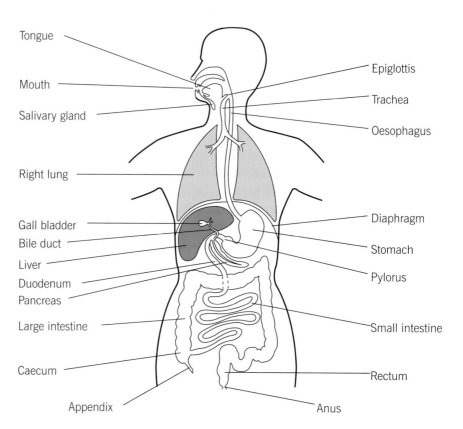

The human digestive system

The essential nutrients

To be healthy, the body needs a combination of different nutrients – protein, fat, carbohydrate, vitamins, minerals and water.

Protein, fat, carbohydrates and water are present in the foods we eat and drink in large quantities. Vitamins and minerals are present only in small quantities, so it is much more common for those to be lacking in a child's diet.

Protein

Protein foods are essential for growth and repair of the body. Protein foods are divided into *first-class* and *second-class* proteins.

Sources of first-class protein include meat, fish, chicken, cheese, milk and milk products. Sources of second-class proteins include nuts and seeds, pulses (e.g. black beans, chick peas, lentils, soya beans, kidney beans), cereals (e.g. rice, cornmeal and oats) and cereal-based foods such as bread, pasta, chapattis, noodles.

Protein foods are made up of *amino acids*. There are ten essential amino acids. First-class protein foods contain all of them, second-class protein foods contain some.

Carbohydrates

Carbohydrates are divided into *starches* and *sugars*, which provide energy for the body.

Sources of starch include cereals, beans, lentils, potatoes, plantain, pasta and yams. Sources of sugar include sugar from cane or beet, fruit and vegetables, honey and milk.

Carbohydrates are broken down into glucose before the body can use them. Sugars are quickly converted and give a quick source of energy, starches take longer to convert to glucose so they provide a steadier longer lasting supply of energy.

Fats

Fats provide energy for the body and contain essential vitamins. They also make food more pleasant to eat and aid its passage through the digestive tract. Fats are divided into *saturated* fats and *unsaturated* fats.

Sources of saturated fat include butter, cheese, milk, lard, meat and palm oil. Sources of unsaturated fat include fish oil, olive oil, sunflower oil, corn oil and peanut oil.

Vitamins and minerals

Vitamins and minerals are present only in small quantities in food, but they are essential for growth, development and normal functioning of the body.

 Progress check

1 Why is food essential?
2 What are the essential nutrients?
3 Why are proteins necessary?
4 What are the different types of protein and what sort of foods are they found in?
5 What is the difference between starches and sugars?
6 Give some examples of the sources of saturated and unsaturated fats.

GASTRO-ENTERITIS

What Is Gastro-enteritis?	Inflammation or infection of the stomach and intestines, gastro-enteritis is the most common condition of the digestive tract in childhood. Fifty per cent of cases affect children under 5 years.

What Causes Gastro-enteritis?

- Bacteria in food and drinks.
- Airborne viruses/bacteria.
- Contact with infected faeces usually via poor handwashing techniques. The rotavirus is thought to be responsible for about half of all cases. Several bacteria cause gastro-enteritis, for example salmonella, escerechai coli (E. coli) and shigella.

How To Recognise Gastro-enteritis

A young child will be miserable and cry, refusing food and not participating in any play. Other signs will follow:

- vomiting
- diarrhoea
- loss of appetite
- high temperature – more common with the rotavirus
- feeling and appearing generally unwell and lethargic.

Immediate Action

- For the first 24 hours offer clear fluids – cooled, previously boiled water – or rehydrating solution to drink.
- If there is no improvement in this time seek medical help.

Ongoing Care

- Gradually re-introduce the usual diet.
- Pay scrupulous attention to hygiene, including personal hygiene.

Possible Complications

Dehydration; lactose intolerance – see page 177.

Hospital admission may be necessary for children who become dehydrated as a result of diarrhoea and vomiting. Intravenous fluids will be given to replace the lost fluid.

Further Information

See p. 163 'Good Practice: Preventing dehydration.

An outbreak in a nursery or school should be investigated by taking stool samples to detect the causative organism. It may then be possible to identify the cause of the epidemic.

A vaccine against the rotavirus is being developed.

Remember

Always contact parents if a child develops gastro-enteritis. An adult who is responsible for a young child should seek medical advice if vomiting and diarrhoea continue for more than 24 hours.

✅ **Progress check**

1 What causes gastro-enteritis?
2 What are the signs and symptoms of gastro-enteritis?

3 What action should a childcare worker take if a child is vomiting?
4 When should the doctor be called?
5 How can childcare staff prevent the spread of gastro-enteritis in a childcare establishment?

APPENDICITIS

What Is Appendicitis? The appendix is not involved in the digestive process – it is a small finger-like tube that is attached to the colon. Appendicitis is an inflammation or infection of the appendix. It is unusual in a child under 2 years of age.

What Causes Appendicitis? There is no known cause for the sudden flare-up of the appendix.

How To Recognise Appendicitis

- It may be difficult to recognise appendicitis because the condition can affect children differently. Sometimes the condition begins slowly with discomfort that comes and goes (this is known as a *grumbling appendix*). However, the following are unmistakable signs.
- Dull pain around the tummy button which gets sharper and more severe.
- Pain moves down to the right lower part of the abdomen.
- Pain increases if the child moves or breathes deeply. The child will lie still, sometimes with the knees raised to take the pressure off the abdomen.
- Raised temperature.
- Loss of appetite.
- Feeling nauseous (sick).
- Constipation OR diarrhoea.

Immediate Action

- Call the doctor and parents immediately. If the pain has been present for more than 6 hours, call an ambulance. Do not give the child anything to eat or drink. Giving paracetamol may shield the pain and make it difficult for the doctor to diagnose the condition.
- If the condition is confirmed, the child will be admitted to hospital for surgical removal of the appendix (appendicectomy). This is one of the commonest operations performed in childhood.

Ongoing Care Children are usually discharged home about 3 days after the operation. They recover much more quickly than adults!

A normal diet can be eaten, and comfortable activities should be

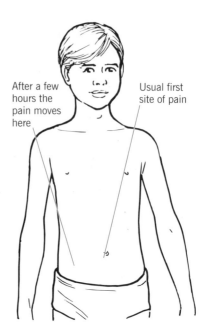

After a few hours the pain moves here

Usual first site of pain

Where the child feels the pain of appendicitis

encouraged, but sport and other vigorous activity should be avoided for about a month after an appendicectomy.

Possible Complications

Peritonitis (inflammation of the lining of the abdomen) will occur if the appendix bursts. This can be fatal if not treated quickly. It causes immense pain in the whole abdomen and is a medical emergency. If this should happen – call an ambulance immediately.

Further Information

For care of children in hospital see Chapter 16.

 Progress check

1 What are the signs of appendicitis?
2 What immediate action should be taken if appendicitis is suspected?
3 How can the childcare worker comfort the child?
4 What treatment will be given if appendicitis is confirmed?
5 What are the possible complications of appendicitis?

THE COELIAC CONDITION

What Is The Coeliac Condition?

Coeliac disease is a rare condition affecting the small intestine which prevents the absorption of nutrients through the wall of the intestines. It is more common in people of European and American origin. The condition was recognised over 100 years ago, but treatment was not established until the 1950s.

What Causes The Coeliac Condition? A sensitivity to a type of protein (gluten) found in wheat, rye, barley and oats results in the lining of the small intestine becoming flattened, so the ability to absorb the nutrients from food is severely reduced. It has been described as an allergy to gluten.

There is an inherited tendency to develop coeliac disease.

How To Recognise The Coeliac Condition Symptoms that usually start soon after weaning is commenced are:

- weight loss – failure to thrive
- pale, bulky stools which float and smell offensive
- breathlessness
- lethargy due to anaemia
- may have a distended abdomen.

The age when children show signs of this illness varies between 9 and 18 months and some may have a slower onset characterised by the following signs:

- lack of growth in height and weight
- iron deficiency anaemia.

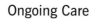

Immediate Action

- A baby/child with the above symptoms will probably have been causing concern for some time before a definite diagnosis is made.
- Any child who is not gaining weight, is constantly tired and/or has fatty, foul-smelling stools should be seen by a doctor. The doctor will take a blood test to detect antibodies to gluten, and a stool sample to measure the amount of fat excreted in the motions. If these are positive then a small sample of the lining of the small intestine (jejunal biopsy) will confirm the diagnosis.

The child with coeliac disease has wasted buttocks and a distended abdomen

Ongoing Care When the child is offered a diet without gluten, recovery is quick and the symptoms disappear within a few weeks. The child will start to gain weight and height, seem happier and have more energy.

Vitamin and mineral supplements may be required for children if the diagnosis has been delayed.

A gluten-free diet will be necessary for life so everyone concerned in the care of the child will need to know exactly what the child can eat – dairy products, eggs, meat, fish, vegetables, rice and corn are gluten-free.

Everything containing flour contains gluten but substitutes are available such as gluten-free bread, flour and pasta. Gluten is found in many foods and The Coeliac Society produce food lists to help those affected to chose the safe options. The crossed wheat is a symbol of a food being gluten free.

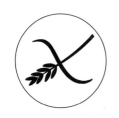

The crossed grain indicates that food is gluten free

Children with this condition should be reviewed regularly and some doctors perform a 'gluten challenge' after 2 to 3 years on the diet. This involves reintroducing gluten into the diet and performing another jejunal biopsy to make sure that the condition is permanent. In most cases the result of the biopsy confirms the original diagnosis.

Possible Complications

The symptoms of the condition may recur if gluten is reintroduced into the diet, accidentally or deliberately.

Iron deficiency anaemia may occur.

Rickets may occur.

There is an increased tendency to cancer of the intestines in people with coeliac disease.

Further Information

Children must be encouraged to keep to the diet. This can be difficult for them at times, when they cannot enjoy a burger or most other convenience, fast-foods. Support groups enable children to meet and share experiences with new friends.

Research shows that there is a link between early weaning with products containing wheat flour and an increased tendency to develop coeliac disease later in life. This is the main reason for the recommendation from health professionals to offer gluten-free foods, such as baby rice, as a first weaning food.

Useful address

The Coeliac Society

PO Box 220

High Wycombe

Bucks HP11 2HY

Activity

Plan a week's diet for a 3- to 4-year-old child with the coeliac condition. Use the Coeliac Society's booklet containing lists of gluten-free products.

- Is this diet suitable for a 'whole family' diet?
- Investigate your local supermarket for the foods listed in the CS booklet. Are they easy to obtain? How does their price compare with similar products which contain gluten?

 Progress check

1 What is the coeliac condition?

2 What happens to the small intestine in the coeliac condition?

3 What are the signs and symptoms of the coeliac condition?

4 What is the symbol for gluten-free foods?

5 What type of foods are gluten free?

6 What is a 'gluten challenge'?

Case study

Amy and Michaela are twins, the youngest children in a family of five. They were both offered only breast milk for the first three months of their lives, and then the breast feeds were complemented with formula milk. Both babies gained weight and remained steady on the 60th centile (see page 111). They were happy and sociable, smiling and laughing at each other and made good developmental progress. They had their immunisations and the health visitor was delighted with their progress. Weaning began when they were $3\frac{1}{2}$ months old and they enjoyed a varied diet of baby food and family meals. When they were weighed at their routine 9-month health check, after their hearing tests, it was clear that Amy was not gaining as much weight as her sister. Her mother told the health visitor that she was miserable and lethargic, not the smiling baby she had once been. She had a good appetite and seemed to eat more than her sister, but her nappies were foul smelling and her stools were pale. The health visitor suspected coeliac disease and suggested that they see the doctor later that day.

1 What signs of coeliac disease was Amy displaying?

2 What may have caused the condition?

3 What is the treatment and when can it be offered to Amy?

4 What difficulties may the family experience with twins on different diets?

DIABETES MELLITUS

What Is Diabetes Mellitus?

Diabetes Mellitus is a metabolic disorder in which the pancreas does not make enough insulin. Insulin is a hormone which enables the body to use and store glucose (sugar). When the body cannot use the glucose taken in the diet, the levels rise in the blood and spill out in the urine.

What Causes Diabetes Mellitus?

1–2 in 1,000 children are affected.

Genetic

There is a family tendency to develop diabetes. A child with two diabetic parents has a 50 per cent chance of developing the disease.

Environmental

Factors in the environment may trigger the onset of diabetes, the most common trigger is infection, for example mumps. Other environmental factors are chemicals and diet for people with a genetic predisposition.

Immune mechanisms

There is an association between diabetes and auto-immune disease of the thyroid and adrenal glands.

How To Recognise Diabetes Mellitus

In 90 per cent of cases in childhood there is an acute (sudden) onset, with signs and symptoms which develop quickly over about a month. In other children the signs are the same but develop more slowly:

- excessive thirst
- frequent passing of urine. Children who have been dry at might may start to wet the bed.
  NB All children with enuresis should have their urine tested for glucose.
- tiredness and lethargy
- loss of appetite
- weight loss of up to 10 per cent of the body weight over 2 to 3 months.
- characteristic smell of pear drops on the breath
- vulval irritation in girls and irritation of the penis in boys due to the sugar-loaded urine.

If the above symptoms are not recognised the condition may proceed to:

- rapid breathing
- drowsiness
- coma.

Immediate Action

- Contact the doctor who will test a urine sample and may take a blood test. If diabetes is the cause of the symptoms, sugar will be present in the blood and urine. The child will be admitted to hospital to stabilise the condition and to assess the individual dietary needs and specific insulin requirements.

Ongoing Care

The child will be discharged on a special diet and needing insulin for the rest of their life.

The aim of the treatment is to maintain the blood glucose levels within the normal range, so a balance is required between the food eaten, the exercise taken and the amount of insulin given.

The diet is usually calculated in 10 gram 'portions' of carbohydrates per day, for example a 3-year-old may need 13 x 10 grams = 130 grams of carbohydrate. Families quickly become proficient at calculating the amount of carbohydrate foods which make up a 10 gram portion.

Blood glucose levels must be taken daily and the insulin dose may be adjusted accordingly.

Insulin is measured in units and parents / carers will be trained to calculate the dose using insulin syringes, guns or pens. They will use various sites on the body for giving the insulin as repeated use of the same area results in thickening of the skin.

Attention to diet will be monitored by a qualified dietician. If a child loses their appetite they should maintain their energy intake by having glucose drinks.

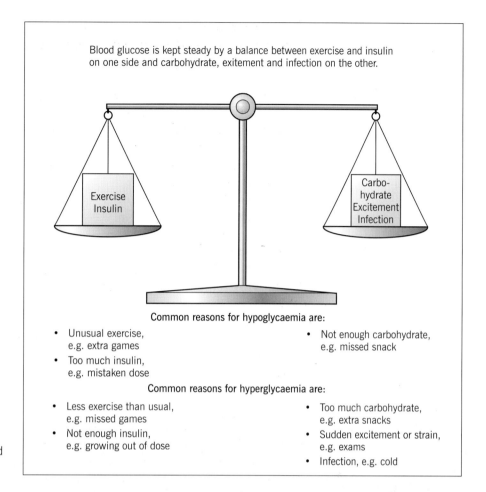

Blood glucose is kept steady by a balance between exercise and insulin on one side and carbohydrate, exitement and infection on the other.

Exercise
Insulin

Carbo-
hydrate
Excitement
Infection

Common reasons for hypoglycaemia are:

- Unusual exercise, e.g. extra games
- Too much insulin, e.g. mistaken dose
- Not enough carbohydrate, e.g. missed snack

Common reasons for hyperglycaemia are:

- Less exercise than usual, e.g. missed games
- Not enough insulin, e.g. growing out of dose
- Too much carbohydrate, e.g. extra snacks
- Sudden excitement or strain, e.g. exams
- Infection, e.g. cold

Blood glucose is maintained by keeping a balance

Possible Complications

Hypoglycaemia

Low levels of glucose in the blood. This may result from too much insulin, not enough food, illness or unusually vigorous exercise.

Signs include:

- irritability and confusion
- loss of co-ordination and concentration
- rapid breathing
- sweating
- dizziness

Management of a hypoglycaemic attack

- Stay with the child.
- Give glucose to drink if the child is conscious and able to swallow, for example Lucozade or dextrose tablets.
- Encourage the child to eat a snack such as biscuits or sandwiches.

If the child is unconscious put them in recovery position and call an ambulance, ensuring that somebody stays with the child at all times.

Parents must be informed of any hypoglycaemic attack because it could indicate the need for adjustment to the diet and/or insulin.

> ### Good Practice
>
> **Always carry glucose tablets or a sweetened drink when accompanying a child with diabetes on a school trip or a swimming lesson.**

If the condition is not well controlled with diet and insulin, complications in later life may affect the function of the following organs:

- eyes
- kidneys
- heart and circulatory system.

Further Information

Most children adjust well after the initial shock. They can learn to be independent and inject themselves and record their own blood glucose levels. This reinforces the need for them to take care with the diet and exercise.

Care Of A Diabetic Child In A Childcare Establishment

Children with diabetes should progress as any other child would. They are not ill and should lead a normal life participating in all activities, outings etc.

Records should be up to date with all relevant contact numbers e.g. home, GP, diabetic nurse etc.

Contact parents immediately if the child becomes unwell and keep them informed of the child's progress.

Children should carry glucose and be allowed to eat snacks as necessary, especially before exercise.

Glucose such as Lucozade and glucose tablets should be available in the establishment with the child's main carer or teacher, and taken with them on school trips, visits etc.

Observe carefully when swimming or climbing.

All staff must be aware of the child's condition and be trained to deal with a hypoglycaemic attack – they should be aware of the signs of hypoglycaemia.

Cooks must be consulted about the child's dietary requirements and the child should eat regularly.

Children may need to test their blood glucose levels at school, so should be given privacy to do this.

Behavioural problems may occur as a reaction to the disorder – children may resent the routines of injections and testing and feel angry about the restrictions caused by the diet. This should be handled with empathy and understanding, and time made to talk to the child.

A child with diabetes who feels unwell should never be left alone.

> ### Remember
>
> If in any doubt about hypo- or hyperglycaemia give the child a sweet drink – it can do little harm if the blood glucose levels are high, and if the levels are low it can prevent the child lapsing into a coma.

Support group
British Diabetic Association
10 Queen Anne Street
London W1M 0BD

> **☑ Progress check**
>
> 1 What is diabetes mellitus?
> 2 What are the signs of diabetes mellitus that may be recognised in a child?
> 3 What is the treatment for this condition in childhood?
> 4 What is the difference between hyperglycaemia and hypoglycaemia and how can you tell?
> 5 What is the role of the childcare worker during a hypoglycaemic attack?
> 6 What action should be taken if you are not sure whether the child is hyperglycaemic or hypoglycaemic?

> ## Case study
>
> Zaira is 6 years old and she is diabetic. Her condition is controlled by insulin injections before school in the morning and after school in the afternoon. She is aware of controlling her diet and knows which foods she can eat and when. Zaira's class have just started to go swimming on Tuesday afternoons and she is very excited; she is so busy chatting about swimming at lunch time that she only eats a small amount of her school dinner. Zaira trips up the top step when getting out of the pool, and is very slow to get her clothes on, buttoning her blouse the wrong way. The teacher notices that her face looks damp when she gets on the bus and that she is breathing quickly. She looks pale and starts to cry quietly.
>
> - What signs of hypoglycaemia is Zaira displaying?
> - What should the childcare worker or teacher give to her to remedy the situation?
> - What has caused this attack?
> - What can the staff of the school do generally to support Zaira and help her to cope with diabetes?

OBESITY

What Is Obesity? A common eating disorder in the Western world where many children are overweight and could go on to be obese.

What Causes Obesity? Often, a family pattern of overeating, or eating the wrong kinds of food, combined with little physical exercise is the cause. Overweight babies can become obese children and adults. Avoiding too many sweet or starchy foods in the early years will lay the foundation for healthy eating patterns for life.

Comfort eating, where babies and children are offered food or sweets as rewards, or to make them feel better, is likely to cause overweight.

Genetic causes are rare.

How To Recognise Obesity

Rolls of fat are obvious on the thighs and arms.

The child weighs 20 per cent more than expected for their height, age and sex when plotted on a centile chart (see page 111).

Immediate Action

- Get dietary advice from the doctor, who will measure and weigh the child, and perform a physical examination to rule out any medical conditions. The health visitor will support the child and family and help to develop an effective diet for the child.
- If this does not help, the child will be referred to a community or hospital dietician.

Ongoing Care

Plenty of exercise combined with a healthy diet will prevent further weight gain.

Provide positive role models such as eating meals in social groups. Offer healthy, fresh food in reasonable quantities. Avoid sugary snacks.

Behaviour therapy may be required to establish healthy eating patterns.

Possible Complications

Carrying too much weight can lead to:
- respiratory illnesses
- heart disease
- joint problems.

Further Information

Overweight children are usually teased mercilessly at school. This can result in psychological problems and unhappiness which can be avoided if the problem is dealt with promptly.

> *Remember*
>
> Children must be told the reasons for their special diet in a way that they will understand. If they are aware of the all foods that they can eat freely, and the foods that are restricted, the diet is more likely to be successful.

ANOREXIA NERVOSA

What Is Anorexia Nervosa?

Anorexia means loss of appetite. Anorexia nervosa is an eating disorder where children (usually adolescent girls) deliberately restrict their intake of food.

What Causes Anorexia Nervosa?

A psychological fear of becoming fat, sometimes due to teasing for being plump, is thought to be the cause.

Adolescents may want to avoid growing up by staying thin and delaying physical development.

Media images of 'thin is beautiful' encourage this disorder.

How To Recognise Anorexia Nervosa

Anorexia has been diagnosed in children as young as 5 years. The child:

- has a distorted body image. Unsightly thinness is seen as beautiful by children with anorexia
- avoids food and family mealtimes
- is a fussy eater
- becomes thin and weak
- has dry skin
- may have fine hair growing on the face and body – this is a sign of starvation.

Immediate Action
- See the doctor.

Ongoing Care

A programme of supervised eating combined with psychotherapy.

Possible Complications

Children can starve to death if the condition continues without treatment.

 Progress check

1 What may cause obesity?
2 How would you recognise that a child was developing a weight problem?
3 How could this be handled sensitively?
4 How can children be encouraged to eat well-balanced meals without developing anxieties about their weight?

Activities

Look at media and television advertisements for food – especially sweets, chocolates, crisps and fizzy drinks. Comment on the ages, sizes and social class of the actors/models.

- Which consumer market do you think that are they aiming for ?
- What strategies are they using, for example do they suggest that buying a certain chocolate bar will make people more popular etc.
- In your placement, ask the children about the adverts they have seen.
- Make a display of your findings
- Write to the manufacturers if you feel that the campaign is targeting vulnerable groups in society.

CONSTIPATION

What Is Constipation? Constipation is passing hard, painful and infrequent stools. Infrequency alone is NOT constipation.

What Causes Constipation?

It may be short term or continue for a long time (chronic).

Short-term constipation may be the result of:

- illness, such as diarrhoea and vomiting which has resulted in temporary dehydration
- some medicines which can cause constipation
- dietary changes when weaning or changing from breast to cows' milk.

Chronic constipation may be caused by:

- not enough fibre or liquid in the diet
- withholding faeces during toilet training probably due to unsympathetic management by parent/carer
- inadequate toileting facilities at nursery or school
- intolerance to certain foods
- emotional problems.

Children who are inactive due to their physical condition may suffer from constipation e.g. in cerebral palsy and spina bifida.

How To Recognise Constipation

- Pain when passing a stool.
- Hard, dry stools.
- Infrequent motions.

Chronic constipation

- Faeces may be impacted (hard and stuck) in the rectum, and watery, brown fluid (liquid faeces) trickles out of the anus, sometimes giving the impression of diarrhoea.
- Pain and excessive straining to pass a stool.
- Blood may be seen on the stools or underwear.
- Loss of appetite.
- The urge to have the bowels open will get less as the lower bowel stretches.

Immediate Action

- Give the child plenty of fluids, preferable fresh fruit juice. Children over 6 months should eat plenty of dietary fibre, for example wholewheat bread, wholewheat cereals, fruit and vegetables as part of a well-balanced intake.
- Regular exercise stimulates the bowels.
- Find the cause of the problem and deal with it. This may require help from a doctor and health visitor.

Remember

After breakfast is a good time of day to empty the bowels. The 'gastrocolic reflex' is stimulated by eating breakfast and this encourages the bowels to open.

Good Practice

Always stress the positive aspects of children's behaviour. A star chart can be helpful as it will encourage the child to use the toilet and record their success.

Ongoing Care — The doctor should be seen if the diarrhoea lasts for more than a week with no improvement. It may be necessary to give the child an enema to clear the bowel and monitor their bowel movements until a normal pattern is established.

Possible Complications — A tear in the wall of the anus (anal fissure) can be caused by hard stools. This creates further pain and so the child deliberately withholds their stools causing chronic constipation. A local anaesthetic cream will reduce the discomfort caused by having the bowels open if there is an anal fissure.

A tear can be treated by curing the constipation with dietary measures. The tear will heal up in about a month and will not be painful when the stools are soft.

Further Information — Children's bowel habits vary considerably from passing a stool 1 to 4 times a day to once every 4 or 5 days. If they are not extremely loose, hard or painful there is no cause for concern.

Constipation can put pressure on the urinary tract and prevent the bladder from emptying completely. This may lead to urinary tract infections.

Remember

Milk is constipating. Do not give more than 1 pint of whole milk a day to a child who is constipated. Children of school age who are eating a balanced diet should be given skimmed or semi-skimmed milk.

Good Practice

Never give laxatives to a child unless it is done under strict medical supervision. Laxatives do not cure the problem of constipation, which should be treated with diet and a 'laid-back' approach to toilet training.

✔ Progress check

- What is constipation and how would you recognise that a child had this problem?
- What causes short-term and long-term constipation?
- What treatments can be offered to resolve constipation?

Case study

Jane has three children and she prides herself on having trained them all to pass their motions on the potty before they were one year old. Her mother says she trained Jane before she was 6 months old.

John is the youngest of Jane's children. He is 18 months and does not like sitting on the potty. He prefers to jump off and run to play with his two brothers who are aged 6 and 4 years. Jane always insists that he comes back and stays on the potty until he has passed a stool.

It has been several days since he passed a motion – then it seemed harder than usual – but Jane was not worried. John cries when he sees the potty and now he seems to have diarrhoea. He has started staining his nappy and today Jane noticed a small blood-stain.

- Why do you think Jane is so keen to train her children early?
- What problems may be associated with toilet training too soon?
- What do you think is the cause of John's diarrhoea?
- What steps can be taken to cure this?
- What advice could Jane be given about managing his toilet training?

HEPATITIS A

What Is Hepatitis A?	Inflammation of the liver.

What Causes Hepatitis A?

It is a virus caught by eating or drinking something which has been contaminated by infected faeces.
Incubation period: 10–40 days.

How To Recognise Hepatitis A

Most hepatitis A infections in children are mild and produce the following symptoms:
- headache, fever and tiredness similar to influenza
- loss of appetite
- nausea and vomiting
- abdominal tenderness (upper right area where the liver is situated).

About a week after the illness begins these symptoms appear:
- jaundice – yellowing of the skin, especially noticeable in the whites of the eyes in all races (see plate 4)
- dark-coloured urine
- pale stools.

Immediate Action

- Call the doctor who will most probably advise that the child should be cared for at home. Occasionally, hospital admission is recommended if the child is very ill.
- The child should be looked after in bed and encouraged to drink lots of fluids to prevent dehydration – hourly drinks especially if the child is vomiting. Small appetising meals can be offered as the child begins to feel better.

Ongoing Care

Jaundice will last about 2 weeks, but the child will not be well enough to return to school or nursery for about a month. Weakness and tiredness can continue for many weeks.

Careful hygiene including regular hand washing, and boiling food utensils will prevent the spread of the disease.

Possible Complications

All family members should be immunised against hepatitis A to limit the spread of the disease.

Permanent damage to the liver is rare.

Further Information

An affected child is infectious for 14 days before and 7 days after the jaundice is apparent.

Immunisation against hepatitis A is recommended before travelling to countries where the disease is common.

> **Remember**
>
> Always call the doctor if a child is showing signs of jaundice whether any other symptoms are present or not.

 Progress check

1 How is hepatitis A transmitted from person to person?
2 What symptoms occur before the jaundice is obvious?
3 What care should be offered to the child to aid their recovery?

Case study

Flowerpots Day Nursery is situated in a leafy green suburb of a southern city. It is a thriving and established business which puts a great deal of emphasis on its high standards of childcare supplied by experienced and qualified staff. Many parents take advantage of the annual fortnight's closure in August to take their children on holiday, and many go abroad.

One morning, early in October, Robyn said that she felt sick. The staff had told her parents that she had not been eating well for a few days, but had put this down to excitement about her fourth birthday party in a few days time. When Robyn started to vomit and had diarrhoea the officer-in-charge contacted her parents and asked them to collect her as soon as possible. The staff continued with their hygiene routines and comforted Robyn while they waited for her father to arrive.

During the next few days four other children were sent home with vomiting and diarrhoea. The following week, Robyn's father rang the nursery to tell the staff that she had been diagnosed with hepatitis A and would not be coming back to nursery for a few weeks.

1 Which other condition may cause similar symptoms?
2 What are the characteristic signs of hepatitis A?
3 How do you think the other children became infected with this condition?
4 How could the staff at the day nursery prevent the continued spread of the disease?

FOOD REFUSAL

What Is Food Refusal?	Consistent and repeated refusal to attempt to eat, chew or swallow food.

What Causes Food Refusal?

Toddler food refusal is common because they are often too busy exploring the world and enjoying their play to stop and eat!

Pressure to eat may create a clash between parent and child, both of whom want to win the battle.

How To Recognise Food Refusal

Toddlers and older children who consistently refuse to eat at family mealtimes.

They may eat snacks and 'junk food' at other times.

Immediate Action

- Carers should be reassured if the child is of normal body weight and height, is thriving and no medical condition is identified by the doctor. Meals should be offered in small portions with no other eating between meals.

Ongoing Care

- The child should be offered food at mealtimes and allowed to eat according to appetite.
- Allow the child to feed himself and remember that mess is to be expected, especially if he is just learning to do this.
- Any remaining food should be removed without fuss.
- The next meal should be offered at the usual time with no snacks given between meals.
- It is important that the child participates in family meals rather than eating in isolation.

Possible Complications

Poor management in the early years can lead to serious eating problems later in childhood, which may require treatment from behavioural psychologists.

Further Information

Mealtimes should not become a battle ground. Eating should be a pleasurable and sociable experience with the family or other groups.

Stimulating the appetite
Never pressurise a child to eat. Providing attractive and appetising food regularly in small quantities should help. The following tips may provide some help.
- Children do not eat as much at one mealtime as an adult, so they need smaller helpings at 5 to 6 meals or snacks a day.
- Food faces or games may encourage eating.

TODDLER'S DIARRHOEA

What Is Toddler's Diarrhoea?	Very loose motions in healthy children between the ages of 1 year and $2\frac{1}{2}$ years

What Causes Toddler's Diarrhoea? Possible poor chewing of food.

How To Recognise Toddler's Diarrhoea
- Recognisable foods e.g. raisins, corn, carrots, peas, are passed in watery stools.
- The child is generally well and usually gaining weight.
- Nappy rash may be present if the child is in nappies.

Immediate Action
- It is best to see a doctor to exclude any other causes of the loose stools.
- Mashing the foods which are difficult to digest will provide a solution, but encouraging the child to chew is the preferable option!

Ongoing Care Children usually grow out of this condition by their third birthday. It is not infectious and is not a reason for exclusion from childcare establishments.

Further Information A stool sample may be taken to make sure that the child does not have an infection or other more serious condition.

 Progress check

1 Why is food refusal common in toddlers?
2 What attitude from parents/carers may make food refusal a more serious condition?
3 What strategies should be used to deal with the condition?
4 Which other condition is associated with inadequate chewing of food?
5 What is the treatment for this condition?

RICKETS

What Is Rickets? Softening of the bones.

What Causes Rickets? Lack of the fat-soluble vitamin D in the diet and/or exposure to sunlight. Vitamin D is produced by the body as a result of the action of sunshine on the skin.

It is sometimes associated with coeliac disease (see page 255).

How To Recognise
Rickets

- Bowing of the legs due to softening of the bones.
- Dental decay may also be present.

Immediate Action

- Consult the doctor who will arrange tests to confirm the diagnosis. A dietician will formulate a diet containing adequate amounts of vitamin D and calcium.

Ongoing Care

- Careful attention to dietary requirements.
- Ensure that the child has exposure to sunlight.

Further Information

Rickets is, fortunately, now rare in this country but is still sometimes seen in Asian children who are not exposed to adequate amounts of sunlight.

 Progress check

1 What causes rickets?
2 Why is vitamin D important in the diet?
3 How else can the body obtain vitamin D?
4 What ongoing care should the child receive?
5 Which other disease is rickets a side-effect of?

Chapter *12* *Problems with the eyes and ears*

This chapter includes:

- ■ Structure and functions of the eye
- ■ Conjunctivitis
- ■ Squint
- ■ Bruised eye
- ■ Foreign bodies in the eye
- ■ Structure and functions of the ear
- ■ Otitis externa
- ■ Otitis media
- ■ Glue ear
- ■ Foreign bodies in the ear

This chapter should be read in conjunction with 'Chapter 4, Screening' hearing (page 98) and vision (page 103).

The ears and eyes are sensory organs and both are delicate mechanisms which require gentle stimulation to encourage their development. Hearing and vision are considered to be the most important senses because they help children to learn about the world. They have an important role in social and emotional development because they help children to use verbal and non-verbal communication.

Vision is essential for normal development. Babies are stimulated to move by their curiosity to reach things that they can see. Walking on two legs is encouraged by a desire to imitate what they see other people doing and to explore the world around them. They learn to name objects which they know by sight and learn sounds by linking the noise with the object which makes it. The detection of visual difficulties is important because treatment will help visual skills to develop normally. Prompt treatment should prevent lasting disability.

Hearing is probably the least developed sense at birth, but babies do respond to sound and soon recognise their mother's voice and learn to identify other familiar sounds. Persistent ear infections can eventually damage the hearing and have an impact on all areas of development, especially speech and cognitive skills.

Children are vulnerable to infection and many have eye and ear infections during childhood. Sometimes they are recurrent problems which will improve as the child grows and the organ matures.

Signs and symptoms of ear and eye disease should never be ignored because of the damage that may be caused to these intricate organs, and the negative effects on development which may result.

Childcare workers must be aware of the signs and symptoms of ear and eye disease, the immediate treatment that they can provide and the importance of medical intervention when necessary.

Structure and functions of the eye

The eye is the most complex sensory organ but a brief examination of the structure will increase understanding about:

- normal visual development
- why and where problems may arise.

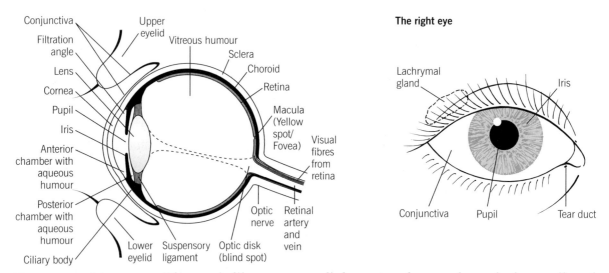

The structure of the eye

The eye is like a camera: light enters the eye through the pupil at the front of the eye and an image is reflected onto the retina at the back. These light rays are then converted into nerve impulses which are carried to the brain via the optic nerve. The brain receives these messages and recognises them as images or pictures.

The *cornea* forms the fixed-focus lens of the eye. Its outer layer is the *conjunctiva* which extends to cover the whites of the eyes and lines the eyelids. The cornea is protected from germs, pollution and dust by a film of tears. Without tears the outer layer would lose its transparency and blindness may result.

The *iris* is the part of the eye which gives it its colour. It is disc shaped with a central hole through which light passes. This hole is the *pupil* – the black spot in the centre of the eye which gets smaller or larger depending on how much available light there is.

The *lens* is a crystal-like disc which focuses the image onto the retina. It thickens or flattens according to the distance away of the object being observed.

The *retina* is the lining of the eye which is sensitive to colour and light. At birth the retina is not fully developed, so new babies have blurred vision and may be colour blind. Vitamin A is important for the healthy functioning of the retina – hence the old saying that eating carrots helps you to see in the dark!

CONJUNCTIVITIS

What Is Conjunctivitis?

Conjunctivitis is an inflammation of the conjunctiva, the delicate membrane covering the eye and the eyelid. One or both eyes may be affected.

What Causes Conjunctivitis?

It is caused by bacteria or a virus. It is commonly associated with the common cold virus.

An allergic reaction may also cause this inflammation of the eye.

How To Recognise Conjunctivitis

- The child will rub their eye(s) because they are itchy and sore.
- Eye looks red, especially the white of the eye.
- Sticky, yellow pus in the corner of the eye and around the eyelashes.
- Eye(s) may be stuck together in the morning or after a day-time sleep.

Immediate Action

- Bathe the eyes if they are stuck together. Moisten a cotton swab with cooled, boiled water and wipe each eye from the inside corner to the outside. Use a single stroke with each swab and then throw it away. Do not contaminate an unaffected eye. Wash your hands carefully after cleaning the eyes.
- See the doctor as soon as possible.
- The condition is easily cured, if caused by bacteria, with the application of antibiotic eye drops or ointment.
- Anti-inflammatory eye drops can be given to reduce the irritation of an allergic reaction. The cause of the allergy should be found, if possible.

Ongoing Care

- Apply the prescribed eye ointment or cream as instructed – possibly 4 times a day.
- Bathe the eyes if they become sticky.
- Encourage the child not to touch their eyes and to wash their hands if they do.
- Keep all washing equipment separate – no sharing of flannels, sponges or towels.
- Conjunctivitis is highly infectious, so children should stay at home until the eyes are back to normal.
- It can take up to a week to clear.
- Allergic conjunctivitis is not infectious.

Possible Complications   Infectious and allergic conjunctivitis do not have a permanent affect on vision.

Good Practice

Conjunctivitis is highly infectious. Encourage parents to keep their child at home until the infection has cleared.

SQUINT

What Is A Squint?   Squint is the inability to move both eyes in the same direction at the same time. It is most common in children, and most babies occasionally squint until about 4 to 6 months of age. After this time a squint is abnormal. A persistent squint is abnormal at any age.

A squint is sometimes described as a 'lazy eye' but this is not entirely correct. A lazy eye is one which has not achieved its full potential – the vision may be blurred and out of focus, but not necessarily squinting. Any condition which prevents an eye from maturing will result in a lazy eye and a squint is the most common cause.

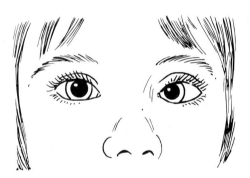

Convergent squint of the left eye

What Causes A Squint?   A squint is caused by an imbalance between the focus of the eye and the muscles which move the eye to look in different directions. There are six muscles which move the eyeball to provide a full range of movements. Some may be underactive and others overactive resulting in abnormal movements in one or both eyes.

Some squints are congenital i.e. present at birth. Most occur between 2 and 4 years of age.

How To Recognise A Squint
- An eye which turns too far inwards (convergent squint) or outwards (divergent squint) when looking directly at an object.
- The child may repeatedly close or cover the affected eye because s/he is experiencing double vision or blurred vision in that eye.

Immediate Action	Any baby or child thought to be squinting should be examined by an ophthalmologist (eye doctor). The GP will refer cases. If the condition is diagnosed there are several treatments which can be used, depending on the age/stage of the child and the type of squint.

Ongoing Care

The child will be reviewed regularly to make sure that the best and most appropriate treatment is offered, which could be the following.

- Patching the unaffected eye to encourage use of the affected eye.
- Glasses if the child has focusing difficulties or long sight.
- Surgical repair of the squint is usually very successful.

Possible Complications

The brain cannot use two images received by eyes looking in different directions (double vision), so it ignores the image from the squinting eye. If this eye is not used it can result in permanent impairment of vision.

Prompt treatment is essential to ensure that visual development continues normally.

Further Information

Normal vision is not achieved until about 5 years of age.

An optician is always available to examine children's eyes and provide expert advice about visual problems.

Tips for caring for children with glasses

- Discourage children from putting glasses down with the lens side down, because they are easily scratched.
- Check that the lenses fit correctly and are not loose or absent.
- Encourage children to take responsibility for their glasses and to wipe them regularly with a lens cloth.
- Observe the child for visual signs, for example screwing up the eyes to focus even with the glasses may mean that their eyes need re-testing and the lens prescription needs adjustment.

Remember

There are different types of squint.

- Latent squint is present only when the child is under stress i.e. tired or ill. Children with this type of squint usually do not need treatment.
- Manifest squint is present all the time. This is never normal and needs treatment.
- Alternating squint means that the child fixates with each eye alternately.
- Pseudosquint is the appearance of a squint caused by broad epicanthic folds – a wide bridge to the nose.

Good Practice

Encouraging a child to wear their spectacles

- Make sure that the glasses fit correctly. If glasses are uncomfortable children will object to wearing them. Children will need new frames as they grow.
- Reflect positive images of children wearing glasses in establishment books and displays. Many childhood idols wear spectacles – show photographs to the child!

Remember

Visual difficulties may lead to delayed development. Make sure that children are offered access to the same opportunities, activities and equipment as their visually normal peers.

 Progress check

1 What is conjunctivitis?
2 What special precautions should be taken to prevent the spread of conjunctivitis in a childcare establishment?
3 How is conjunctivitis treated?
4 What is a squint?
5 What may cause a squint?
6 How would you recognise a squint?
7 When is normal vision acquired?
8 What effect will an untreated squint have on a child's vision?

Case study

When he was a baby, Arthur's mother, Daisy, was concerned about his eyes because she thought that they sometimes looked in different directions. Nobody else seemed to understand – her husband and her mother thought that she was imagining it. Arthur's eyes looked perfectly alright to them and they told her so. She mentioned her concern to the health visitor who thought that the squint was more pronounced when Arthur was tired. She advised Daisy to see the GP and ask to be referred to the ophthalmology department at the local hospital. Daisy did this and she and Arthur went to the hospital for his first appointment when he was 9 months old. The specialist watched Arthur pick up hundreds and thousands with a pincer grasp and examined his eyes. He explained to Daisy that Arthur was squinting slightly. By the time he went for his next appointment, 6 months later, his squint was pronounced. The specialist decided to patch his good eye to encourage the weaker eye to focus and strengthen the muscles. He explained that it may be necessary for Arthur to wear spectacles. If the squint worsened he may need an operation. Daisy was devastated but felt that she had done the right thing by taking Arthur to the doctor when nobody else believed her!

1 What is the difference between a squint and a lazy eye?
2 Why do you think that Arthur's father and grandmother did not notice his squint?
3 When may the squint have been detected as part of the screening programme, if Daisy had not noticed it?
4 How could you reassure Daisy about the long-term effects on Arthur?

BRUISED EYE

What Is A Bruised Eye? A bruised eye is a collection of old blood beneath the skin. It is commonly called a black eye.

| What Causes A Bruised Eye? | The tissue around the eyes is very soft, and any injury to the face or scalp which causes bleeding beneath the skin tends to drain towards the eyes. |

- Accidental injury caused by falls or knocks. However, the face is not the usual sight for bruising in childhood – children usually put out their arms to protect themselves as they fall.
- Non-accidental injury.

| How To Recognise A Bruised Eye | The skin around the eye looks yellowy at first, turning purply-blue before fading after a few days. It is obvious in fair-skinned children and the skin looks darker in black-skinned children. The eye may be partly closed due to swelling. |

Immediate Action

- Reassure the child and encourage them to remain calm.
- Look at the eye to check for injury to the skin or a foreign body.
- Apply a cold compress on the eye to relieve discomfort.
- Try and find the cause of the bruising.
- If the injury occurs at a childcare establishment the parents should be informed and the Accident Book should be completed immediately.

Ongoing Care

It is advisable for the child to be checked over by a doctor to ensure that there is no further injury, or damage to the eye.

Bruised eyes tend to look worse before they get better.

Possible Complications

Two bruised eyes is unusual and can only be caused by injury to the nose or directly between the eyes. Permanent damage to the eyes can result from trauma.

Further Information

Repeated bruising needs investigating. If there is concern, report these to the officer in charge of an establishment who may talk to the parents, contact the health visitor or contact the Social Services Department.

FOREIGN BODIES IN THE EYE

What Is A Foreign Body?

A foreign body is any object which is not usually found in the eye (see plate 4).

What Causes A Foreign Body?

It could be any of the following:

- an eyelash
- a flying insect
- dust, sand or gravel blown in the wind
- chemicals which can burn or irritate the eye.

How To Recognise A Foreign Body

- The eye will be painful and look red and sore.
- The child will rub their eye to relieve the discomfort.

■ The eye may be watering.
■ The child may complain that s/he cannot see out of one or both eyes.

Immediate Action If anything is sticking into the eye do not attempt to remove it and *do not cover the eye*. The child should go to hospital immediately.
■ Reassure the child.
■ Send someone to call an ambulance.
■ Encourage the child to remain still and quiet looking straight ahead. Movement can cause more serious damage.
If a foreign body can be seen on the conjunctiva follow the steps to remove it (below), but do not attempt to remove an object which is embedded or sticking to the eye.

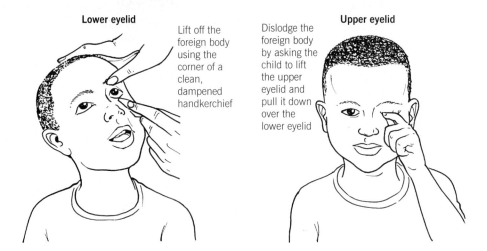

Lower eyelid

Lift off the foreign body using the corner of a clean, dampened handkerchief

Upper eyelid

Dislodge the foreign body by asking the child to lift the upper eyelid and pull it down over the lower eyelid

Removing a foreign body from the eye

Ongoing Care Most children will immediately feel better when the offending object has been removed.
Continue to observe the eye for signs of infection.

Possible Complications *Corneal abrasion*
This is a scratch to the cornea, which needs treatment from an accident and emergency department. It is extremely painful but tends to heal quickly after being patched for up to a week.

Further Information *Removing a foreign body from the eye*
Baby/Toddler
■ Wrap the child in a blanket to restrain the arms, talking and reassuring the child all the time.
■ Look into the eyes by gently opening the lids with the fingers.
■ If a foreign body can be seen, fill a feeding cup or eye wash bottle with cooled, boiled water.
■ Wash the eye by pouring the water onto the affected eye from the inner to outer corner. Tilt the toddler onto their side to allow the water to drain.
■ If the foreign body remains, take the child to hospital.

Older child

- Tilt the head back to look for the foreign body by gently opening the eyelids with the fingers. If it can be seen on the lower lid or the white of the eye, gently lift it off with the damp corner of a tissue or clean handkerchief. Great care must be taken not to scratch the eye or drag the foreign body.
- Then wash the eye as for a baby or toddler (see page 278).
- If the foreign body can be seen on the upper lid, ask the child to pull the upper lid down to dislodge the object.
- If the foreign body remains, take the child to hospital.

<table>
<tr><td>

Remember

Some important do nots when dealing with eye injuries or infections

- **Do not** self-treat children's eye disorders by getting remedies from the chemist. They can cover up important signs and possibly damage the eye.
- **Do not** delay in getting medical advice.

</td></tr>
</table>

Good Practice

Children should never run with sharp objects in their hands. Teach them how to carry scissors and pencils safely.

✓ Progress check

1 What may cause a bruised eye?
2 What immediate action should be taken if a child injures their eye?
3 Why might you be concerned if a child came to nursery with two bruised eyes?
4 Which foreign bodies may irritate the eye?
5 What action should a childcare worker take if a child has an object sticking out of the eye?
6 What is corneal abrasion and how is it treated?
7 How can an adult try to remove a foreign body from the eye of a toddler?
8 What should be done if the attempt is unsuccessful?

Structure and functions of the ear

The ear is composed of three distinct parts, each performing a specialised function in the transmission and interpretation of sound.

The outer ear conducts sound to the middle ear.

The middle ear conducts the sound via three tiny bones called the ossicles (the hammer, anvil and stirrup) to the inner ear.

The inner ear senses the sound and relays the message to the brain via the auditory nerve.

When a sound is made it is carried through the air by sound waves. These enter the outer ear through the *pinna* into the *external auditory meatus* (a bony canal through the skull). The eardrum (*tympanic membrane*) which is at the end of the *external auditory meatus*, now vibrates and stimulates movement in the *ossicles* in the middle ear.

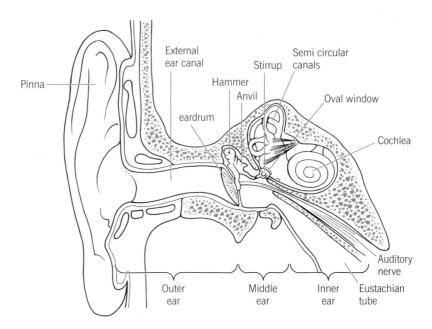

The structure of the ear

The ossicles are attached to the eardrum at one end of the middle ear and at the other they are attached to the *oval window*, which leads to the inner ear. These tiny bones transmit and amplify the vibrations through the oval window to the inner ear, which is composed of the *cochlea*, also called the organ of hearing. In the cochlea vibrations are picked up and transmitted to the hearing centre which is situated in the temporal lobe of the brain.

The *external auditory meatus* is lined with a special skin containing tiny hairs called cilia which produces wax. Wax is wafted along the tiny cilia and to keep the canal clean and protected from dirt and infection.

The *Eustachian tube* connects the middle ear to the back of the throat and keeps the air pressure in the middle ear the same as the outside air. It also drains fluid from the ear and should keep it healthy. In childhood the Eustachian tubes are short and narrow and so infection easily passes up from the throat to the ear. They are also easily blocked when a child has a cold or an ear infection.

Any concerns about a baby's or child's ability to hear should be referred to the doctor or health visitor. If concern continues, the parent/carer can themselves refer the child to an audiology (hearing) clinic.

OTITIS EXTERNA

What Is Otitis Externa? Otitis externa is an inflammation or infection of the outer ear canal (the external auditory meatus).

What Causes Otitis Externa? It can be caused by:
- bacterial infection
- seborrhoeic dermatitis
- eczema.

The risk of infection is increased if the canal is in water for long periods, for example swimming, if it has been scratched by a foreign body or poked with a pencil or cotton bud etc.

How To Recognise Otitis Externa
- Pain in the ear – a baby will rub their ear(s) and cry.
- Discharge of mucus, blood or pus from the ear (see plate 3). This discharge usually smells offensive.
- Crusting around the ear or blisters may be seen.
- Hearing loss – especially if the ear canal is impacted with wax.

Immediate Action
- Call the parents who will call the doctor and reassure the child.
- Paracetamol will reduce the pain.
- The doctor will look at the ear with an auriscope to find the cause e.g. foreign body, wax, infection, eczema etc.

Ongoing Care Infections will be treated with antibiotic drops and eczema or dermatitis will be treated with drops to relieve the inflammation and itching.

Paracetamol may be required for 48 hours while the condition settles down. Holding a warm cloth or warm, covered, hot water bottle to the ear may relieve the discomfort. Never use a hot water bottle with a baby who cannot push it away if it is too hot.

Lying flat often increases the pain, so propping children up on pillows may help.

Children should not swim or get the ear wet until the infection has cleared. Hair can be sponged while the child wears a shower cap during a bath or shower.

With treatment otitis externa usually clears up quickly, within 1–2 weeks.

Possible Complications Children with eczema and dermatitis may suffer from recurrent infections, but prompt treatment as soon as the first signs appear, should prevent lasting damage.

Excessive wax production can be improved by using prescribed drops to stop the wax from hardening and encouraging it to drain away.

Further Information *Administering ear drops* (see page 344)
- Wash your hands.
- Lie the child down with the affected ear upwards.
- Gently lift the pinna towards the back of the head, and with the other hand insert the drops into the ear taking care to give the prescribed number.
- Gently rub the area around the ear canal.
- The child should lie still for 1–2 minutes after the drops have been inserted. Wipe away any residue with a tissue when the child sits up.

OTITIS MEDIA

What Is Otitis Media? Otitis media is an inflammation or infection of the middle ear which is very common in children until 7 or 8 years of age. The short Eustachian tube in young children makes them vulnerable to infection spreading from the throat/nose to the middle ear.

What Causes Otitis Media?
- Virus or bacteria, usually following an upper respiratory tract infection, for example cold or sore throat.
- Enlarged adenoids may block the eustachian tubes.
- Infection in the middle ear produces fluid and pus which cannot drain away if the tube is inflamed or blocked by large adenoids.

How To Recognise Otitis Media
- Severe earache – babies will rub or pull the ear and cry.

Sometimes children will not complain of earache, because they cannot describe or localise the pain. They may show other signs of illness such as:
- raised temperature
- vomiting
- lack of sleep
- general lethargy
- behaviour changes caused by hearing loss.

If the eardrum bursts the pain will stop and there will be a discharge from the affected ear.

Immediate Action
- Contact the parents if the child is not at home. Call the doctor immediately if a child has earache. The child should be seen as soon as possible.
- Paracetamol will relieve the pain.
- The doctor will look in the ears. In otitis media the eardrum looks red and bulging. Oral antibiotics will improve the pain and clear the infection quickly.

Ongoing Care Continue steps above to relieve earache (see Good Practice: Relieving earache on page 283).

Hearing loss may persist, because there is still fluid in the middle ear. The hearing should be checked after about 3 months. If it is still below the expected level, the child will be referred to the hospital's Ear, Nose and Throat Clinic and to a Children's Hearing Assessment Unit.

Possible Complications
- A burst eardrum can heal quickly but may result in permanent scarring. There may be some residual hearing loss.
- Glue ear – see page 284.

Further Information

Remember

Children with otitis media will not always complain of earache or show signs of an ear infection. A child who is obviously unwell with a raised temperature should have their ears checked by a doctor or practice nurse. Untreated otitis media can lead to permanent scarring and can cause deafness.

Good Practice

Relieving earache

Give paracetamol to relieve the pain with the parents' consent.

Lying flat often increases the pain, so propping children up on pillows may help.

Holding a warm cloth or warm, covered, hot water bottle to the ear may relieve the discomfort.

Never use a hot water bottle with a baby who cannot push it away if it is too hot.

Remember

Never put ear drops into a child's ear unless their ears have been examined by a doctor and the drops have been prescribed for that child.

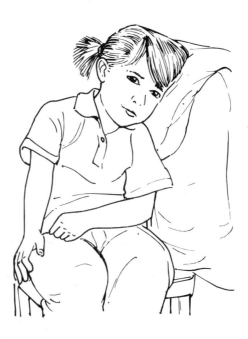

Relieving the pain of earache

Activity

Prepare a display for your establishment explaining the difference between glue ear and otitis media. Include illustrations of the ear and describe the:

■ signs and symptoms of each condition
■ specific care
■ possible treatments
■ effects on hearing.

GLUE EAR

What Is Glue Ear? Glue ear is the presence of thick, sticky mucus in the middle ear. This interferes with the movement of the eardrum and the ossicles and prevents sounds from being transmitted to the inner ear. It results in conductive hearing loss.

What Causes Glue Ear? The sticky mucus produced in the middle ear cannot drain away efficiently because of blocked Eustachian tubes. Glue ear is usually a complication of recurrent attacks of otitis media. It can sometimes occur unexpectedly in a child with no history of ear infections.

How To Recognise Glue Ear Hearing loss may be permanent or intermittent (come and go). This can result in any or all of the following.
- Failure to develop age-appropriate speech with indistinct sounds and words.
- Behaviour problems. Typically, a child with glue ear finds it difficult to concentrate and can range between being disruptive or very quiet when their hearing is impaired.
- Deteriorating work at school. Children with glue ear often display signs of slow learning and may be labelled as 'naughty' by carers who are not aware of their problem.
- Reading difficulties.

Immediate Action Because pain is not usually associated with glue ear, it takes an observant and intuitive carer to notice the signs. Discuss your concerns with a senior member of staff who will talk to the parents. The doctor should be consulted and the condition can be diagnosed by looking into the ear with an auriscope. Referral to an ear, nose and throat specialist in the hospital's out-patients department will follow.

Ongoing Care The movement of the eardrum will be tested. If the condition does not improve within a few months, the child will be given an operation to remove the mucus and insert tiny tubes (grommets) into the eardrum(s). This should assist the drainage of fluid from the middle ear. Grommets fall out within 2 years of the operation and the hole in the eardrum usually heals quickly.

Speech therapy may be required if the child has language delay, or difficulty with pronouncing sounds.

Regular hearing tests will be performed and further treatment will be offered as necessary.

Possible Complications Permanent hearing loss.

Further Information Any child who is disruptive, aggressive, overly clingy or quiet, struggling with speech or finding it difficult to concentrate, should have their hearing tested. Labelling children as having behaviour problems when, in fact, they have a hearing disorder does them a serious disservice and damages their educational opportunities. The GP, health visitor or school nurse will be able to arrange an appropriate test.

Good Practice

Working with children with a hearing loss

1 Make sure that the child can see your face when you are speaking and speak clearly in sentences.
2 When they find it difficult to concentrate, check that they understand the task or the activity they are attempting to achieve.
3 Provide as much one-to-one and small group time as possible.
4 Be aware that their hearing may be better some days than others.
5 Reassure them – it is bewildering for children who find it difficult to make sense of what is happening around them.
6 Try to keep noise to a minimum especially when important instructions are given, and at storytime etc.

✔ Progress check

1 What is otitis media?
2 Why is it more common in children under the age of 7 years?
3 What signs and symptoms would make you suspect that a child has otitis media?
4 How can earache be relieved?
5 Why should the hearing be tested after an attack of otitis media?
6 What is the difference between otitis media and glue ear?
7 Why are children prone to glue ear?
8 What effects can glue ear have on development?
9 What is the usual treatment for glue ear?
10 How can childcare staff support children with a hearing loss in a childcare establishment?

Case study

Rowan is a 5-year-old child who has just started school in the infant class of a large primary school. His development has followed an average pattern. His parents have taken him for all the screening checks and he has achieved all of the expected developmental milestones. His behaviour is becoming a cause for concern because although he can speak quietly, on some days he shouts, disrupting some of the other children. His new teacher has noticed that Rowan has difficulty in concentrating and can get frustrated with himself and others. He has thrown a pot of paint on the floor and refused to join the other children doing a collage activity, insisting on playing in the sand tray. Some days he will not sit still to listen to the story and insists on playing in the home corner, but at other times he participates fully in the story and songs.

1 What condition is Rowan showing signs of?
2 Why do you think that Rowan's behaviour is more acceptable on some days than it is on others?
3 What should the teacher say to the parents?
4 What may they have noticed about his behaviour at home?
5 What course of action should be taken by the parents and school staff?
6 Why should all children with challenging behaviour have their hearing tested?

FOREIGN BODIES IN THE EAR

What Are Foreign Bodies?	A foreign body is any object which is in the external auditory meatus.
What Causes Foreign Bodies?	These are usually objects pushed by children into their own or other children's ears, for example beads, sweets, small pieces of Lego, pen tops, etc. Insects may fly or crawl into the ear.
How To Recognise Foreign Bodies	The child may: ■ complain of mild or severe earache depending on what is in the ear ■ have temporary hearing loss ■ tell you that they have put something in their ear.
Immediate Action	■ Take the child to hospital to have the object removed. ■ Attempting to remove it from the ear may push it further in and damage the eardrum. ■ Insects may be washed out using warm water.
Ongoing Care	Parent/carer must look for any signs of infection e.g. continuing earache, raised temperature, continued hearing loss, and seek medical help as necessary. Children should be warned about the dangers of pushing things into their ears – but they do not usually want to repeat the experience.
Possible Complications	■ Damage to the eardrum. ■ Infection if the foreign body is not removed promptly or completely.

✅ *Progress check*

1 What objects may a child push into their ear?
2 How would a childcare worker or other adult know that a child had pushed something into their ear?
3 What immediate action should be taken?
4 How can children be discouraged from pushing things into their ears?

Chapter *13* *Conditions affecting the respiratory tract*

This chapter includes:

- **The structure and functions of the respiratory tract**
- **The common cold**
- **Influenza**
- **Epiglottitis**
- **Tonsillitis**
- **Enlarged adenoids**
- **Sinusitis**
- **Bronchitis**
- **Pneumonia**
- **Asthma**
- **Allergies**
- **Cystic fibrosis**

Respiratory tract conditions affect children more than any other illnesses. Amongst them bacterial and viral infections are the most common, followed by allergic disorders.

In childcare establishments the children work, play, eat and receive care in close proximity with each other. The circulating air in a busy playroom or classroom is laden with pathogenic organisms from the children and adults present. Many diseases are spread by droplet infection including all the respiratory tract infections. These environmental conditions, combined with children's immature immune systems, mean that they are vulnerable to infection most of the time. It is not really surprising that they are subject to respiratory infections.

Children attending playgroup, nursery or school for the first time are especially likely to contract a respiratory tract infection. They are exposed for the first time to a variety of bacteria and viruses to which they are not yet immune.

Childcare workers can reduce the risk by ensuring access to fresh air and sunlight via good ventilation and provision for outdoor play; being positive hygienic role models by using handkerchiefs and tissues and encouraging children to do the same; and by discouraging parents from bringing obviously poorly children into the establishment. Despite these precautions children will still pick up infections. The role of the carer is to comfort the child and ease their symptoms, to know when to contact the parents, whether to contact the doctor or send for an ambulance. The information in this chapter will increase understanding of these common childhood conditions.

The structure and functions of the respiratory tract

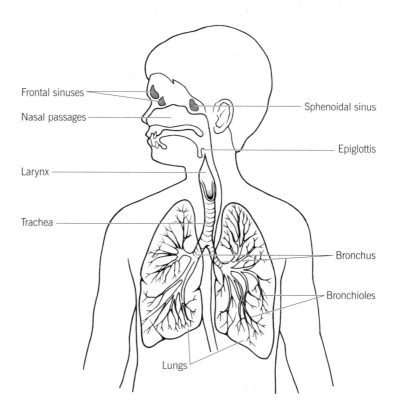

Frontal sinuses

Nasal passages

Sphenoidal sinus

Larynx

Epiglottis

Trachea

Bronchus

Bronchioles

Lungs

Cross-section of the respiratory system

Air is inhaled (breathed in) through the nose and/or mouth and passes over the tonsils, uvula and epiglottis – a flap of cartilage acting as a valve to separate the trachea and the oesophagus – to the trachea or windpipe. The trachea contains the larynx (voice-box) and carries the air into the lungs. The trachea divides into two bronchi – one goes into each lung. The bronchi branch off into progressively smaller airways, the bronchioles. The alveoli are at the end of the bronchioles and this is the area where the exchange of gases takes place. Oxygen in the inhaled air is passed into the blood and taken to the heart to be pumped around the body. Carbon dioxide from the blood returning to the lungs is filtered through the alveoli into the lungs to be exhaled (breathed out) with the next breath.

THE COMMON COLD

What Is The Common Cold? The common cold is a simple infectious illness of the upper respiratory tract which occurs frequently in children. Most children have 4 to 6 colds each year.

| What Causes The Common Cold? | The common cold is caused by virus passed by droplet infection. There are about 200 different viruses known to cause the common cold, so it is unlikely that children will be immune to them all! |

How To Recognise The Common Cold

- Sneezing.
- Runny nose and watery eyes.
- Blocked nose which may make feeding difficult for a baby.
- Sore throat.
- Cough which prevents infection spreading down to the lungs.
- Raised temperature sometimes.

Immediate Action

- Offer plenty of fluids and an appetising balanced diet rich in vitamin C.
- Allow the child to rest, and humidify the atmosphere (see page 185).
- Give paracetamol for a raised temperature and to relieve any aches.
- Call the doctor if a baby is having problems feeding or breathing.

Ongoing Care

With the above care colds should clear up completely in 7 days.

Possible Complications

- The infection may spread to the lungs and cause:
  - bronchiolitis in a baby (see page 186), or
  - bronchitis in an older child (see page 297), or
  - pneumonia (see page 299).
- Otitis media (see page 282) may result if the infection spreads to the middle ear.
- Conjunctivitis (see page 273).
- A cold may trigger an asthma attack (see page 300).

> ### Remember
> Avoid giving cough suppressants to children with a cold. Coughing is a valuable reflex which gets rid of infected mucus and prevents infection spreading further down the respiratory tract.

INFLUENZA

What Is Influenza?

Influenza is an infection of the upper repiratory tract. More common in the winter, it is spread by droplet infection and direct contact. There are usually small epidemics each year.

Influenza is not 'a bad cold'.

What Causes Influenza?

Influenza is caused by the influenza virus.

How To Recognise Influenza

- Raised temperature of 40°C or above.
- Complete lethargy and weakness.
- Headache and sometimes a sore throat (pharyngitis).
- Loss of appetite and refusal to drink.
- Muscular aches all over the body, especially in the joints.

Immediate Action	■ Call the doctor for a child under 2 years.
	■ Give paracetamol for the aches and pains and to control the temperature.
	■ Care for the child in a well-ventilated and humidified room.
	■ Encourage plenty of warm, soothing drinks and a light, nourishing diet.

Ongoing Care — Call the doctor if there is no improvement in 48 hours. See Good Practice box (below).

Possible Complications

■ Pneumonia.

■ Bronchitis.

■ Sinusitis – see below for these three conditions.

Good Practice

■ Plenty of drinks, especially warm soothing liquids such as honey and lemon, will help.

■ Humidifying the atmosphere by putting a damp towel on a warm radiator will help breathing.

■ Avoid overheating the room as this dries out the atmosphere.

■ Offer prescribed doses of cough linctus to soothe a cough.

Activity

Conduct some research in your childcare placement to establish how many children are affected by the common cold over a 3-month period in the winter. Use the nursery or infant class you are working in as a sample.

■ Prepare a questionnaire for parents.

■ Record absences yourself and enquire about the reasons for absence.

■ Note all the children who show signs and symptoms of the common cold and remain in the placement.

Evaluate the research.

■ How many children had more than one cold in this period?

■ Do your findings support the belief that all children have 5 to 6 colds a year?

■ Were there any children who were not affected with a cold at all?

■ Why do you think this was? For example was it dietary factors, fresh air, exercise, length of time at school etc?

Case study

Christina, aged 4, came to nursery for the morning session with Joan, her child-minder, as usual. She looked a little pale and was unusually tearful when Joan said goodbye. Joan said that she had been the same when her mother left her that morning and that she had refused her breakfast. The nursery staff reassured Joan that they would call her immediately if Christina seemed unwell. As the morning progressed, Christina opted out of all the activities and flopped on a bean bag in the book corner. She refused to drink her milk because she said that her throat hurt and her legs hurt too. The nursery teacher felt her forehead – it was very warm – and decided to call Joan because Christina was obviously unwell. Joan collected her and took her home.

1 What signs and symptoms was Christina displaying?
2 What action should Joan take?
3 How can Christina be cared for to ensure a full recovery?

EPIGLOTTITIS

What Is Epiglottitis? Epiglottitis is a very serious condition affecting the epiglottis (cartilage at the entrance to the larynx). The epiglottis swells quickly and obstructs the airway.

What Causes Epiglottitis? Epiglottitis is caused by the bacteria, haemophilus influenzae.

How To Recognise Epiglottitis The symptoms start very suddenly and the child may have great difficulty breathing within a few hours of the onset.
- Sore throat.
- Croupy/barking cough – like a seal.
- Difficulty in swallowing.
- Dribbling because swallowing is increasingly difficult.
- Breathing becomes difficult – noisy breaths will quieten as the illness gets worse.
- Blueness around the mouth.
- The child will quickly become exhausted.

Immediate Action This is a medical emergency.
- Reassure and comfort the child. Sitting up leaning forwards slightly, will help the breathing.
- Get the child to hospital as quickly as possible, by car or ambulance.
- The child will be admitted and given antibiotics and may be intubated (a tube inserted into the windpipe to keep it open). Some children need artificial ventilation.

Ongoing Care Most children recover within a week, with the right hospital treatment.

Possible Complications Death because of airway obstruction.

Most children who recover from epiglottitis never suffer from the infection again because they have developed antibodies.

Further Information Haemophilus influenzae type B (HIB) immunisation is offered to all children in the primary immunisation schedule. This has reduced the incidence of the disease and the number of deaths from epiglottitis.

 Progress check

1 What is the difference between the common cold and influenza?
2 Why is it inadvisable to give a cough suppressant to a child with a cold or influenza?
3 What is the difference between a cough linctus and a cough suppressant?
4 How should a child with a cold be cared for?
5 What are the possible complications of:
   ■ the common cold
   ■ influenza?
6 What is epiglottitis?
7 How could you recognise the condition?
8 How could you assist the child to breath?
9 Why have the number of cases of epiglottitis fallen?

TONSILLITIS

What Is Tonsillitis? Tonsillitis is inflammation of the tonsils. The tonsils are the body's first line of defence against infection and are active in childhood before shrinking in size as the child matures.

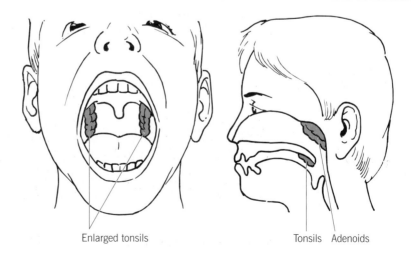

Position of the tonsils and adenoids

Enlarged tonsils   Tonsils   Adenoids

What Causes Tonsillitis?	Tosillitis is caused by streptococcal bacteria and viruses passed by droplet infection.
How To Recognise Tonsillitis	■ Raised temperature. ■ Inflamed and sore throat – the tonsils look red and swollen, sometimes with white patches (see plate 3). ■ Swollen and tender glands in the neck. ■ Refusal to eat due to the pain experienced when swallowing. ■ Earache. ■ The breath may smell unpleasant (halitosis).
Immediate Action	■ Call a doctor if the symptoms continue for more than 24 hours or get more severe. Antibiotics will be prescribed for a bacterial infection. ■ See Good Practice: Comforting a sore throat (below and page 295). ■ Give lots to drink and paracetamol to control the temperature
Ongoing Care	The child is infectious for about 3 days after the start of the sore throat and contact with other children is best avoided. Children should recover fairly quickly, especially from a bacterial infection treated with antibiotics.
Possible Complications	*Quinsy* An abscess may form around a tonsil. This will make swallowing increasingly difficult and may need drainage in hospital. Tonsillectomy may be performed when the infection has cleared. Rare complications may result if the bacteria or virus attacks other parts of the body: ■ rheumatic fever – joint inflammation which can also affect the heart ■ nephritis – inflammation of the kidney.
Further Information	Some children suffer from recurrent attacks of tonsillitis which affects their general health and school work. Doctors now try to delay removing the tonsils unless it is absolutely necessary because of their role in defending the body against infection. However, tonsillectomy (surgical removal of the tonsils) is performed on children who have frequent, severe attacks, develop a quinsy, or have a large and deeply scarred tonsil.

Good Practice

Comforting a sore throat
Sore throats are usually the result of pharyngitis (inflammation of the throat associated with the common cold) and tonsillitis. The following remedies should help to relieve the discomfort:
1 Give liquid paracetamol to relieve the pain.

> **Remember**
> Never give aspirin to a child under 12 years old because of the risk of Reye's syndrome which results in brain and liver damage following a simple viral infection.

2 Give lots of cold drinks and soft food to eat, for example yoghurt, fruit mousse, ice-cream etc. Ice lollies will soothe the throat.
3 Give throat pastilles or lozenges if the child is old enough to suck. Never leave a child alone whilst sucking a hard lozenge to the risk of choking.
4 Diluted antiseptic can be gargled if the child can do this.

ENLARGED ADENOIDS

What Are Enlarged Adenoids?

Enlarged adenoids are adenoid glands which have increased in size to block the back of the nose. The adenoids are composed of lymphatic tissue, which fight infection.

What Causes Enlarged Adenoids?

Enlarged adenoids are caused by:
- viral infections
- allergies e.g. to house dust mite, pollen, animals etc.

How To Recognise Enlarged Adenoids

- Snoring when sleeping.
- Waking at night due to breathing difficulties.
- Constantly blocked nose.
- Breathing through the mouth which results in a dry mouth and unpleasant breath (halitosis).
- Eating with the mouth open.
- Difficulty with pronouncing sounds, for example 'm' and 'n', and a nasal voice.
- Ear infections if the Eustachian tubes are blocked.

Immediate Action

- Humidify the air in the bedroom at night to help breathing.
- Encourage sleeping on the side or front to discourage snoring.
- Mild symptoms do not reqire urgent treatment. BUT if the child has speech problems or recurrent ear infections, the child should be seen by a doctor and referred to ear, nose and throat doctors, who will provide the appropriate treatment. They may conduct allergy tests.

Ongoing Care

If the cause is an allergy then the offending allergen must be found, if possible and removed from the child's environment as far as it is practical to do (see Allergies on page 305).

Children with enlarged adenoids may require adenoidectomy (surgical removal of the adenoids). Doctors are reluctant to recommend this at an early age because the adenoids tend to shrink in size from the age of 7 years. Postponing an operation may mean it will not be necessary as the child has grown out of the condition!

Possible Complications
- Glue ear (see page 284) and hearing problems.
- Speech delay.
- Sinusitis (see below) – this usually affects children over 10 years.

Case study

Jaganjeet had been a healthy child until she started playgroup when she was 2½ years. She missed more sessions than she attended because of sore throats, so her mother decided to keep her at home until she was old enough to go to nursery. The health visitor explained that it was better to continue at playgroup so that Jaganjeet could build up resistance to the infections. When she started nursery at 4 years of age she settled quickly and enjoyed the company of the other children. Within a few weeks she had another sore throat – the doctor diagnosed tonsillitis and prescribed some antibiotics. Jaganjeet quickly recovered but within a few days of returning to nursery she was complaining of a sore throat again. This pattern continued until Jaganjeet was nearly 5 years old. The doctor then referred her to the ear, nose and throat specialists requesting that she should be considered for a tonsillectomy.

1 Why do you think Jaganjeet's sore throats started when she began playgroup and then continued at nursery?
2 Why did the doctor wait until she was nearly 5 before referring her to hospital?
3 How can Jaganjeet be supported to if she has a lot of absences when she starts mainstream school?

SINUSITIS

What Is Sinusitis?
Sinusitis is inflammation of the lining of the sinuses (air filled cavities around the nose). Mucus membrane lines these air holes.

What Causes Sinusitis?
Sinusitis is caused by bacterial infection, often after a cold. Mucus is constantly produced in the sinuses and is usually drained out through narrow passages into the nose and throat. During a cold, these passages may be blocked by inflammation, resulting in bacteria multiplying in the mucus in the sinuses.

How To Recognise Sinusitis
- Green/yellow discharge from the nose.
- Headaches.
- Pain in the cheeks and forehead.
- Pain in the back teeth.

Immediate Action	■ See the doctor who will prescribe antibiotics if the sinuses are infected.
	■ Give paracetamol for the pain.
	■ Encourage the child to blow their nose regularly.
	■ Encourage plenty of fluids.

Ongoing Care	The infection usually improves within 7 days.

Good Practice

Inhalations

Breathing in the steamy vapours of Vic or tincture of benzoin helps to relieve a stuffy nose quickly. Great care must be taken to protect the child from scalds or burns. Sit with the child, place the inhalation bowl on a stable table with the child sitting in front of it. Let them breath in the vapours without touching the bowl.

 Progress check

1 Why are the tonsils and adenoids important in childhood?
2 What are the signs and symptoms of tonsillitis?
3 What care should be offered to a child with tonsillitis?
4 Explain what a quinsy is.
5 Why do doctors try to avoid removing the tonsils and adenoids?
6 How can an adult help to soothe a child's sore throat?
7 Why should children NEVER be offered aspirin?
8 What are the two main causes of enlarged adenoids?
9 What would make you think that a child may have enlarged adenoids?
10 How can the symptoms be relieved?
11 What are the possible complications of enlarged adenoids?
12 What is sinusitis?
13 How would you recognise this condition?
14 What are the benefits of inhalations and what special care must be taken?

BRONCHITIS

What Is Bronchitis?	Bronchitis is inflammation of the bronchi (the main airway).

What Causes Bronchitis?	Bronchitis is usually a viral infection following a common cold or flu. Occasionally, it is a bacterial infection.

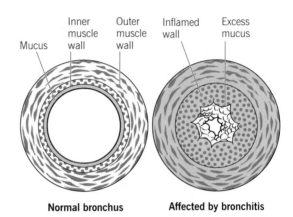

Mucus | Inner muscle wall | Outer muscle wall | Inflamed wall | Excess mucus

Normal bronchus   **Affected by bronchitis**

How bronchitis affects the airways

How To Recognise Bronchitis

- Constant and persistent chesty cough which may cause vomiting.
- Green or yellow phlegm coughed up from the lungs.
- Shortness of breath and rapid breathing (40 or more breaths a minute), even when resting.
- May wheeze.
- Raised temperature.
- Feeling very unwell.
- Blueness around the lips and mouth.

Immediate Action

- Call the doctor if the child finds breathing difficult, has a temperature over 39°C or is not improving in 24 hours. Antibiotics may be prescribed.
- Allow the child to rest quietly – sitting up is best to help breathing.
- Humidify the air in the room.
- Give paracetamol to reduce the temperature.
- Rub the back during a coughing attack (see Good Practice: Soothing a cough, below and page 299).

Ongoing Care

Recovery should be complete within a week.

Possible Complications

Some children have recurrent attacks of bronchitis but they have usually grown out of it by about 5 years of age.

Remember

Call for an ambulance immediately if a child is:
- unable to talk or make any sounds
- blue around the mouth or tongue.

Good Practice

Soothing a cough
- Plenty of drinks, especially warm soothing liquids such as honey and lemon, will help.
- Humidifying the atmosphere by putting a damp towel on a warm radiator may help to loosen phlegm in the airways and relieve the cough.

- Avoid overheating the room as this dries out the atmosphere and irritates the cough.
- Cough linctus may be prescribed by the GP and should be given according to the prescribed dosage.
- Do not use cough suppressants if children are producing mucus – this needs to be expelled from the lungs.

Case study

Aiden is 3 years old and has developed a wheezy cough whilst on a weekend break by the sea-side with his grandparents. They think that the bracing March air will do him good and so they take him for a walk along the sea front. Aiden's condition worsens and he vomits during an extended coughing bout. They comment on his pink face, thinking at first that it is due to the fresh air, but soon realise that he is flushed with a high temperature. They notice that his breathing is very rapid, even when sitting in his buggy. After a long discussion they decide to return home. During the journey, Aiden continues to cough and produces yellow phlegm. He lies on the back seat, grunting as he breathes, and his lips begin to turn blue.

- How can his breathing be helped?
- What other action should the grandparents take?
- What respiratory conditions could Aiden be suffering from?

PNEUMONIA

What Is Pneumonia? Pneumonia is infection of the lung tissue. It may affect both lungs or just one. It is most common between the ages of 4 and 12 years.

What Causes Pneumonia? Pneumonia is usually caused by a viral infection following the common cold, influenza or chickenpox.

Children with cystic fibrosis (see page 308) are very vulnerable to pneumonia.

How To Recognise Pneumonia
- Constant and persistent chesty cough which may cause vomiting.
- Green, yellow or blood-stained phlegm coughed up from the lungs.
- Shortness of breath and rapid, difficult breathing (40 or more breaths a minute), even when resting.
- Wheezing, rattling or grunting may be heard and the child may complain of chest pain.
- Headache.
- Raised temperature.
- Feeling very unwell and refusing to eat or drink.
- Blueness around the lips, tongue and mouth.

Immediate Action	■ Call the doctor who may take a throat swab or blood sample to identify the cause of the infection. ■ Allow the child to rest quietly – sitting up is best to help breathing. ■ Rub the child's back during a coughing attack (see Good Practice: Soothing a cough, pages 298–9). ■ Humidify the air in the room. ■ Give paracetamol to reduce the temperature and relieve the headache.

Ongoing Care

If the infection is severe the child may be admitted to hospital and given a chest X-Ray and oxygen therapy.

Most children will recover in about a week and fresh air is recommended, but vigorous exercise should be avoided for 7–14 days.

Possible Complications

Bronchopneumonia – rare in childhood but may occur after whooping cough or measles.

Remember

Call an ambulance if a child is showing signs of severe pneumonia i.e. blueness around the lips, tongue and mouth and/or drowsiness.

 Progress check

1 What is the difference between bronchitis and pneumonia?
2 What causes bronchitis?
3 How would you recognise this condition?
4 When should an ambulance be called for a child with bronchitis or pneumonia?
5 What can be done to help to comfort a child with a severe cough?
6 How would you recognise pneumonia?
7 What treatment will a child with pneumonia need?
8 For how long should vigorous exercise be avoided?
9 What are the possible complications of pneumonia?

ASTHMA

What Is Asthma?

Asthma is a chronic disease of the lungs which results in narrowing of the airways. 1 in 7 children are affected by asthma and most have their first attack before the age of 4 years. Children who receive incorrect treatment will not grow to their full potential.

About 50 children each year die during an asthma attack. It is not an infectious condition.

What Causes Asthma?

Children with asthma usually come from families with a history of allergic conditions e.g. eczema, hay fever and migraine.

Asthma is the narrowing of the bronchioles (small airways) as the result of:

- increased secretion of thick, sticky mucus due to inflammation
- the airways going into spasm
- the walls of the airways swelling.

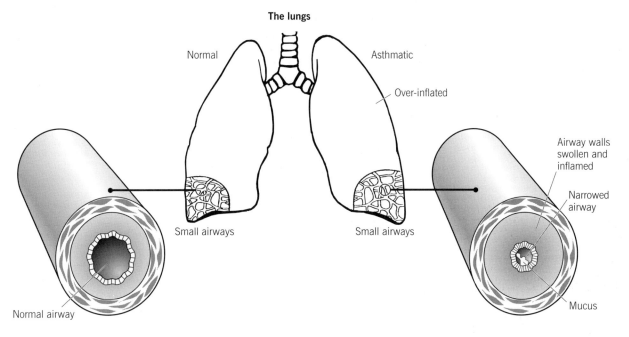

The lungs

Normal · Asthmatic · Over-inflated · Airway walls swollen and inflamed · Narrowed airway · Small airways · Small airways · Mucus · Normal airway

How asthma affects the lungs

The airways of children with asthma are hypersensitive to the following.

Environmental trigger factors

- Cold air.
- Infection e.g. common cold.
- Smoking.
- Exercise.
- Stress or excitement.
- Chemicals and fumes e.g. car exhausts, pollution, busy city streets, strong cleaning fluids, paint.

Allergens

- House dust mite.
- Furry or feathery animals.
- Grass pollen.
- Food e.g. peanuts, milk eggs.

Many children with asthma have other allergic conditions.

How To Recognise Asthma

- Night-time coughing is sometimes the first sign of asthma.
- Coughing after, and/or during, exercise.
- Wheezing.
- Shortness of breath.
- Feeling of tightness in the chest.
- Reluctance to join in any physical activity.

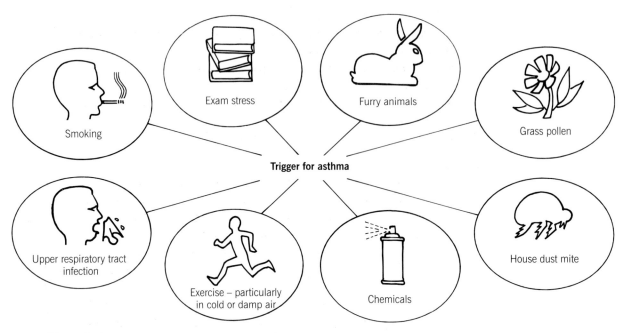

Trigger factors

An asthma attack

This is a terrifying experience for a child. The main difficulty is exhaling (breathing out). The typical picture is of a child leaning forwards with a hunched posture, gasping for breath – taking air in but unable to blow it out. Speech is impossible during an attack.

Immediate Action	■ If a child is suspected of having asthma a doctor should be seen within 24 hours.
	■ If an undiagnosed child has an asthma attack call an ambulance. In the meantime follow the steps below.

Management of an asthma attack

1 Reassure the child.
2 Encourage relaxed breathing – slowly and deeply.
3 Loosen tight clothing around the neck.
4 Sit the child upright and leaning forward, supporting themselves with their hands or any comfortable position.
5 Stay with the child.
6 Give the child their bronchodilator to inhale – 2 doses – if they are known asthmatics.
7 Offer a warm drink to relieve dryness of the mouth.
8 Continue to comfort and reassure. DO NOT PANIC as this will increase the child's anxiety which will impair their breathing even more.
9 When the child has recovered from a minor attack s/he can resume quiet activities.
10 Report the attack to the parents when the child is collected. If the child is upset by the episode they should be contacted immediately.

When to call an ambulance

Call an ambulance immediately, or get someone else to do so if:

- this is the first asthma attack
- the above steps have been taken and there is no improvement in 5–10 minutes
- the child is unable to talk and becoming increasingly distressed and exhausted
- the lips, mouth and face are turning blue.

Ongoing Care

Drugs And Medicines

Treatment aims to get rid of symptoms by regular use of:

- **preventer** medicines which can be corticosteroids and non-steroids e.g. Intal which reduce inflammation, swelling and mucus in the lungs. These are usually in a brown/orange inhaler
- **relievers** which are bronchodilators (which dilate the airways) for episodes of wheezing and before exercise. These are usually in a blue inhaler.

Inhalers and *spacer* devices are used in asthma so that the drug can immediately enter the lungs, where it works directly on the airways.

A spacer is a large plastic chamber into which the inhaler is sprayed so that the child can breath in the drug.

Nebulizers are used for babies. These deliver the drug in a fine mist via a mask.

Rotohalers, spinhalers and autohalers are also used in the treatment of asthma.

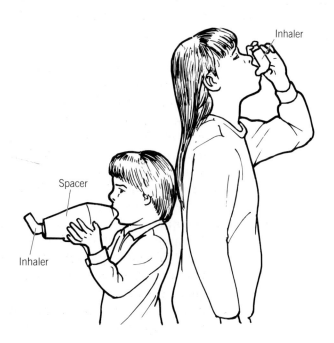

Inhaler

Spacer

Inhaler

Spacers make it easier for young children to inhale their treatment drugs

Daily life

Asthmatic children can enjoy all the activities that their non-asthmatic peers do. Apart from taking their medication regularly as prescribed, and avoiding known trigger factors, life should continue as normal.

Physical exercise and sport

Regular exercise is important – swimming and cycling are especially beneficial. Exercise in short bursts, rather than prolonged exertion, is recommended. Children should take their reliever inhaler before participating in a vigorous sporting activity.

Peak flow meters

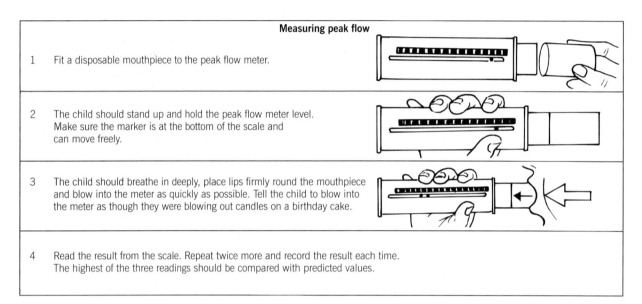

	Measuring peak flow	
1	Fit a disposable mouthpiece to the peak flow meter.	
2	The child should stand up and hold the peak flow meter level. Make sure the marker is at the bottom of the scale and can move freely.	
3	The child should breathe in deeply, place lips firmly round the mouthpiece and blow into the meter as quickly as possible. Tell the child to blow into the meter as though they were blowing out candles on a birthday cake.	
4	Read the result from the scale. Repeat twice more and record the result each time. The highest of the three readings should be compared with predicted values.	

How to use a peak flow meter

Peak flow meters measure how fast children can blow out. The measurement will monitor the severity of the asthma. The school nurse may record peak flows on a termly basis and carers may also be involved in recording peak flow.

A single reading is not adequate, children need to learn how to use the device to provide an accurate measurement. This is not usually achieved until the child is about 6 years old.

Possible Complications

Persistent attacks of asthma can result in permanent lung damage. This should not happen with careful and controlled treatment.

Further Information

Further information and/or support can be supplied by the following organisations:
- National Asthma Campaign
- School Health Service
- GPs, health visitors and specialist nurse practitioners
- Health Promotion Units
- Local voluntary and self-help groups.

Good Practice

Caring for an asthmatic child in a childcare establishment

- Ask parents what the trigger factors are for an attack in their child. Be aware of them and avoid the child's contact with them if possible, for example keep the child indoors when the pollen count is high if the child is allergic to grass pollen etc.
- Find out about the child's asthma treatment. Talk to the parents, and school nurse if the child is at school.
- Make sure that the child can easily access their medication. Ideally, children should carry their own inhaler (certainly by the age of 7 years). If this is not possible their personal carer or teacher should have the inhaler and spacer within reach at all times.
- Inform other staff about the child's condition and treatment.
- Tell the school nurse if the child is absent a lot with chest problems.
- Tell the parents about how the child is coping with general activities and exertion and whether frequent medication is used.
- Make sure that the child takes their medication regularly if this is prescribed, especially before any exercise.
- Reassure the child when they have an asthma attack.
- Include the child in everything that is happening!

If a child is asthmatic as a result of house dust mite or has an allergy to house dust mite, the following precautions may provide some relief:

- keep house dust to a minimum with regular damp dusting
- treat all carpets with insecticide to kill mites
- enclose the child's mattress with a plastic cover
- avoid feather pillows and/or duvets
- keep all rooms well ventilated.

ALLERGIES

What Are Allergies?

An allergy is a condition in which the immune system responds inappropriately to a usually harmless substance.

An allergic reaction is the result of the immune system producing antibodies to that substance (called an allergen). On the first contact with the allergen there is no obvious reaction – the immune system registers its presence and begins to make antibodies for the next encounter. When the second contact occurs the response is quick and dramatic.

What Causes Allergies?

Allergies can be caused by:
- chemicals on the skin
- food which has been swallowed
- drugs which have been injected or swallowed
- insect bites
- particles inhaled in the air.

Some common allergens are:
- house dust mite
- furry or feathery animals
- grass pollen
- food e.g. peanuts, milk, eggs.

How To Recognise Allergies

Symptoms range from very mild to extremely severe e.g.anaphylactic shock (see below).

Allergies may affect the skin, nose and/or eyes or be widespread with a reaction that involves more than one system or part of the body.

Symptoms may include:
- rash
- sore or itchy eyes
- blocked nose
- coughing
- diarrhoea and vomiting.

Immediate Action

- Treat the symptoms and reassure the child. Antihistamines may help.
- If there is no improvement in 24 hours see the doctor.

Ongoing Care

Identify the cause of the allergy and remove it from the child's environment.

Possible Complications

Many allergies get less severe as a child grows into puberty.

Anaphylactic shock
Allergies can lead to a generalised reaction to an allergen. Anaphylactic shock may occur in extreme cases. This is very dangerous because:
- the mouth and face will swell
- breathing becomes laboured as the airways swell
- swallowing is difficult
- it can be fatal.

Immediate Action for Anaphylactic Shock

Call the doctor or take the child to the accident and emergency department of the nearest hospital if this will be quicker. Support the child in a semi-sitting position to ease the breathing. Children who have had this type of allergic response should wear a bracelet indicating their allergy, and parents and teachers may have adrenalin to inject in case of an emergency.

Further Information   It is possible to test children with various allergens in a carefully controlled environment to find out precisely what they are allergic to. A programme of de-sensitisation may help to cure the allergy.

Allergic rhinitis

This is an inflammation of the lining of the nose resulting from an allergy. This is also called hay fever if the reaction is due to grass pollen.

 Progress check

1 What is asthma?
2 What are the possible trigger factors for asthma?
3 How would you recognise asthma in a young child?
4 Explain what happens during an asthma attack and how you would manage it.
5 Explain how a child with asthma can be supported in a childcare establishment.
6 How can the effects of house dust mite be kept to a minimum for an asthmatic child?
7 What is an allergy?
8 Give an example of 4 common allergens which can be inhaled.
9 How could you comfort and offer practical help to a child with an allergy?
10 Describe anaphylactic shock.

Case study

John, aged 5, and his family had recently moved into a new house. They were all very excited because it was on the edge of a new estate and backed onto a field – it was like having an enormous garden! John had spent most of the summer holidays playing with his new friends in the corn and had visited the stables with his dad to help with the horses. His mother was concerned about his night-time cough. She was getting up several times at night to give him a drink to soothe him back to sleep. In the daytime he was his usual lively self and did not seem ill at all, but she noticed that he was quickly out of breath when their new puppy escaped and they had to run after him. She decided to take him to see the GP to see if she could find anything wrong with John.

1 What illness is John showing signs and symptoms of?
2 What new circumstances in John's life could have triggered an illness?
3 What treatment may help him?

CYSTIC FIBROSIS (CF)

What Is Cystic Fibrosis?

CF is a very serious disease which affects mainly the respiratory and digestive stystems.

Effects on the respiratory tract
The secretions produced by the lungs are thick and sticky and cannot flow through the airways freely. Eventually the airways become clogged which makes breathing difficult and increases the risk of infection.

Effects on the digestive tract
The pancreas is responsible for producing digestive enzymes which break down food and help absorption.

In CF the ducts in the pancreas also become clogged with mucus and this prevents the enzymes from helping to digest food. Fats are not absorbed and the child does not gain weight adequately.

What Causes Cystic Fibrosis?

CF is inherited and affects 1 in 2,000 births. The defective gene is carried by 1 in 20 in the white population. Although it is present from birth the disease may not be diagnosed for several months, occasionally years.

How To Recognise Cystic Fibrosis

At birth
- Meconium ileus – most babies pass their first stool (meconium) within a few hours of birth. In CF, babies usually have a thick plug of meconium blocking the intestine. All babies who do not pass meconium within 24 hours of delivery should be tested for cystic fibrosis.

Guthrie test
- All babies are given a heel prick blood test for phenylketonuria, hypothyroidism and *cystic fibrosis* on the sixth day of milk feeding.

Early months
- Failure to thrive due to malabsorption.
- Persistent coughing.
- Recurrent chest infections.
- Diarrhoea and very offensive, fatty stools.

Immediate Action

- A doctor must be consulted if a baby/child has ANY of the above symptoms.
- The child will have a sweat test because in CF the concentration of salt in the sweat is much greater than normal.
- Genetic tests will confirm the diagnosis.

Ongoing Care

Physiotherapy
Regular, aggressive chest physiotherapy to loosen the chest secretions and enable the child to cough up the mucus. Keeping the lungs clear will help to prevent infection.

Exercise
Regular exercise is encouraged because it increases the capacity of the lungs and boosts children emotionally – it helps them to feel good!

Antibiotics
Antibiotics prevent chest infections.

Pancreatic enzyme supplements
These pancreatin tablets will be taken with every meal to replace the enzymes normally produced by the pancreas.

Diet
Low fat, high protein and carbohydrate diet with vitamin supplements is recommended for CF. A dietician will work with the family to achieve the most satisfactory diet for the child. High energy snacks are very good for the child.

Possible Complications

- There is no cure for CF, but with constantly improving treatment most sufferers survive into adulthood.
- Some children/young adults benefit from a heart/lung transplant.
- Early death.

Further Information

- The Cystic Fibrosis Research Trust, Alexandra House, 5 Blythe Road, Bromley, Kent BR1 3RS offers support and advice.
- It is very important that children with CF are immunised for all the childhood conditions.
- Genetic counselling (see page 40) is available to all families with a child who has CF.

✔ *Progress check*

1 What effects does cystic fibrosis have on the respiratory tract?
2 How can the disease be recognised in the early months of life?
3 What treatment will a child with cystic fibrosis require?
4 How do you think that caring for a child with CF will affect the family?
5 How will CF affect all round development?
6 How could you support a child with cystic fibrosis at nursery or school?

Chapter 14 Life-threatening conditions

This chapter includes:

- AIDS
- Hepatitis
- Childhood cancer
- Leukaemia
- Duchenne muscular dystrophy
- Sickle cell anaemia
- Thalassaemia

This chapter should be read with Chapter 16, 'Coping with Chronic Illness'.

There are many conditions which affect children and are potentially life-threatening if the correct treatment is not given before the disease becomes serious. Several examples of these are contained in the previous chapters of this book, for example meningitis and epiglottitis. Other life-threatening conditions affecting specific parts of the body are also explained earlier in the book, for example cystic fibrosis.

This chapter is concerned with other conditions which may be terminal and will affect the growth and development of the child who is unfortunately affected despite the treatment and care which is provided.

Some of the conditions are genetic – passed from parent(s) to child – and are thus present at the time of birth, for example muscular dystrophy and thalassaemia. There are no cures for these genetic conditions. Some other conditions occur during childhood for no apparent reason, for example leukaemia and other forms of cancer.

Childcare workers may be involved in the ongoing care of a child with a serious illness, and must be aware of the effects of the illness on the child's specific and global development, and the inevitable effects on family life.

AIDS

What Is AIDS? Acquired – it is the result of an infection which is transmitted by direct contact.

Immune – the disease affects the immune system.

Deficiency – the immune system cannot work properly, so it is deficient.

Syndrome – a collection of particular signs and symptoms is a syndrome.

AIDS is the result of infection with the Human Immunodeficiency Virus (HIV).

What Causes HIV and AIDS?

Infection with HIV always occurs before AIDS develops.
Human – the virus only affects humans.
Immunodeficiency – it results in the immune system getting weaker.
Virus – the infection is viral.

Most viruses affect only specific types of cells in the body (e.g. the influenza virus affects the upper respiratory tract). HIV infection affects the T4 cells in the immune system. T4 cells are important in fighting infection – they are responsible for activating the immune system, and as they are damaged the immune system gets weaker. Eventually, it is not able to fight some infections that would normally have been destroyed. This process usually takes years. Infection with HIV progressively damages the immune system and leads to AIDS.

Children may be infected with HIV by the following.

■ *Transmission of the virus from their mother:*
1 through the placenta in pregnancy
2 during birth. There is about a 10–14 per cent risk of an infected mother passing the infection to her baby before or during birth, but with a caesarian delivery and not breast feeding the risk is reduced to 5 per cent
3 breast feeding. There is about a 10 per cent risk of passing the virus from mother to baby in breast milk. HIV positive mothers are advised not to breast feed their infants to reduce this risk.
■ *Transfusions with infected blood or blood products*:
although this risk is now very small (all donated blood is tested for AIDS), many haemophiliacs were infected with HIV during the 1980s, when their injections of Factor 8 were contaminated with HIV from foreign donors.

HIV can also be spread by:
■ sexual contact
■ using contaminated needles for injecting substances, or sharing equipment with somebody who has the virus.

HIV is transmitted only by body fluids – blood, seminal and vaginal fluid and breast milk – entering into the blood stream. It cannot be caught by normal social contact such as touching, kissing, using the same cups, plates and cutlery or from toilet seats. Swimming pools, towels and washing equipment cannot spread the infection either.

How To Recognise HIV and AIDS

Children who have been infected during pregnancy or the birth process, will usually show some symptoms by the time they reach their second birthday. However some take several years to display any signs at all.

The signs of HIV infection developing into AIDS in children are wide-ranging and include the following:
■ enlarged, swollen glands

- frequent infections
- pneumonia
- failure to thrive
- delayed development sometimes.

Symptoms will appear only when the immune system is sufficiently weakened to allow infections to become rampant, these are called opportunistic infections.

The disease may also cause tumours on the skin called sarcomas. The virus may attack the brain.

Immediate Action
- Consult a doctor if there is any concern that a child may have been born with HIV, or may have been infected at some later time. A decision must be made about whether to perform an HIV antibody test, in consultation with the child's parents.
- Careful medical treatment is required from a team of specialists.
- A mother who is HIV positive may pass her HIV antibodies to the child and they may remain in the baby's bloodstream for a year or more. The baby is not diagnosed as HIV positive until it produces its own antibodies as a result of contact with the virus.

Ongoing Care

Counselling for the parents and child
Decisions will be made about who to inform of the child's HIV status, and how to cope as the child gets older. Parents do not have a legal obligation to inform the child's school or day care setting that their child is infected with HIV. The risk of transmission is very small and non-existent if the correct hygiene routines are followed. There have not been any recorded instances of HIV being transmitted in a childcare setting.

Drugs
- Anti-viral drugs e.g. AZT, zidovudine to attack the virus and slow down the progress of the disease.
- Antibiotics e.g. cotrimoxazole (Septrin) to prevent and/or treat infections such as pneumonia.
- Gamma globulin injections help to improve the efficiency of the immune system.
- New treatments are always being developed and the hope is that eventually HIV and AIDS will be curable.

Complementary medicine
Acupuncture has been used to alleviate the illness.

Relaxation and massage can help to reduce the stress of the situation and promote a feeling of well-being.

Children infected with HIV are very vulnerable to the common childhood illnesses e.g. chickenpox and these conditions can be life-threatening for a child who is HIV positive, or has full-blown AIDS.

Remember
A child with HIV should be treated in exactly the same way as any other child. Physical contact is important for ALL children. HIV cannot be spread by touching.

Good Practice

Implement a high standard of hygiene practices with all children. Treat any blood or body fluid spillages as though they are contaminated with a blood-borne infection (see below).

The following guidelines should be implemented at all times:
- skin injuries should be covered with a waterproof dressing
- staff should wear disposable latex gloves when in contact with bodily waste i.e. blood, faeces, urine
- cover spillages with a paper towel
- blood should be covered with a 1% hypochlorite solution to destroy the virus – it can then be wiped up with a disposable cloth which should be discarded in a sealed bag.
- hands should be washed with an antiseptic soap
- floor mops should be soaked in a solution of 1 part bleach to 10 parts water and dried
- nappies, dressings, disposable cloths and used latex gloves should be placed in a sealed bag before placing in the appropriate bags for incineration
- designated areas with covered bins for different types of waste should be provided

If body fluid should contact damaged or broken skin, encourage the wound to bleed and wash the area immediately with an antiseptic solution. Urgent medical aid will be required.

Possible Complications

Few children infected with HIV make a full recovery, although several children infected at birth are now reaching their teens without any signs of developing AIDS.

AIDS ultimately results in death from infection because of the weakened immune system; pneumonia is often the cause of death.

Further Information

The first cases of AIDS were detected in the early 1980s. Since then about 400 babies have been born in the UK infected with HIV – approximately half of them have died. Some of the surviving children are now reaching their teens having moved from primary to secondary education.

Helpline
The National Aids Helpline: 0800 567123
A freephone number offering confidential advice about any aspect of HIV and AIDS.

Useful Address
Terence Higgins Trust
52–54 Grays Inn Road
London WC1X 8JU
Tel. 0171 8310330

Progress check

1 What does AIDS stand for?
2 What does HIV stand for?
3 How may children be infected with HIV?
4 How can HIV infection be recognised?
5 What are the signs of AIDS?
6 What ongoing care should be offered to a child who is HIV positive?
7 What precautions should be taken in a childcare establishment with regard to the disposal of bodily waste products?

Case study

Edward was born and had been breast fed for 9 months before his mother Lorraine was tested for HIV antibodies. His father, Hugh, was contacted by an HIV/AIDS contact tracer to be told that one of his previous girlfriends was HIV positive. Hugh and Lorraine both tested HIV antibody positive. 18 months after Edward's birth he, too, was tested. The result was positive. The family were devastated but decided that life must carry on as normally as possible for Edward's sake. They thought that with all their love and skill as parents they could protect him from ignorance and prejudice. When Edward started playgroup, Lorraine and Hugh decided that the playgroup leader should be informed in confidence of Edward's HIV status, mainly because parent helpers did not always use the correct procedures when a child needed first aid. They thought that the leader could make sure that everyone wore disposable gloves to deal with all the children's cuts and grazes. Unfortunately the information was not treated confidentially – the playgroup committee met and all the parents were informed. They were very supportive and Edward continued to be without symptoms. However, when Edward went to primary school in a different area, some parents heard about his condition. Several of them campaigned aggressively to have him removed from the school because of the risk to their children's health and safety.

1 Do you think that the staff of childcare establishments have a right to know about any HIV positive children in their care? Give reasons for your answer.
2 How could staff at Edward's primary school reassure these parents and convince them that he is not a hazard to their children?
3 Which policies should be in place in all childcare establishments for the protection of children and staff regardless of their HIV status?

HEPATITIS

What Is Hepatitis? Hepatitis is an inflammation of the liver. There are two main types.

Hepatitis A is also called infective hepatitis and has an incubation period of 10–40 days. It is transmitted via contact with infected faeces. See page 266.

Hepatitis B is also called serum hepatitis and has an incubation period of 60–160 days. It is the more serious of the two and can cause death due to liver failure.

What Causes Hepatitis? Hepatitis is caused by several strains of virus.

Hepatitis B can be contracted via the same routes as HIV and AIDS:

- transmission of the virus from their mother i.e.
  1 through the placenta in pregnancy
  2 during the birth process
- transfusions with infected blood or blood products
- sexual contact
- using contaminated needles for injecting substances, or sharing equipment with somebody who has the virus.

How To Recognise Hepatitis
- Fever.
- Headache.
- Generally feeling unwell.
- Tiredness.
- Loss of appetite.
- Nausea and vomiting.
- Tender abdomen – the upper right area where the liver is located.

About a week after the first symptoms the child will become jaundiced, with yellowish skin and yellowing of the whites of the eyes. This is accompanied by dark urine and pale-coloured stools. The infected liver cannot metabolise the waste products, so a build-up of bilirubin in the blood occurs which causes the jaundice.

Immediate Action The child should be seen by a doctor. If the first signs occur in the childcare establishment, the parents should be contacted and encouraged to seek medical advice. The child should rest and drink if possible.

Ongoing Care
- The child should be cared for in bed or wherever s/he feels most comfortable.
- Plenty of fluids to prevent dehydration and small, light appetising meals to tempt the poor appetite.
- Scrupulous attention to hygiene is required.

Possible Complications   People who have recovered from hepatitis B continue to be carriers of the infection. They are well themselves but carry the virus in their bloodstream and can pass the infection to others.

Further Information   Immunisation against hepatitis B is available for people believed to be at risk from the infection e.g. health carers.

 Progress check

1 What is the difference between hepatitis A and hepatitis B?
2 How could a child contract hepatitis B?
3 What are the signs and symptoms of the illness?
4 Why does jaundice occur?
5 What teatment should be offered to a child with hepatitis B?

Activity

Read the Health and Safety policy in your establishment or placement. Check the procedures for disposal of body fluids and hazardous waste.
Do you think that the policy is thorough?
Are the procedures displayed in the establishment?
Are they carried out efficiently and reliably?
Is there anything else that should be included in the policy?

CHILDHOOD CANCER

What Is Childhood Cancer?   Cancer is a malignant growth (tumour) which can occur in any part of the body. It is fortunately quite rare in childhood.

In childhood the body is developing quickly and cells are constantly produced to enable this growth to occur. Cells are also being replaced as they wear out. Usually this cell production takes place without problem, because cells are produced and replaced by a process of cell division which is programmed into the body by its genes. Occasionally the process loses control. Cells are produced too quickly creating abnormalities which continue to reproduce and overpower the normal cells. The function of the affected area of the body is damaged.

What Causes Childhood Cancer?   There have been many suggestions for the causes of cancer in childhood, many scientists believe that there is an inherited (genetic) tendency to cancer in some children. There is not a single, known cause for cancer but current thinking is that there are a variety of factors which may trigger cancerous cells to be produced. Some of these are listed below.

■ Radiation.

■ Viruses which cause cells to behave in an unusual way.
■ Chemicals.

How To Recognise Childhood Cancer

Signs and symptoms of the many different types of cancer will depend upon which area of the body is affected. However, there are some signs which always need investigating.
■ Weight loss.
■ Excessive tiredness and lethargy.
■ Unexplained lumps anywhere on the body.
■ Looking pale and possibly anaemic.
■ Generally unwell and lacking energy despite a good diet and plenty of sleep.

Signs And Symptoms Of Cancer In Specific Areas Of The Body

AREA OF THE BODY	SIGNS AND SYMPTOMS
Brain and central nervous system	■ irritability ■ headaches – especially on waking in the morning ■ nausea and vomiting due to raised pressure inside the skull ■ weakness of the muscles and/or loss of co-ordination ■ loss of sensation in some areas of the body ■ convulsions
Kidney (Wilm's tumour) and urinary tract	■ abdominal swelling ■ blood in the urine
Lymph system	■ nausea and vomiting ■ night sweats ■ enlarged lymph glands ■ recurrent infections ■ anaemia
Bone	■ unexplained lump on the affected bone ■ pain in the area

Immediate Action

Any suspicion of a malignancy should be taken seriously and the doctor consulted. Usually it is a false alarm, but immediate treatment will commence when the diagnosis has been confirmed. The treatments for cancer depend upon where in the body the tumour is sited, how extensive it is and whether it has spread from the original site. Some types of cancer are successfully cured by a combination of treatments. The main types of therapy are as follows.

Surgical removal
Tumours can be successfully removed if they are confined to one area of the body and have not spread to other organs. They may also be removed to improve the quality of life for a child, even though the

condition cannot be cured. Surgery is usually followed by one or both of the following treatments to destroy any cells which may remain after the operation.

Radiotherapy

Carefully calculated doses of radiation are directed at the site of the cancer over a period of time. The result may be a reduction in the size of the tumour which will relieve the symptoms. Occasionally it may be used to cure the condition. There are inevitable complications of this invasive treatment:

- tiredness
- nausea and vomiting
- inflammation of the skin around the treatment site (radiation burns are possible but should be prevented by skilled radiotherapists)
- loss of hair from the treated area

Chemotherapy

Powerful drugs can be used to destroy the malignant cells, but unfortunately they can also destroy some healthy tissue. Cytotoxic therapy (drugs such as vincristine) destroys cells which are multiplying rapidly. They are usually given intravenously in hospital in a controlled environment and the treatment usually lasts several weeks, with the child going home between treatments. The side-effects from the therapy can be very severe e.g.

- anaemia and tiredness
- diarrhoea and vomiting
- hair loss from the entire body
- children having chemotherapy are very vulnerable to infections, because the drugs can destroy some of the bone marrow which produces white blood cells. Antibiotics are sometimes given to prevent secondary infections occurring.

Ongoing Care

The success rate for curing childhood cancer continues to increase.

Children and their parents should be offered counselling and support to cope with the disease and its treatment.

School, nursery etc. should be kept well informed of the child's progress and encouraged to maintain contact by visits, tapes and letters.

A normal routine should be continued as far as practically possible: the child can return to school when s/he feels well enough – even between treatments.

Possible Complications

Complications include the side-effects of the treatments, recurrence of the original tumour and the risk of the cancer spreading to other parts of the body.

Progress check

1 What is cancer?
2 What is the current thinking about the causes of cancer?
3 How may you recognise cancer in a child?
4 What are the signs and symptoms of a tumour in the brain?
5 What are the main types of treatment for cancer?
6 Describe the possible side-effects of all types of treament for cancer.
7 What on-going care will a child require?

LEUKAEMIA

What Is Leukaemia?

Leukaemia is a malignancy (cancer) of the blood. The bone marrow normally produces the required amounts of healthy white blood cells which enable the body to fight infection. In leukaemia many abnormal white cells are produced which are too immature to function effectively.

There are several different types of leukaemia which are named according to the type of white blood cell that is affected. Leukaemia can also be acute (rapid onset becoming serious very quickly) or chronic (slow development, progressing slowly). Acute leukaemias are most common in childhood and the most common type is acute lymphoblastic leukaemia.

What Causes Leukaemia?

There is no specific cause for leukaemia which has been proven. However, there may be several triggers which affect children who have a genetic predisposition to leukaemia.

Congenital Factors
Children with Down's syndrome have an increased risk of leukaemia, as do children with a parent or sibling who has had the condition.

Viruses
Leukaemia may be triggered by a viral infection. The body manufactures more white cells during an infection, and this may be an abnormal response – the white cell production gets out of control.

Radiation
Areas in the country with a higher than usual level of radiation have a higher than average number of childhood leukaemias per head of population than areas within the normal range.

X-rays of the embryo or fetus during pregnancy can increase the risk of leukaemia after birth.

Chemicals
Exposure to certain toxic chemicals in childhood may result in leukaemia.

**How To Recognise
Leukaemia**

Different types of leukaemia may produce slightly different signs and symptoms, but the following are characteristic of leukaemia in general.

Too many white cells
Excessive amounts of white cells being produced may result in inadequate production of other blood cells, too few red cells will result in anaemia which is lack of haemoglobin in the blood. This will result in:
- pale skin – black skin looks dull and paler than usual
- lack of energy, tiredness.

Too few platelets
Platelets are necessary for clotting the blood. In leukaemia too few are manufactured resulting in:
- bruising – widespread or irregular marks which appear easily
- pinkish/purple flat spots on the skin
- bleeding from the gums.

Reduced resistance to infection
The immature white cells cannot successfully fight infection so a child with leukaemia is very vulnerable to infection. The following characteristic signs of infection may be noticed:
- swollen lymph glands
- fever
- loss of appetite resulting in weight loss
- painful joints, especially in the arms and legs – there may be general aching in the bones. White cells are produced in the bones and their over production may result in pain.

Immediate Action

Consult the doctor at once if there is even a slight suspicion that a child has leukaemia. The child will be given a blood test to confirm the diagnosis. If the test is positive they will be admitted to hospital for a bone marrow biopsy. Cells from the bone marrow will be taken for examination to detect the type of leukaemia because this will influence the type of treatment which is offered.

Ongoing Care

Treatment will depend upon the type of leukaemia, but generally follows two stages.

Stage 1
Drugs are given which will destroy the affected abnormal cells. This treatment lasts for several weeks. Another bone marrow biopsy is taken and when no abnormal cells are seen the child is in remission.

For about two years the child will have further drug treatment to kill any leukaemic cells which may still be present in the body.

Stage 2
Bone marrow transplants from a suitable donor may be performed if conventional treatment does not cure the condition.

There is an increasingly high success rate for childhood leukaemia. About 70 per cent of children with acute lymphoblastic leukaemia achieve full recovery.

Possible Complications

Children with leukaemia who are having drug treatment are very vulnerable to infection. They should be kept away from viral infections such as chickenpox and measles.

Hearing loss as the result of some drugs used in the treatment of leukaemia e.g. vincristine.

✔ Progress check

1 What are the characteristic signs of leukaemia?
2 What immediate action should be taken if leukaemia is suspected?
3 What are the two stages of treatment?
4 What is a possible complication of this treatment?

Case study

Michelle was always tired and complaining of her legs aching and soreness in her joints. Her legs were constantly bruised and when some bruises were beginning to disappear others appeared. Her mother thought that this was due to starting school at the beginning of that term, and reassured Michelle that she would feel better when the summer holidays started. Michelle had always been a pale-skinned child but seemed to look paler than ever. Her mother noticed that when she cleaned her teeth her gums bled slightly. The dentist could not find any cause for the bleeding and thought it may be due to a milk tooth which was loose. When the school holidays started Michelle did not improve, she did not want to go out to play or to go out to her favourite fast-food restaurant. She slept most of the days away. When the GP saw her, and heard about her signs and symptoms, he took some blood tests which confirmed leukaemia.

1 Would any of Michelle's symptoms on their own make you suspect leukaemia?
2 What support could be offered to this child from the children and staff at her new primary school during her treatment?
3 How could Michelle and her family be prepared for her treatment?

DUCHENNE MUSCULAR DYSTROPHY

What Is Duchenne Muscular Dystrophy?

Duchenne muscular dystrophy is the most common of several muscular dystrophies. It is a degenerative disease of the muscles which affects only boys. The condition gets progressively worse as the muscles get weaker and weaker. About 2 boys per thousand are affected. As walking becomes difficult, a wheelchair will be necessary – usually by 9 to 12 years of age. The respiratory muscles and heart muscle will also weaken and the respiratory tract is very vulnerable to infections. Affected boys do not usually survive beyond their early twenties.

What Causes Duchenne Muscular Dystrophy?

The abnormal gene for muscular dystrophy is carried on the X chromosome. The condition is inherited from the mother, so boys can be affected and girls can be carriers of the disorder. Each pregnancy has a 1 in 4 chance of producing an affected male. Each boy has a 1 in 2 (50%) chance of having the disease and each girl has a 1 in 2 (50%) chance of being a carrier.

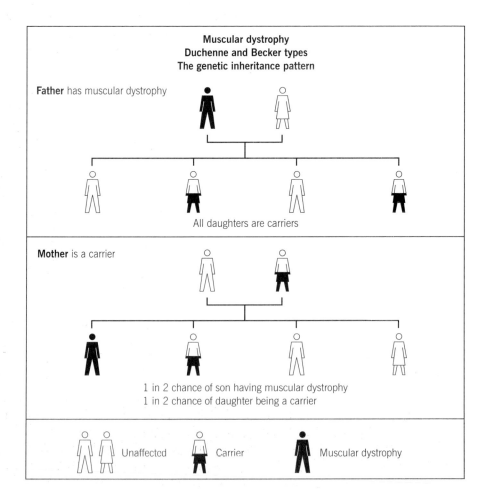

The genetic inheritance pattern for Duchenne muscular dystrophy

How To Recognise Duchenne Muscular Dystrophy

There may be a family history of the condition, although the mother may be unaware of the reason for the death of male relative(s) from earlier generations. In some cases a gene mutation has occurred in this pregnancy, so there is no history of the condition.

There are no obvious signs of Duchenne at birth. Affected boys usually walk and make slow but acceptable progress in gross motor development in the early years. It is with hindsight, after the diagnosis has been made, that parents may realise that their son had shown earlier clumsiness or delay.

There are characteristic signs.

- Late walking.
- Difficulty in climbing stairs.
- Frequent falls.
- Awkward and difficult running posture.

A boy with Duchenne may enter pre-school care before diagnosis is made. He is the child who is last to reach the exciting activity he wants to get to, he cannot keep up with his friends in outdoor play, he falls often and his walking posture is a wide-legged waddle.

Carers may also notice the following.

- Difficulty in standing up after a fall – the boy will roll over onto his front and use his hands to walk up his legs to return to an upright posture. Weak leg muscles result in the child needing to push against the ankles, knees and thighs to get up.
- Inward curvature of the lower spine – lordosis.
- Enlarged calf muscles.

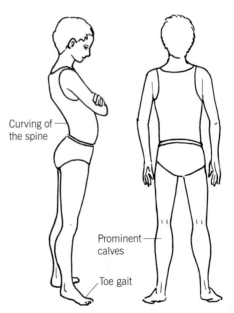

Curving of the spine

Prominent calves

Toe gait

The typical Duchenne posture shows curvature of the spine, prominent calves and a wide-legged stance

Immediate Action

If any of the above signs are noticed by carers or teachers in a childcare establishment, a senior member of staff should discuss their concerns with the parent and arrange a medical with the school doctor. Parents should take their child to the family doctor who will arrange a hospital appointment where tests can be conducted to provide a diagnosis. The tests include creatinine kinase levels (an enzyme produced in muscles) and a muscle biopsy (a small sample of muscle tissue is taken to check for any abnormalities).

Ongoing Care

Mobility

Physiotherapy will help the child to keep as mobile as possible and also maintain fitness. Several hours each day may be spent exercising.

Diet must be carefully monitored to prevent the child from becoming overweight. Too much weight will reduce their activity and put a greater strain on weakened muscles.

Maintaining independence

Self-esteem is very important, and children with Duchenne should be supported and encouraged to do as much as possible for themselves. Eventually feeding and washing will be difficult for them, so great tenderness and care must be given in supporting them to keep their independence in the everyday tasks which are most important to them.

Support

Families inevitably find it difficult to tell their child about the condition and its likely effects. They will be experiencing a range of emotions themselves (see Chapter 16). In general, any questions from the child should be answered honestly and in a way that he will understand i.e. related to his age and stage of development. Parents and health professionals must be consulted to make sure that everyone is telling the same story – beware of giving too much information or talking about the future months and years. However, as the child gets older he may ask for this information.

Possible Complications

Because of the possibility of late diagnosis, more children may be born into the family with the condition, before the first child has been diagnosed.

Further Information

Women who are carriers for Duchenne will be offered pre-natal testing of each pregnancy and offered a termination of affected boys. This is obviously a difficult decision for parents who should be treated with empathy and understanding.

 Progress check

1 Describe Duchenne muscular dystrophy.
2 What is the inheritance pattern?
3 How can DMD be recognised?
4 What should a childcare worker do if they suspect DMD?
5 What are the most important aspects of the treatment?
6 How can support be offered to these boys and their families?

Case study

Liam Wilson was 3 years old when his mother produced a baby brother, Ben, for him. He was delighted and insisted that Ben should come to his nursery so that all the children could see him. The nursery teacher was pleased to hear that Ben and his mum were coming in to visit – she had been meaning to have a word with Mrs Wilson about Liam. She had noticed that he was falling over a lot and needed help to climb the ladder on the nursery slide. Some of the older children were beginning to notice his awkwardness and were calling him Mr Clumsy. Liam's mum said that she too had thought that he was having difficulties and said she would talk to the doctor when Ben went for his 6 week check. Liam was referred to the local hospital where tests confirmed that he was affected with Duchenne muscular dystrophy.

1 What are the chances that Ben will also be affected?
2 What tests could have been offered during this pregnancy if Liam had been diagnosed earlier?
3 What extra support can be offered in the childcare establishment to help Liam and his parents to cope with his condition?
4 How could the childcare workers deal with unkindness of the other children?

SICKLE CELL ANAEMIA

What Is Sickle Cell Anaemia?

Sickle cell anaemia (also known as sickle cell disease and sickle cell condition), is a serious disorder of the blood in which the normally round red blood cells become distorted into a sickle shape. Haemoglobin is part of the red cells which carries oxygen around the body. Affected red cells carry abnormal haemoglobin – haemoglobin S – which collapses when oxygen has been given up to the cells in the body. This is when the characteristic sickle shape occurs. The awkward shape of these sickled cells means that they can clump together and get stuck in the tiny blood vessels. As a result the blood supply to affected parts of the body is reduced or cut off completely.

These red blood cells do not live as long as normal red cells.

What Causes Sickle Cell Anaemia?

The condition is inherited via a recessive pattern of inheritance.

Sickle cell anaemia
Both parents pass an abnormal gene to the child and the child has the full-blown disease.

Sickle cell trait
One parent passes an abnormal gene to the child, and the child is a carrier for the condition and may have very mild symptoms.

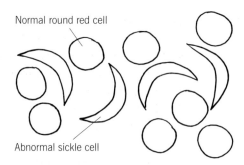

Normal round red cell

Abnormal sickle cell

Sickle-shaped red blood cells and normal blood cells

Sickle cell disease affects mainly people of African-Caribbean descent; people from Mediterranean countries, Asia and the Middle East may also be affected. This geographical distribution has probably arisen because sickle cell trait offers some protection to malaria. Children born to parents from mixed races may have sickle cell trait or sickle cell disease.

How To Recognise Sickle Cell Anaemia

In a baby

Affected babies usually appear healthy and well at birth. After a few months they may display the following signs:

- excessive tiredness and lack of energy
- poor blood supply to the extremities i.e. hands and feet, which may look blue and feel very cold
- numerous infections e.g. colds, coughs – the baby is never 100 per cent well.

Older children

If the condition has not been detected and treated in infancy, the following signs and symptoms will be noted in childhood.

- Pain. When the sickled cells get stuck, they prevent normal blood flow. The blockages cause pain in the arms, legs, back and stomach – the pain can be severe. This is called a sickle cell CRISIS. Swelling of the hands and feet, and stiff, painful joints are also characteristic of the condition. Vital organs (e.g. heart, lungs, kidneys, spleen) can be damaged if their blood supply is affected.
- Anaemia. This is due to the rapid destruction of red blood cells – not due to a lack of iron. The child will be pale, tired and lethargic.
- Jaundice. This yellowness of the whites of the eyes and the skin is due to the rapid breakdown of red blood cells. Jaundice can be difficult to see on black skin.
- Infections. The child is more prone to coughs and colds.

Immediate Action

- Any suspicion of sickle cell disease should be reported to a doctor who can arrange the necessary blood tests and refer the child to a hospital consultant specialising in the condition.
- If a child is having a crisis, supporting the affected limb in an elevated position and keeping it warm will help until the ambulance arrives.

Ongoing Care

Treatment

The usual treatment includes:

- folic acid supplements to reduce the severity of the anaemia
- penicillin to prevent infections
- immunisation against pneumococcal and meningococcal infections
- blood transfusions when the anaemia is severe
- analgesics to control any pain.

Children will be admitted to hospital if they have a painful crisis. They will be treated with a combination of blood transfusions, oxygen, lots of fluids, antibiotics and painkillers

Preventing Crises

Certain conditions make attacks (crises) more likely, so the following guidelines will help to keep the child in a healthy state and reduce their vulnerability to a crisis.

- Immunisations – the child should be fully immunised according to the immunisation schedule.
- Keeping warm – avoid extreme temperatures and make sure that the child does not get chilled when swimming, going outdoors.
- Preventing dehydration – ensure that the child drinks plenty of fluids to help the circulation. This will mean regular visits to the toilet or nappy changes. It may also result in enuresis (bed-wetting), which should be handled sensitively.
- Avoid stress – careful preparation for any change in the child's life will help to reduce worry and anxiety e.g. starting nursery or school, moving house etc.
- Prescribed medicines – folic acid, antibiotics etc. should be given as often as prescribed. Painkillers can be given as required.

Possible Complications

- Infections – pneumonia
- Damage to the vital organs will affect their function – some children may suffer cerebro-vascular accidents (strokes), due to damage to the blood supply to the brain.

Further Information

- Bone marrow transplants are sometimes offered to children who are severely affected, if a suitable, compatible donor can be found. If this is successful then the cure is complete.
- Call the parents or doctor if the child has a painful attack with a fever, sudden loss of colour, vomiting, diarrhoea, difficult or rapid breathing or lack of energy.
- Blood tests are available to detect the abnormal gene for sickle cell disease for people at risk. A couple who both have the gene are offered genetic counselling before starting a pregnancy. This will enable them to weigh up the risks of having an affected child and whether they want to proceed with starting a family. Pre-natal testing (chorionic villus sampling – CVS) is available, and parents who decide to check whether or not the embryo/fetus has sickle-cell disease are offered the option of a termination of an affected pregnancy.

Remember

Sickle cell crises can be induced by infection, stress, cold temperatures, strenuous physical exercise and dehydration. Try to protect a child with sickle cell disease in your care from any of these conditions.

> ### *Good Practice*
>
> A child with sickle cell disease may become unwell very quickly. If a child complains of severe pain in the abdomen or chest, headache, neck stiffness or drowsiness call the parents immediately. The child needs urgent hospital treatment.

THALASSAEMIA

What Is Thalassaemia?

Thalassaemia is a condition affecting the blood resulting in a particular type of anaemia. It is a serious, crippling illness in which the body cannot produce normal haemoglobin (the pigment in red blood cells which carries oxygen to the tissues in the body). The red blood cells are small and fragile and easily destroyed which results in severe anaemia.

What Causes Thalassaemia ?

The condition is inherited via a recessive pattern of inheritance.

There is a geographical pattern to the incidence of thalassaemia – it occurs mainly in people of Mediterranean, Asian and African origin.

Thalassaemia major
Both parents pass the abnormal gene to the child and the child has the full-blown disease.

Thalassaemia minor (Trait)
One parent passes the abnormal gene to the child and the child has a much less severe form of thalassaemia – the red blood cells are slightly smaller than usual.

How To Recognise Thalassaemia

There are major symptoms of anaemia which begin in the first year:
- very pale skin
- shortness of breath
- tiredness and lethargy – a baby will probably sleep excessively, feed poorly and fail to thrive.

Immediate Action

Any child with signs and symptoms of anaemia should be seen by a doctor, especially if there is a family history of thalassaemia.

Ongoing Care

Monthly blood transfusions to treat the anaemia.

These regular blood transfusions can result in damage to the internal organs, as they become overloaded with iron. This may be resolved with a special drug – desferrioxamine – given regularly by infusion.

Overnight drug pumps may be used to administer this treatment, so that it can be carefully controlled. This is painful and inconvenient – it is difficult for children and their families to adjust to this condition and its treatment, but there is no cure for this inherited condition.

Good Practice

Observe a child with thalassaemia carefully for signs of tiredness and structure activities to meet their needs.

Possible Complications   Thalassaemia is a debilitating condition which requires a lot of careful support and may result in death if the correct treatment is not given.

Further Information   As with sickle cell disease, blood tests are available, for people at risk, to detect the abnormal gene for thalassaemia. A couple who both have the gene are offered genetic counselling before starting a pregnancy. This will enable them to weigh up the risks of having an affected child and whether they want to proceed with starting a family. Pre-natal testing (chorionic villus sampling – CVS) is available, and parents who decide to check whether or not the embryo/fetus has thalassaemia are offered the option of the termination of an affected pregnancy.

 Progress check

1 What is the difference between sickle cell anaemia and thalassaemia?
2 How are these conditions inherited?
3 What are the signs and symptoms of sickle cell anaemia in a baby and an older child?
4 How can a sickle cell crisis be prevented?
5 How can childcare establishments support children with this condition?
6 What action would you take if you thought a child was having a sickle cell crisis?
7 When do the symptoms of thalassaemia begin and what are they?
8 What is the main form of treatment for thalassaemia?
9 How can families at risk of these diseases be helped with genetic counselling?
10 Sickle cell anaemia and thalassaemia are conditions that many people have either not heard of, or know very little about. Why do you think this is?

Part 3: Caring for the Sick Child

Most children are ill at some time in their childhood. When they are ill they need care from someone they know well and trust, who can meet their individual needs. Childcarers need to know how to provide that level of care, how to treat symptoms and to prevent complications. Children sometimes become ill in childcare settings. The responsibilities of the staff in these circumstamces is explained, including treating children with empathy and sensitivity and contacting the parents and doctor if necessary. The case studies used throughout this section highlight particular aspects of care.

Each year many children are admitted to hospitals as planned or emergency admissions. Their anxieties will be reduced if they have been prepared for the experience. Preparation for hospital includes offering **all** children the relevant knowledge and experience of hospital.

When children are seriously or terminally ill there are inevitable social and emotional effects on the child and the family. The available services and resources which may help them to cope with practical issues are described. Childcare workers may need to support the child and family through some difficult experiences. Understanding the nature of loss and the range of reactions should help carers to cope, and provide the level of assistance required by the child and their family.

Chapter 15 Caring for an ill child

This chapter includes:

- Meeting needs
- Treating symptoms
- Medication
- Caring for a sick child in day care
- Children in hospital
- Preparation for hospital
- Play in hospital
- Care of the child in hospital

This chapter stresses the importance of good care for sick children to aid their speedy recovery and promote their overall health and well-being. All childcarers will be expected to care for ill children at home and/or in childcare establishments at some time in their careers. Knowing the general and specific needs of ill children, and how to provide for them, will enable carers to supply the necessary nurturing environment. The values of record keeping and report writing are reinforced in this chapter to enable childcare workers to keep parents accurately informed about their child and to give correct details to medical staff. Preparing all children for hospital is important because many children are admitted to hospital without warning as the result of accidents or sudden illness. Their response to the situation is more positive if they are familiar with the setting and staff. The importance of providing play opportunities in hospital and an insight into the effects of hospitalisation on development is also included.

This chapter should be read in conjunction with 'Chapter 6, Recognising illness in a child'.

Meeting needs

The care of children who are ill revolves around meeting their particular needs, just as caring for children who are well means responding to their individual needs. See page 23 for meeting needs. Children prefer to be cared for by familiar people whom they trust. They will recover much more quickly if offered care by these adults at home. Most childcare establishments do not offer care to sick children knowing that they will recover more quickly at home, and also to prevent the spread of illness around the establishment.

Meeting physical needs

Children should be allowed to stay where they feel comfortable, this could mean staying in bed or lying on the sofa with a quilt and pillow.

Food and fluids

Appetite is usually suppressed during illness (see page 164) and returns again when the child feels better. In a usually healthy and well-nourished child a temporary reduction in food intake is not important. Small, appetising meals of easily digested food should be offered. Children with conditions which are treated with a special diet, for example diabetes, will need careful monitoring during illness to prevent complications. If the illness is long-term (chronic), then a careful nutritional strategy is required because children have low reserves of energy and nutrients. During illness the body requires extra nutrition because episodes of fever and infection increase normal energy requirements. Children will lose weight (with protein loss and muscle wasting) when they are ill if their calorie intake is reduced for a period of time. This will lead to tiredness, lethargy, poor wound healing and an increased risk of infection.

Children with a temperature must be encouraged to drink as much as possible because fluids help to reduce the fever. Offering any drinks that the child likes is generally satisfactory. Nutritious drinks such as fortified milk and fruit juice are preferable if the appetite has been poor for a period of time. Fluids are especially important to prevent dehydration if a child is suffering from sickness and diarrhoea. Using a feeding beaker or straw may encourage a child to drink, or providing plain or flavoured ice-cubes or ice-lollies will make sure that some fluids are taken.

Allow the child to choose their favourite foods – during illness it is better that they eat something rather than nothing at all! The senses of smell and taste may be impaired during illness, so ensure that the food is attractive – lemon may enhance the flavour of savoury dishes and honey will improve the flavour of desserts. Some children may prefer puréed food – purées of fruit and vegetables are excellent sources of nutrients which are easy to eat and digest. Offer small meals and snacks regularly and keep the child company when they are trying to eat.

Table of suitable drinks for children during illness

LIQUID	CALORIES	CARBOHYDRATE	PROTEIN	FAT
200ml whole milk with 40g ice cream	196	19.4	8	10.2
200ml whole milk with 20g Complan	218	20.4	10.6	10.8
200ml whole milk with 25g Build Up	217	26.4	12.2	7.9
100ml whole milk with 150ml tomato soup	180	23.2	10	9.1
150ml whole milk with mashed whole banana	177	26.3	6.1	6
100ml whole milk with 100ml fruit yoghurt	160	22.6	8.1	4.8

Temperature control

Control of the body temperature and the environmental temperature are both important. Children who are ill usually have a raised body temperature so they should not be cared for in a hot room. The air should be cooled to try to reduce the child's temperature.

Rest and sleep

Children should be encouraged to rest as much as possible when they are feeling unwell. This may be in bed, or wherever they feel comfortable. Comfort is important, especially if the child is in bed. Pillows should be arranged to support the child's body if s/he is sitting up. A triangle arrangement with 3 or 4 pillows is preferable. A child with a cough will be more comfortable if s/he is propped up with pillows.

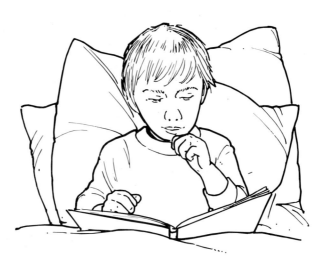

A comfortable position is important

Restful activities will reduce anxiety and encourage recovery. Children may need the additional reassurance of sleeping with an adult at night. This insecurity will pass when they are feeling better.

Exercise and fresh air

Most children will not feel like running around and playing when they are not well. Recovery from some conditions may be encouraged by gentle exercise.

Rooms should be kept well ventilated because of the positive effects of fresh air. Sitting outside or taking a walk is beneficial if the child feels well enough and is dressed for the weather.

Hygiene

Regular washing, brushing the hair and cleaning the teeth will help to make the child feel better. A daily bath or shower may be preferred by some children but is not essential – attention to washing the hands, face and bottom is sufficient.

A bed bath may be required if a child is too poorly to be taken to the bathroom for a few days:

- ensure that the room is warm enough – close the windows during the bedbath
- remove the nightie or pyjamas
- cover the child with a sheet and remove the top bedding
- place a towel under each part of the body as it is being washed
- start washing with the face and upper body
- wash the bottom and genitals last using a different flannel or sponge.

Clothes will need regular changing – at least once a day. If the child is in bed, sheets and pillowcases should be changed regularly – twice daily if the child has a temperature.

Toileting

Children may need help with toileting as they will probably experience a change in bowel habits associated with their illness. Diarrhoea may result in accidents and the child will need reassurance and gentle washing and changing. Using a cream such as zinc and castor oil will prevent soreness around the anus. Constipation due to reduced fluid and food intake will resolve itself when the appetite returns to normal.

Children with a temperature may have a reduced output of urine due the combination of lack of fluids taken in and the body trying to reduce the temperature. Consult a doctor if a child has not passed urine for 12 hours.

Safety

Children should be supervised at all times when they are ill. Their condition can change very quickly, so carers must be vigilant.

- Keep all medicines out of reach of children, even if they seem too poorly to be inquisitive.
- Observe for any change in the child's condition which may be caused by medication or treatment.
- Be aware of any complications of the condition and look for early signs.

Medical care

Prescribed medicines should be given according to the doctor's instructions (see page 340).

Call the doctor if the child does not seem to be recovering as expected.

Meeting intellectual needs

Regression

Children who are unwell usually experience regression – when they are ill they perform at a slightly earlier developmental stage. They may need to wear nappies again if they have recently become clean and dry, or drink from a feeding cup again. A preference for playing with familiar, non-challenging toys which are usually of no interest to them is to be expected. Children should not be pressurised into taking part in activities which they are not comfortable with. Neither should they be made to feel that their behaviour or development is unacceptable. An attitude of caring tolerance will aid their recovery.

Appropriate activities

Children who are unwell will have a short attention span and will probably be unable to entertain themselves. This requires gentle encouragement and understanding from parents and carers.

The following activities and resources provide suggestions for appropriate activities whilst a child is too ill to return to their usual daily routine, or is confined to the home. A table or a tray with legs across the bed will enable the child to play, eat and complete projects if confined to bed or the sofa!

- Playing board games, dominoes and card games with relatives and friends will provide social contact. The child can play alone if preferred.
- Pictures, diary recordings, photographs, flowers etc. provide the opportunity to create a scrapbook or personal journal, with the help of an adult if required.
- Magazines, coloured paper, shells, even pasta and rice etc and equipment such as scissors, glue and card can be used to make collages and mobiles.
- Model kits can be made and painted.
- Books provide gentle stimulation and offer a feeling of security, especially if they are familiar stories. New tales may be preferred for the child to read alone or to be read by an adult.
- Videos, games, cartoons, documentaries and feature films provide amusement.
- Jigsaw puzzles on a tray can be returned to several times before completion.
- Soft dough offers the opportunity to be creative and is an outlet for feelings of anger and aggression.
- Crayons and coloured pens with a pad of paper may encourage drawing and writing.
- Painting – a plastic sheet or table cloth and an overall will protect the child and furniture from the inevitable splashes and spills!

> **Remember**
> Sick children cannot concentrate for long, so offer different activities regularly and allow plenty of time for rest.

Language

Sitting and talking to the child, reading stories and looking at books together will help the child to feel secure – books and stories, songs and rhymes and games are all activities which will encourage language. Looking at photograph albums together will encourage conversation about favourite and amusing memories. Audio cassette story tapes and radio will provide gentle stimulation for the child.

A positive attitude from the carer will be reinforced by their conversation.

Meeting emotional and social needs

Emotional

Children need the security of their main carers when they are ill. Even when they are older and developing more independence, they will probably be frightened during an illness and will need constant reassurance from a trusted adult. Children are very vulnerable and deserve consistency of care from someone who will always offer encouragement and support. Their feelings of security will be enhanced if their carer is honest with them and always tells the truth, knowing how much they are able to understand and without inflicting unnecessary anxiety.

Social

Contact with family should be constant for the child who is cared for at home. Although reasonable care must be taken to prevent transmission if the disease is infectious, family members will usually have been exposed to the condition before the symptoms have appeared.

As the recovery process begins, children need to maintain contacts with the outside world when they are confined to the home due to illness. Contact can be encouraged with visits and letters from friends and school peers which will reassure the child and boost their morale. They will know that that they are not forgotten, and will be welcomed back into the establishment as soon as they are well enough to return.

 Progress check

1 What type of diet is most appropriate and acceptable to a child who is ill?
2 Give some suggestions for nourishing drinks for children who have lost their appetite.
3 How can a child be helped to feel comfortable when they are ill?
4 What are the beneficial effects of fresh air?
5 How would you ensure good hygiene for a child confined to bed?
6 What particular toileting requirements may a child need when they are poorly?
7 Explain what regression is and how a sick child may be affected?
8 List seven appropriate activities for a child confined to bed.
9 How can language development be maintained?
10 Describe the social and emotional needs of sick children and how they can be provided for.

Treating symptoms

The symptoms a child experiences depend upon the particular condition they are suffering from. Descriptions of signs and symptoms can be found in Chapter 6 and include pyrexia, swollen glands, coughing, vomiting, changes in bowel habits, convulsions, pain, skin changes, behaviour changes, alteration in sleep habits and loss of appetite.

Remember

1 **Never** give paracetamol to a baby of less than 3 months unless a doctor has prescribed the drug.
2 **Never** give any medicine to a child without the parent's consent.
3 **Never** give aspirin to a child under 12 years because of the dangers of Reye's syndrome.

Good Practice

Reducing a raised temperature
The following action points should be put into practice promptly if a child has a raised temperature

- Offer cool drinks.
- Remove excessive clothing. Reduce bedding to a cotton sheet if the child is in bed.
- Give paracetamol elixir, e.g. Calpol, if parents have provided the medicine and given their consent that it should be used in case of such an emergency. If not, contact the parents and get their verbal consent – arrange for them to collect the child as soon as possible and suggest that a doctor's advice is sought. Always follow the instructions on the container and give the correct dose.
- Lower the room temperature, if possible, to about 15°C (60°F).
- Fan the child if possible.
- *Tepid sponging*. Removing the child's clothes and sponging them with tepid (lukewarm) water will reduce the temperature. Placing them in a lukewarm bath will have the same effect. BUT BEWARE – reducing the temperature too quickly can result in shock. For this reason some medical practitioners no longer recommend this action, but it may be effective as a last resort. It may be recommended for a child who has previously had a febrile convulsion.

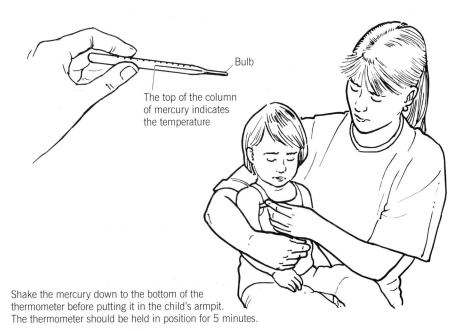

Bulb

The top of the column of mercury indicates the temperature

Taking the temperature with a mercury thermometer (see page 137)

Shake the mercury down to the bottom of the thermometer before putting it in the child's armpit. The thermometer should be held in position for 5 minutes.

Complications

Some childhood illnesses may result in complications i.e. further illness or disability caused by the original illness. Childcare workers should be aware of the possible complications of the:

1 particular disease affecting the child e.g. mumps may lead to meningitis

2 specific symptoms produced by the illness e.g. a child with a high temperature may have a febrile convulsion if attempts are not made to reduce the temperature.

Complications can usually be avoided by:

■ offering the most appropriate care e.g. providing lots of fluids to a child who is vomiting may prevent dehydration

■ ensuring prompt medical attention and treatment for the illness in its early stages – consult the doctor or health visitor as soon as possible (see page 165, 'When To Call A Doctor') e.g. early antibiotic therapy will reduce the risk of bacterial infection progressing to other parts of the body

■ observing the child closely for signs and symptoms of the illness progressing and providing the necessary care and treatment. This may involve getting medical help.

 Progress check

1 What are complications of illness?

2 What type of complications should the childcare worker be aware of?

3 How can the childcare worker try to prevent complications of childhood illness?

Medication

Most children will require some form of medication when they are ill. All medicines are drugs which are potentially very dangerous if they are not treated with caution and respect. Medicines can be purchased over the counter in pharmacies, corner shops and supermarkets as well as being prescribed by the GP or hospital doctor. Childcare workers should not offer drugs to children unless they have been prescribed by a doctor and/or the parent's written consent has been obtained. It is, therefore, important for childcare workers to feel confident about the administration of medicines and prescribed treatments.

Most medicines are given once, twice (every 12 hours), three times (every 8 hours) or four times (every 6 hours) a day depending on how quickly the drug works and how long it is effective for. Never wake a child to give medicine unless the doctor clearly states that this should be done. The doses can usually be incorporated into the child's waking day, if the first dose is given on waking and the last just before going to bed.

Remember

It is very important that children finish the prescribed course of medicines and antibiotics. Parents and carers should not stop as soon as the child feels and seems better. This will lead to resistant bacteria and/or a possible recurrence of the condition.

Medicines

DRUG	USE	EFFECTS
Analgesic	Painkiller e.g. paracetamol	Reduces pain and helps to control the temperature
Antibiotic	Kills bacteria – some antibiotics are more effective against specific bacteria	Controls infection The course must be completed – do not stop the medicine if the child seems to be better
Antiemetic	Anti-sickness	Helps to reduce nausea and vomiting
Antifungal	Kills fungi	Relieves fungal infections e.g. athlete's foot, ringworm
Antihistamine	Anti-itch	Reduces irritation in some skin conditions Can have a sedative effect
Antiparasitic	Kills parasites infesting the body	e.g. kills threadworm
Bronchodilator	Dilates the breathing passages	Assists breathing e.g. in asthma
Corticosteroid	Reduces the inflammatory response in some conditions	e.g. controls eczema and asthma
Laxative	Softens faeces	Assists the painless passage of softer stools in severe constipation.
Sedative	For relaxation	Relaxes the child and reduces anxiety

Good Practice

Rules for handling medicines in the home and childcare establishment
1 Ensure that the parents' written consent has been obtained.
2 Always read the directions carefully on the medicine container and give the exact dose for the age/weight of the child according to the instructions.
3 NEVER give a medicine to a child which has been prescribed for somebody else.
4 Do not give or take medicines in the dark.
5 Ask the doctor and parents if medicines are safe to be used together e.g. giving paracetamol with another medicine prescribed by the GP.
6 Always complete the course as instructed.
7 Dispose of surplus prescribed medicines by returning them to the pharmacy.

Methods of administering medicines

There are several different ways for medicines to be given and the doctor will decide which is most:
- appropriate for the child
- effective to treat their condition.

Before administering any medicines the carer should:
- wash their hands carefully
- record the time and dosage of the treatment

■ explain to the child exactly what is going to happen and that they should feel better as a result
■ use language which the child will understand
■ remain calm and relaxed. If you are tense the child will quickly pick up your anxiety and resist the medicine
■ use distraction techniques if necessary (see below).

After the treatment the hands should be washed. The successful completion of the treatment must be recorded with the time and dosage.

Oral medicine

Most medicines for children are given in elixirs by mouth. This obviously means that the child must swallow them.

Most oral medicines are best given just before a meal because they will be absorbed into the bloodstream more quickly (most drugs are absorbed through the wall of the stomach). The child is less likely to vomit then as the stomach is empty. Read the instructions carefully because some medicines should be taken with, or after, food.

The child should be asked to sit down, preferably on a carer's knee.

The bottle should be shaken well and the dose must be measured carefully. Some children find it easier to take medicine from a syringe placed in their mouth pointing towards the cheek. Never point the syringe towards the back of the mouth as this may cause choking.

Offer a drink to wash the medicine down.

Bribery is acceptable for a reluctant child, for example offering to read a favourite story, or a sweet or piece of chocolate may do the trick !

A firm approach may be needed for some children who refuse to take the medicine, but never lose your temper with them. A determined, business-like approach works well with the help of a colleague who holds the child while the medicine is put into the mouth. This should be avoided if possible, as the child may spit it out or choke.

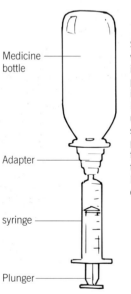

Medicine bottle

Adapter

syringe

Plunger

Shake the bottle well. Fit the adapter into the bottle and push the syringe into the adapter. Hold the bottle upside down and slowly pull the plunger out until the syringe contains the required dose. Measure the dose carefully.

Giving medicine with a syringe

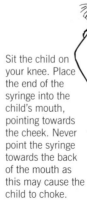

Sit the child on your knee. Place the end of the syringe into the child's mouth, pointing towards the cheek. Never point the syringe towards the back of the mouth as this may cause the child to choke.

If the child is persistently unco-operative do not try to deceive the child or trick them into taking the medicine in a disguised form. It may work the first time but is not successful in the long-term and the child's trust is lost.

If resistance continues, ask the parents if the doctor can prescribe the medicine in an alternative form. A different flavour or texture may be more successful.

Eye drops and eye ointment

Putting drops into the eyes usually requires two people. The child should lie on their back on a comfortable surface with the head extended backwards.

- Fill the dropper with the medication.
- Pull down the lower lid with one hand.
- Ask the child to keep their eye open for as long as possible.
- Place the other hand on the child's forehead and count the required number of drops into gap between the lower lid and the eyeball.
- With ointment, squeeze a line of cream along the inside of the lower lid.
- The child will close their eye and some liquid will escape which should be wiped away with a clean tissue. Encourage the child to remain still and keep their eye closed.
- Take care not to touch the eye(s) with the dropper.

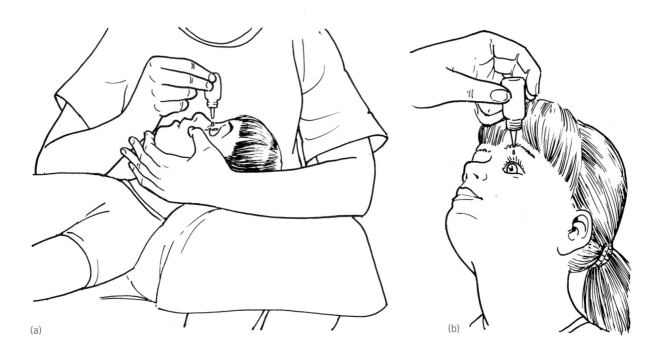

(a) (b)

Administering eye drops to (a) a very young child; and (b) an older child

Ear drops

The child should lie on one side, or tilt their head to one side, with the affected ear uppermost.

- Pull the pinna gently backwards towards the back of the head, this straightens the ear canal slightly.
- Release the required number of drops into the ear.
- Gently massage the base of the ear.
- Encourage the child to remain in that position for 2 to 3 minutes.
- Place a fairly large piece of cotton wool into the outer ear to prevent unnecessary leakage. Do not pack it tightly as it may be painful and difficult to remove.

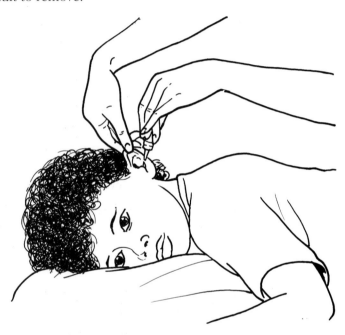

Administering ear drops

Nose drops

Ask the child to blow their nose and to lie down on a comfortable surface, with their head and neck extended over a pillow placed under the shoulders. A baby or toddler will be more comfortable lying on the carer's knee with their head extended over the thigh.

Place the tip of the dropper just into the nasal cavity and release the prescribed number of drops into the nose. Encourage the child to stay in that position for 1 to 2 minutes.

Creams and ointments

Skin conditions are often treated with creams which are applied directly to the affected area. These usually bring relief, so children are generally quite happy to have their cream put on. Preferably, carers should wear disposable gloves to prevent them absorbing the drugs into their system.

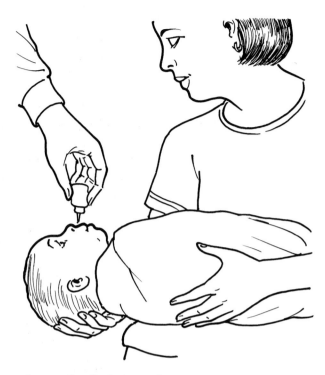

Administering nose drops

Injections and rectal administration

Qualified medical staff usually give drugs which need to be given by injection or by suppositories into the rectum. Childcare workers would need special training and extra support to use these therapies if it was absolutely necessary.

✔ Progress check

1 In what circumstances is it acceptable for childcare workers to give children their medication?
2 Why is it important for children to complete the course of medicine, even if they are feeling better?
3 What different types of medicines may help a child who is feeling sick?
4 How can a child with an allergy that is making the skin itch be comforted?
5 What should be done with unused medicines?
6 What strategies can be adopted to encourage a child to take their oral medicine?
7 Describe how ear drops should be administered.
8 How could a child be prepared for having eye drops for the first time?

Caring for a sick child in day care

Children quite frequently show the first signs and symptoms of illness when they are at playgroup, nursery or infant school, with the nanny etc.

In these situations it is important that childcare workers are aware of the correct procedure to follow in alerting others to the child's illness; this will ensure that the illness can be treated correctly and appropriate care offered.

In a school or playgroup setting, any concerns should be reported to a senior member of staff so that they can decide whether or not the parents should be contacted. A nanny or child-minder would normally be able to contact the parents immediately. All carers should have current information about every child's personal details so that contact is immediate.

Establishment records

Details about each child should be readily available so that emergency contact can be made with parents/carers. Every child's records should contain the following information.

1 Full name.
2 Date of birth.
3 Names and addresses of child's main carers.
4 Address and telephone number of child's home.
5 Address and telephone number of parent's/carer's place(s) of work.
6 An additional emergency contact number – possibly another relative.
7 Telephone number and surgery address of child's GP and health visitor.

Recording symptoms

Records of a child's illness should be kept so that accurate information can be given to the parents or the doctor. These records should include:

- when the child showed signs of illness
- what the symptoms were
- what action was taken e.g. sitting quietly with the child, taking the temperature etc.
- whether any further symptoms have developed and/or whether the original symptoms have become more severe.

Practical help

Offer practical support to the child and keep them comfortable as they wait to go home. Incidents of sickness and/or diarrhoea may distress the child greatly, and should be cleared up with as little fuss as possible to help the child to retain their dignity. Most establishments have a supply of spare clothing for such eventualities. A quiet area with toilets nearby and offering a sick bowl will help to provide reassurance.

A carer should keep the child company and use language that the child will understand – an ill child should never be left alone, physically or emotionally, in a childcare establishment or in the home.

Expectations

When children are unwell, their behaviour and development usually regress. This is sometimes the first sign that all is not well. Childcare staff must be aware of the possible effects of illness on the child and reduce their expectations accordingly.

Giving medicines

When a child has an illness which means that they are well enough to come to playgroup, nursery or school the childcare worker may be asked to give any prescribed medicines during the session. If this is the case the following precautions should be taken to ensure the safety of the child and the carer.

Obtain the parent/carer's written consent for prescribed medicines and paracetamol. Preferably, this consent should be on a pro-forma which contains the:

- name of the child
- name of the medicine
- precise dose to be given
- time it should be given and/or circumstances for giving irregular medicines i.e. parents should write down the precise symptoms which the child should display before the medicine is given
- how it should be given e.g. eye-drops, oral medicine, nose drops, inhaler etc.
- parent's name and signature.

Make sure that the medicine has been prescribed for that child and is labelled with the child's name.

Paracetamol can be purchased over the counter, but a separate bottle should be kept for each child, carefully labelled with the child's name.

Follow the dosage instructions carefully. (See Good Practice on page 341) It is preferable to have a colleague who will witness the procedure and check that the child, medicine and dosage are correct.

Maintain a written record (chart) of medicines given including dose, method of administration, date and time and whether the child took the medicine.

Store medicines safely in a secure place, preferably in a locked cupboard out of the reach of children, except for inhalers which should be close to the child at all times.

✔ Progress check

1 Why is it important for childcare workers to be aware of the correct establishment procedure to follow when children become ill?
2 Who should the first signs and symptoms of illness be reported to?
3 What information about each child should be kept in each establishment?

4 What information should be included when recording the signs and symptoms of illness in a childcare establishment?
5 What sort of practical help can be offered to a sick child in day care?
6 What specific information should be included on a parental consent form for giving medicines?
7 What procedure should be followed when giving medicine in a childcare establishment?
8 Which medicines should be kept close by the child at all times?

Children in hospital

Most children will have personal experience of hospital in their early years. This could be the result of a visit to the Accident and Emergency Department after an accident or an appointment at the Outpatient Department after being referred by their GP. Either of these routes may lead to hospital admission as an in-patient on a children's ward. Every year 1 million children are admitted to hospital, half of these (500,000) are under the age of 5 years. Other children will experience hospital as visitors to friends or relatives who are ill or needing hospital care e.g. during pregnancy or childbirth.

Why children may be admitted to hospital

There are two main types of admission to hospital.

Emergency admissions

Children may be admitted to hospital as the result of an accident or sudden, unexpected disease. Long-term planned preparation is not possible because of the nature of the injury or illness. Examples of emergency admissions are as follows.

Accidental injuries
- road traffic accidents
- falls
- burns
- poisoning
- swallowing or inhaling foreign bodies e.g. pen tops, batteries, coins, Lego etc.
- non-accidental injuries.

Infections
- meningitis
- bronchitis
- pneumonia
- gastro-enteritis.

Acute abdomen – intense abdominal pain
- appendicitis
- urinary tract infection.

Breathing difficulties
- asthma attack.

Convulsions
- febrile convulsion
- epilepsy.

Diabetic coma
- diabetes.

Parents and children will need a great deal of support in these circumstances. They will usually make first contact with the hospital in the Accident and Emergency Department having arrived in an ambulance or via their own transport. They will not be prepared for the experience, so a gentle, tactful explanation of the situation, treatment and likely outcome will be vital if the family is to come to terms with the situation.

Planned or routine admissions

In these cases children and their families know that a hospital admission will occur and are usually given a period of notice and a date for the planned admission. Children may have been placed on a waiting list for surgery or a given date to attend for a medical procedure or therapy. Most will have visited the hospital before – usually the Outpatients Department – perhaps on more than one occasion. They may have been invited to an organised pre-admission programme of visits to the paediatric wards.

Examples of reasons for planned admissions are as follows.

Routine surgery
- tonsillectomy
- insertion of grommets
- circumcision
- hernia repair.

In these cases it is preferable if the child can be treated as a day case which will reduce the psychological trauma, worry and stress for all concerned.

Congenital disorders – conditions that a child has had since birth
- talipes – club foot requiring multiple operations
- spina bifida / hydrocephalus.

Cancer

Children with malignancies are usually admitted on numerous occasions for surgery, chemotherapy and/or radiotherapy (see Chapter 14).

Respite care

Some hospitals have facilities for caring for children to have a long-term illness or disability, to review their care and treatment and also to give their main carers a break.

Preparation for hospital

It is good practice for all childcarers to familiarise children with hospital so that they are not bewildered or frightened when they enter the hospital.

This is more straightforward when an admission to hospital is planned, a child may need an operation for the insertion of grommets for example, so that the family and carers have plenty of notice of the child's admission date. This allows them to prepare the child emotionally and physically. On the contrary, an emergency admission by its very nature is unexpected, and does not allow for the luxury of planning. Many admissions to hospital in childhood are emergencies. All children must be prepared for this as much as possible.

General preparation

Home

Most children will have some toys that relate to hospitals, for example a doctor's set, dressing-up clothes such as a nurse's uniform, a toy ambulance or a Playmobil hospital. These provide lots of opportunities for talking about hospitals and the work of doctors and nurses.

Extending their play in this area at home could include bandaging dolls, teddies, the nanny and all the family! Temperatures can be taken with toy thermometers and lots of care given to poorly toys.

Books about hospitals are available to read to children and to explain the illustrations to them. A familiar character visiting hospital is especially useful for younger children, for example Spot and Pingu. Local libraries usually have a selection of children's hospital books.

Travelling on the bus or in the car may take families past the local hospital. This should be pointed out to children so that they become familiar with the building. Children often want to know where they were born and if this hospital was the place of their birth, it will increase their interest.

Remember
Hospital should never be threatened as a form of punishment for unacceptable behaviour.

Childcare establishment

Preparation for hospital should be included in all pre-school and early years establishments. Positive images of hospital and medical personnel will help to reduce anxiety and encourage children to talk and discuss their concerns.

Role play

Setting up a 'children's ward' play area in the nursery or infant classroom can help children to overcome their fears about going into hospital by enabling them to:

■ share experiences with those who have no first-hand knowledge of hospital
■ broaden their experiences
■ play through their anxieties and worries about hospital.

Children can participate in designing the area and making suggestions for equipment which should be included. Creating a reception area, making registration cards and signs and posters and gathering resources help the children to 'own' the area. Giving injections, bandaging and caring for each other within their role play is good preparation for hospital admissions.

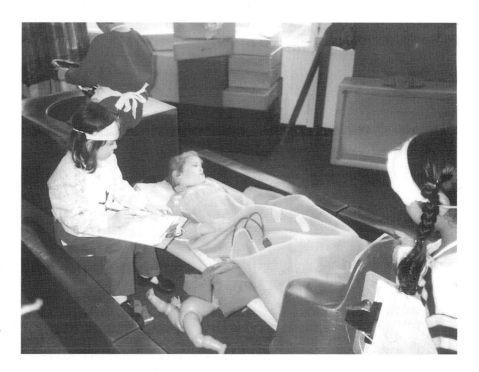

Role play at the nursery can help children overcome their fears

Puppets

Creating puppets and performing puppet shows related to hospital, gives the opportunity to discuss hospital and enables information to be given to other children.

Storytime
Books and rhymes related to hospital introduce new words and concepts.

Displays
Using the children's work about hospital to create a display will reinforce the concept and include all the values of display. Interest tables could include some 'real' equipment, photographs and books.

Visitors
The health visitor, school nurse or doctor may visit the establishment to talk to the children about preparing for hospital and being admitted to hospital.

Preparation for a planned admission

Children are admitted to hospital only if it is absolutely necessary and if adequate care and treatment cannot be successfully provided at home. Children who have been prepared for their admission will cope better than children who have had no preparation, and they will recover more quickly.

Parents will usually be notified about a child's admission several weeks beforehand. General conversations about hospital and role play at home form a gentle introduction and provide the opportunity to resolve any fears the child may have. Keeping the admission a secret from the child until a few days beforehand does not usually work because children are astute and pick up clues. These can increase their anxieties because their carers are not being honest with them.

More intensive preparation can be left until 7 to 10 days before the admission date. Most hospitals will send children a pre-admission booklet which contains important information, often with many pictures of children and toys which reassure the child. It will include details of the:
- role of parents when their child is in hospital
- ward routine e.g. mealtimes, doctor's visits etc.
- playroom
- hospital school
- items to take into hospital.

Hospital visit

Most hospitals offer a pre-admission visit to children and their families. These are very successful in reducing anxiety. It is always preferable to actually see inside the hospital and meet the staff, than imagining something terrible!

The child tours the wards and goes into the playroom. They will see the beds and lockers, see where the toilets are and be reassured to see parents with their children. A great fear for some children is to be separated from their carers. They will meet some of the staff who will care for them, especially the hospital play worker. Most children's wards will have a permanent play specialist who is usually a qualified nursery nurse who has completed some extra training in hospital play. The children will be encouraged to play with some of the toys in the play area and some centres show a video about a child's experiences in hospital.

A few days before admission

Tell the child very clearly and honestly what will happen on the day of admission and about how you are going to prepare together for going to hospital.

Answer any questions clearly and honestly.

Reassure the child that a parent/carer will stay with them all the time, staying overnight.

Arrange to go shopping for a new toothbrush or pair of pyjamas!

The age of the child will influence how much detail can be given in a meaningful way.

The day before admission

The child can pack their own bag. They must be involved as much as possible in all preparations. The contents of their hospital bag will include:

- some special toys
- comfort blanket if the child uses one
- photograph of family and home
- washbag (toothbrush and toothpaste, soap, flannel, brush/comb)
- pyjamas
- dressing gown
- slippers
- Parent Held Child Health Record
- tissues
- squash or cordial to drink
- any other personal items required by the child.

> **Remember**
> Some hospitals encourage children to dress in their own clothes at all times during the day. The hospital booklet should make clear what type of clothing/nightwear is required.

Admission to hospital

On the day of admission the child will be taken to the allocated ward. A named nurse will help the child to settle in and make them feel comfortable by introducing them to other patients and finding them toys to play with. The child will be encouraged to unpack their bag into their locker. They will be shown where their parent will be sleeping – sometimes next to them on a Z-bed!

If the child is going to theatre for an operation, a theatre nurse may visit to explain to the child what will happen later that day or the following day. S/he will explain about the special gown, hat and socks they may wear and encourage the child to dress their doll/teddy in similar clothes. Magic cream (EMLA cream), which is used to anaesthetise the skin on the injection site for the anaesthetic, will be explained and the child will be encouraged to role play this as well. The child will be reassured at all times and encouraged to ask any questions. Parents are allowed to accompany the child to the anaesthetic room and to stay with them until they are anaesthetised. They are usually invited to accompany the nurse who collects the child after the operation to return them to their bed in the ward.

Pre-admission unit

Some children may be invited to a pre-admission unit a few days before their admission, so that they can be examined before they are admitted onto the ward or the day care unit. Staff who are trained in the care of children help them to feel at ease and provide toys and equipment to enable them to familiarise themselves with hospital.

Children should always be told the truth and their questions should be answered honestly. Telling a child that something will not hurt when in fact it is very uncomfortable, will destroy their trust in adults being honest and dependable. It is much better to tell the child that something will be uncomfortable, but that you will stay with them and it will soon be over. They will usually readily accept this truthful explanation.

Day care surgery

Many children are treated in day care units. They are admitted in the morning, a few hours before the surgery takes place and as soon as they have recovered sufficiently they can be taken home. This care is preferable for minor surgery for many reasons.

- Stress is reduced for child and parents. The child will not suffer a great loss of independence and will not be so concerned about possible separation. Parent(s)/carer(s) can stay for the duration of the treatment and take the child home that day.
- Family disruption is prevented, which may occur when one parent stays with a child in hospital as an in-patient.
- Children are discharged home on the day of the surgery and recover more quickly in their familiar home environment
- It is a cost-effective method of care. More children can be treated for a lower cost compared to admitting them to a ward.

Good Practice

Before admission to hospital

- Talk to the child about hospital – this will provide information and give the child the opportunity to ask questions and express fears.
- Encourage 'hospital play'.
- Reassure the child that going into hospital is commonplace for many children. It is to help them to feel well. It is not a punishment or because their behaviour has been unacceptable!

When discharged home

- Observe for signs of infection, for example fever, lethargy, loss of appetite. Call the doctor if the child is unwell.

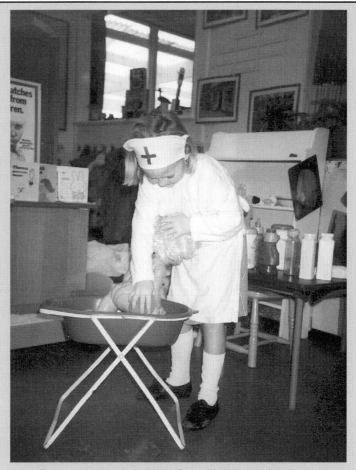

Encourage hospital play before admission to hospital

- **Expect some regression in their behaviour and development – offer extra support, understanding and encouragement.**
- **Be positive about the child's achievements in hospital and the improvement in their health. Many children are eventually more self-confident and independent after a successful hospital experience.**
- **Expect the child to continue their play at home with a hospital theme! This therapeutic play is psychologically healing.**

✅ *Progress check*

1 Why is it good practice to prepare children for a planned or an emergency admission to hospital?
2 How can adults prepare children in general terms for admission to hospital?
3 What sort of activities in a childcare establishment will increase children's awareness about hospitals?

4 What is the value of role play?

5 Describe how adults can prepare children for a planned admission to hospital.

6 What will happen on the day of admission?

7 What is the value of a pre-admission visit to the hospital?

8 What are the advantages of day-care surgery?

9 What good practice points should the carer be aware of before admission to hospital?

10 How can carers assist a rapid recovery when the child has been discharged home?

Activity

You are the nanny for Jenny, a four-year-old child, who has just been discharged from hospital after an operation to remove a birthmark from her face. Jenny's parents have been with the child throughout her hospital stay, but must now return to work, leaving her in your care.

Using the information contained in this chapter describe how you would provide:

- appropriate care at home
- play therapy
- the opportunity for the child to be re-established back at nursery school.

Play in hospital

Play is an essential part of every child's day. It is especially important in hospital because it can aid recovery by helping the child come to terms with their experience, and by enabling them to understand what is happening to them.

Providing good facilities for play in hospital is very important for the welfare of the child. Most wards have a playroom with a wide variety of toys and activities, and many hospitals also provide an outdoor play area for children. Specialised staff supervise play in these areas and are also responsible for taking activities to the child if they cannot get to the play areas because of their condition. Play is invaluable in minimising distress in hospital.

The type of activities offered will depend upon:

- the age and stage of the child
- their range of movements and mobility
- the participation of others.

Children must feel secure before they can begin to play, so the following factors must be taken into account before play begins:

- emotional stage of development
- intellectual (cognitive) development

- previous experience
- individual fears
- physical position
- cultural background and first language.

Types of hospital play

Pre-procedural play: play preparation

This type of play is used by play specialists and other professional hospital staff to help children to prepare for medical or surgical procedures, for example a blood test, an operation or an X-ray. It can help in the following ways.

- To show children what will happen to them so that they know what to expect and what will be expected of them.
- To provide information in advance for children in a way that they will understand.
- To answer any questions which children may have and reassure any fears.
- To identify their anxieties and help them to resolve them.

Children will be able to acknowledge their fantasies and have their questions answered. Parents can be involved here too, as they may also have fears and misconceptions about the treatments and tests. Children can deal with pain more effectively if they are aware of what is happening to them and have become familiar with the procedures. Play preparation should be provided before all investigations and procedures and before all changes in treatment.

Activities
Dolls with injection sites, intra-venous infusions which can be used with coloured water, puppets, small world play such as Lego, Playmobil, books, videos and photographs are all useful activities.

Post-procedural play

This type of play allows children to play out their experiences after the medical or surgical treatment. It enables children to be reassured and encourages them to accept their treatment, positive attitudes are reinforced if children are praised enthusiastically after the procedure. Staff can assess the child's understanding of their treatment and can see if the child seems to be coping with the experience. The child is in control of the play process.

Activities
Specially adapted dolls, puppets, books, photos and medical equipment are useful. It is not unusual to see children reassuring their dolls about the treatment they themselves have experienced!

Distraction techniques

When children are going through a particular procedure, play by distraction can relieve their anxiety. It does not intend to pretend that the procedure is not happening but helps children to cope with the situation.

> **Remember**
> A well prepared and informed child is less vulnerable and better able to cope with hospital.

Activities

Musical instruments, bubble blowing, yo-yos, spinning tops, blowing whistles, noisy sound books and imaginatively thinking about holidays and playgrounds are good activities

Therapeutic play

This type of play encourages exercise and feelings of well-being. Children with breathing impairment such as asthma or cystic fibrosis may be encouraged to blow bubbles or play a recorder. Swimming and other forms of physiotherapy help children with movement.

Activity

You are a playleader on a children's surgical ward. Explain how you provide play therapy for:

- a six-year-old child who has come into hospital with suspected appendicitis, who may need an operation to remove the appendix;
- a three-year-old child who has come into hospital for a routine tonsillectomy.

Suitable child-centred hospital activities for children of varying ages

AGE	ACTIVITY	TYPE OF PLAY & VALUE OF EQUIPMENT	BENEFITS FOR THE CHILD
1–8 YEARS	Dolls	Role play. Dolls can be used to demonstrate procedures and show the child how to behave. Children play out their experiences	■ Children easily identify with dolls ■ Allows the child to use their memory of sights and sounds ■ Concrete thinking is translated into play
2 YEARS AND OVER	Books and leaflets	■ Books provide information for children and their parents if they use them together ■ They increase understanding of specific medical treatments, roles of professionals and reactions to hospital	■ Children can use books and/or leaflets at any time and in most situations ■ They can control how often and how much they look at a book or leaflet
3 YEARS AND OVER	Playmobil and other hospital toys	■ Role play ■ Playmobil can be used to demonstrate routines and procedures and show the child what to expect ■ It can encourage discussion and increase the child's knowledge ■ Fears and anxieties can be expressed	■ Familiar small world toys which the child can identify with ■ Children can play out their experiences

Suitable child-centred hospital activities for children of varying ages *continued*

AGE	ACTIVITY	TYPE OF PLAY AND VALUE OF EQUIPMENT	BENEFITS FOR THE CHILD
6–8 YEARS	Photo-diary	Children can make their own as a record of their personal experience, or use a diary which has been produced by the hospital. These diaries: ■ encourage discussion ■ provide an in-depth explanation of a procedure	■ Childrens own diaries are valuable because they are a permanent and personal record of their hospital experience ■ They can be shown to their family, friends and school ■ They may be used to reassure other children who are going to have hospital treatment
6–8 YEARS	Video	Videos provide detailed information about general and/or specific topics. They can promote discussion with adults and other children.	■ Children who are reluctant to play can be helped by a video which they can control. They can see as little or as much as they like, as often as they like ■ They can watch alone if they prefer to do so

Remember

All activities and equipment for hospital play should be:
■ appropriate for the age and stage of the child
■ provided to meet individual needs.

 Progress check

1 What are the values of play in hospital?
2 What factors about the individual child should be taken into account when planning play in hospital?
3 What is pre-procedural play?
4 List three ways that this play will help the child.
5 Explain what post-procedural play involves.
6 What sort of distraction techniques may be used?
7 Describe therapeutic play.
8 What are the benefits of small world toys for children in hospital?
9 How can understanding of specific medical treatments be increased?

Activity

You are a qualified nursery nurse who has recently applied for a job as playleader on a paediatric ward at your local hospital. You are delighted to receive a letter inviting you to attend for an interview. The letter asks you to prepare a 5–10 minute presentation for the interview panel. The title is 'The Importance of Play in Hospital'.

Prepare for your interview in the following ways.

1 Prepare the presentation – decide which visual aids to use e.g. overhead projector transparencies, examples of play equipment etc.
2 Produce an A4 handout for the panel containing suitable play activities for children of various ages in hospital, giving reasons for your choice.

Care of the child in hospital

When a child is in hospital their care and treatment will be provided by nurses, doctors and a range of other professionals. Parents should always be encouraged to stay with the child.

The importance of parental involvement

In the 1950s and 1960s two child psychiatrists, James and Joyce Robertson, observed several children who were separated from their mothers during hospital stays or in residential nurseries. They noted that during periods of separation, many of the children went through a similar sequence of behaviour. This process, which occurs if children are separated and do not receive adequate care, is referred to as the *distress syndrome.*

The distress syndrome

The distress syndrome followed a pattern of behaviour shown by the children.

- It started with a period of *distress* or protest, shown by crying, screaming, and other expressions of anger at being left.
- This gave way to a period of *despair* when the children, apparently fearing their carer might not return, became listless, needed more rest, were dull, disinterested and refused to play.
- Finally there was a period of *detachment*: if the children became convinced that their carer would never return they appeared to try to separate themselves from any memory of the past. They were unable to make any deep relationships. Their behaviour lacked concentration; they flitted from one thing to another. Behaviour was also erratic; the children sometimes seemed dull and lifeless, sometimes highly active and excitable.

The Robertsons also noted the difficulty children experienced in linking up and relating to their mothers or carers when the separation ended. They followed up the children after separation and noted changes in their behaviour. They found that the separated children cried more than previously, had tantrums and did not show as much affection as before the separation. The Robertsons concluded that these separation experiences might have long-term effects.

As a result of this research many professions concerned with children have changed their practices to avoid the unnecessary separation of children from their parents.

These changes include parents being encouraged to remain with their children in hospital, and the provision of facilities for them to stay overnight

Support for parents

Parents must be made aware of their importance to the child while s/he is in hospital. Although many parents would be as distressed as the child at the thought of separation, separation anxiety should be explained to those parents who seem unaware of the effects of separation. They also need to know about what will happen whilst their child is in hospital and the way the child may react to the experience. The child's reaction will be helped by honesty from everyone involved in their care, especially parents, whose reactions are important. Hospital staff may gently tell them about the effects of their own anxiety on the child, and the need for a stress-free environment for the child.

Settling in to hospital – the role of the play leader

It is often the responsibility of the nursery nurse or play leader to welcome the child and the family to the ward. The following list highlights important factors in the settling-in process.

- Show the child their bed and locker and explain the ward routine as much as possible.
- Take the child on a guided tour of the ward include the playroom, toilets etc.
- Introduce them to other children on the ward and encourage social contact. Older children often like to look after the younger ones, and these relationships are beneficial to everyone.
- Find out from nursing colleagues how much the child has been told about her/his condition and treatment. This will make sure that you do not say anything inappropriate to the child or family.
- Explain everything clearly and never hide the truth. Be honest if a procedure will be uncomfortable. Children can deal with pain more successfully than they can cope with a dishonest adult.
- Ask the parents and nurses if the child has a special comforter, or if there are any special words or phrases which the child uses to explain their needs.
- Introduce play therapy which is appropriate for each individual child.
- Try to keep to the child's usual routine as much as possible – this can be very difficult in a hospital setting !

Good Practice

When caring for children childcare workers should remember the following points:
- children under 3 years benefit from a one-to-one relationship with a specific person
- the particular needs and background of children need to be known
- children's comfort objects should be readily available to them
- children should be provided with activities appropriate to their developmental age and stage, especially play that encourages the expression of feelings
- honest reassurance should be given
- children's parents or carers should have access whenever possible and appropriate
- children should have reminders of their parents or carers, such as photographs, and positive images of them should be promoted.

Meeting needs in hospital

Nursing care will be offered by qualified paediatric nurses and care assistants, who will find out about the child's usual routines from the parents. These will be continued as far as possible, although there will be inevitable changes to adapt to the hospital stay. Information from the parents will include:

- dietary needs and preferences
- sleeping habits, for example comforters, sleeping position and usual times of rests
- language including the child's stage of development and special words
- hygiene, for example how independent the child is at home, and in use of bath or shower
- toileting requirements, for example whether the child is in nappies, needs a nappy at night, or is fully toilet trained, or has any special words.

Hospital school

When children of compulsory school age are admitted to hospital, they should be given the opportunity to continue their education if they are well enough to do so. Most hospitals which care for children provide this service run in conjunction with the local education authority.

The hospital school should be staffed by qualified teachers and nursery nurses who are trained to provide the relevant educational opportunities, and have the necessary facilities to cater for children who are suffering from a variety of conditions.

This usually involves liaising with the teachers at the school the child usually attends if they are of statutory school age. Activities are provided to meet the requirements of the National Curriculum (Key Stage 1 for 5–7 year olds) and the Desirable Outcomes for children of nursery age.

Charter for children in hospital

ASC (Action for Sick Children) is a voluntary organisation which was created to promote the interests of children in hospital. The charity was set up after the publication of the Platt Report on The Welfare of Children In Hospital in 1959. It was previously known as NAWCH (National Association for the Welfare of Children in Hospital) which produced The Charter For Children In Hospital (see page 364). ASC tries to ensure that children's needs are considered at every level of the health service and that those needs are represented to the general public as well as to government. They recognise that children's health needs are a priority.

1 Children shall be admitted to hospital only if the care they require cannot be equally well provided at home or on a day basis.
2 Children in hospital shall have the right to have their parents with them at all times provided this is in the best interests of the child. Accommodation should be offered to all parents and they should be helped and encouraged to stay. In order to share the care of their

child, parents should be fully informed about ward routine and their active participation encouraged.

3 Children and/or their parents shall have the right to information appropriate to age and understanding.

4 Children and/or their parents shall have the right to informed participation in all decisions involved with their health care. Every child shall be protected from unnecessary medical treatment and steps taken to mitigate physical or emotional distress.

5 Children shall be treated with tact and understanding and at all times their privacy shall be respected.

6 Children shall enjoy the care of appropriately trained staff, fully aware of the physical and emotional needs each age group.

7 Children shall be able to wear their own clothes and have their own personal possessions.

8 Children shall be cared for with children from the same age group.

9 Children shall be in an environment furnished and equipped to meet their requirements, and which conforms to recognised standards of safety and supervision.

10 Children shall have full opportunity for play, recreation and education suited to their age and condition.

Activity

Using the information contained in the above charter, produce an information sheet for parents which tells them about the general principles of care their child will receive in hospital. Include:

■ what they can expect from the hospital staff
■ what their child can expect of them.

A child's eye view of hospital

Action for Sick Children (ASC) has conducted some research into children's perceptions of hospital. The following list of questions are those most commonly asked by children before they go into hospital and when they have been admitted.

■ What will they do to me?
■ Will I get better?
■ What will the doctor do/be like?
■ What will the nurse do/be like?
■ I want to go home!
■ Will I be blamed? – or laughed at?

These insecurities can be reduced with good preparation and play therapy.

Investigations

All of the investigations listed below, and any others which may be performed on a child in hospital or at a doctor's surgery require adequate preparation. The child must be told truthfully about what is going to happen. They should be with a trusted adult, usually a parent, and distraction techniques may be used.

Investigations

TYPE OF INVESTIGATION	WHAT HAPPENS	WHAT IT IS
Throat swab	The child will be asked to open the mouth for the doctor to look at the throat. The tongue is gently pressed down and a small swab is used to quickly brush the throat	A sample of the throat for bacteriological examination in the medical laboratories (pathology labs) The type of bacteria or virus causing an infection will be identified and the most suitable treatment (an antibiotic for a bacterial infection) will be provided
Blood tests	The doctor will insert a needle into a suitable vein – maybe in the back of the hand – and withdraw sufficient blood for the required test. EMLA cream should be used to reduce discomfort	Blood samples may be taken for a variety of reasons – the doctor will ask the laboratories to conduct specific tests e.g. haemoglobin levels if anaemia is suspected. The results will tell the doctor if the diagnosis is correct or if further tests are necessary
Urine sample	The child will be asked to provide a specimen of their urine if they are old enough to be able to do so at will. They will be asked to provide a midstream specimen (MSU). They should start to pass water into the toilet or bedpan, and then provide the specimen in a clean container. Babies and young children will wear a urine collecting bag until the sample has been obtained	Samples of urine may be sent for examination in the pathology labs (if an infection is suspected) or tested by the nursing and medical staff using equipment on the ward or in the doctor's surgery. Results will reveal the nature of the abnormality e.g. sugar in the urine suggests diabetes, protein in the urine may be caused by infection, blood requires further investigation
Sputum sample	If a child has a productive cough i.e. they are coughing up mucus from the chest, they will be asked to cough the mucus out into a specimen pot. This is difficult with young children as the natural reflex is to swallow	Samples of sputum will reveal the presence and type of infection, which can then be treated
Stool specimen	Samples of faeces are collected form the nappy, potty or bedpan and placed in a specimen pot for sending to the pathology laboratories	Examination will reveal the existence of some types of disease e.g. cause of diarrhoea, presence of blood, etc
Lumbar puncture	The child curls into a ball (fetal position) as the doctor first inserts a local anaesthetic into the lumbar region, and withdraws a specimen of cerebro-spinal fluid (CF) into a syringe	The sample of cerebro-spinal fluid (CSF) will confirm whether or not the child has meningitis and the type of pathogenic organism causing the illness. Bacterial infections can be treated with antibiotics and the most effective drug can be given to the child

The Children's Charter

The Children's Charter was published in 1996 and proposes new standards for child health services in England. The following recommendations have been adapted.

- Children and their parents have a right to express things in their own way and to be involved in decision making.
- Children should have impartial access to treatment and facilities that are available within the hospital for them.
- Children have a right to considerate and respectful care, which maintains their dignity at all times.
- Children and their parents have rights of privacy and confidentiality.

- Children have the right to be treated in a safe environment.
- Communications should be clear and in plain language. An understanding by the child as well as the parents is important. Help should be given to those with communication difficulties.
- Parents are welcome to participate in the care of their children when appropriate. Nursing staff will give adequate support.
- Parents have the right to stay with their child during the hospital stay. Accommodation or sleeping facilities will be provided.
- Children have the right to appropriate education and play facilities during their stay in hospital.
- Children and parents are entitled to know the name and the professional status of each person providing a service for them.
- Children and their parents have a right to be consulted about care being given or involvement in teaching and research.
- Children and their families are entitled to expect communication and liaison between hospital, community health services and other caring agencies.

 Progress check

1 Describe the distress syndrome.
2 Explain what can be done to prevent children experiencing such distress related to a hospital admission.
3 What support can be offered to parents to help them to cope with their child's admission to hospital?
4 What is the role of the playleader when a child is admitted to hospital?
5 What good practice points should the childcare worker be aware of when a child is in hospital?
6 How will the nursing staff try to meet the child's needs?
7 What is the role of the hospital school?
8 Explain the priorities of ASC contained in their charter.
9 What types of investigation may be conducted on children in hospital?
10 How can the playleader help the child to cope with these intrusive procedures?
11 Write a paragraph to explain the main points of the Children's Charter.

Key terms

You need to know what these words and phrases mean. Go back through the chapter and find out.

analgesic	antiparasitic
antibiotic	ASC (Action for Sick Children)
antiemetic	bronchodilator complications
antifungal	Children's Charter
antihistamine	corticosteroid

day care surgery
distraction techniques
distress syndrome
emergency admissions
EMLA cream
hospital school
laxative
lumbar puncture
medication
play specialst
post-procedural play

pre-admission unit
pre-procedural play
rectal administration
regression
respite care
sedative
sputum sample
stool specimen
tepid sponging
therapeutic play

Chapter 16 Coping with chronic illness

This chapter includes:

- **Effects on the family**
- **Support for families**
- **Effects of long-term illness on development**
- **Terminal care**
- **Dealing with sudden infant death in a childcare establishment**

This chapter should be read in conjunction with Chapter 5. Some childhood diseases and disorders are long-term (chronic) and require childcare workers to have a special degree of knowledge and understanding to support the child and family through some very difficult times. In order to do this effectively, carers must be able to offer, not only the appropriate care for a particular disorder, but empathy and understanding of the social and emotional effects of the situation on the child and the family.

The available support networks which will help families to cope are described. Accessing some assistance from the range of services provided by health professionals and social services will reduce the burden of practical care which families experience at this time.

The effects of long-term illness on development are many and varied. This chapter aims to highlight the different situations and experiences which may impact on development. Childcare workers must ensure that all needs are met so that the negative effects of illness are minimised.

Children may be so severely affected that their illness is terminal. This chapter will provide the childcare worker with valuable insight into the nature of loss and the range of reactions to such circumstances. Recognising the needs of the child and the coping strategies which may help families come to terms with their loss is invaluable for carers who are involved.

This knowledge should help to enable her/him to supply professional and effective care.

Effects on the family

When a baby is born, parents and families naturally expect that their son or daughter will grow and develop through childhood and into adulthood, perhaps ultimately having children of their own. Chronic illness or disability is not in this plan and as a society we are unprepared for dealing with the trauma of long-term illness and possible death in childhood. The birth of a baby with a serious disability, or the onset of a chronic disease during childhood, may produce similar reactions. Unless there is a family history of a genetic condition, illness and disability are always unexpected, something that may happen to 'other' children but not to our own.

Breaking the news

Some types of news will always bring pain and shock. The news that a child is suffering from a chronic, life-threatening illness or is terminally ill are examples. However, the way that the news is broken will affect the way that the parents come to terms with their situation and also their ability to cope.

Some parents of chronically ill children have never recovered from the way that they were told about their child's illness.

Professionals who tell parents that their child is very ill should remember that parents are very vulnerable at this time. They must continue to value the child and respect the parents by offering information and understanding that the initial shock may make the parents unreceptive to anything else that is said. Some parents report being 'dumbstruck' and unable to absorb the news. Contact between the parents and professionals should be maintained so that questions can be asked and answered when the parents are able to take information in. Sometimes the same information needs to be given several times before the parents can accept it.

Family reactions to chronic and terminal illness

When parents are told that their child has a serious or potentially life-threatening disorder they will experience a range of emotions. At this time parents usually experience the stages of grief associated with loss, i.e. the death of a person close to them.

The grieving process can be divided into early grief, acute grief and subsiding grief – parents will experience many conflicting feelings, not necessarily in the order below which suggests a systematic process to be worked through. If the child seems to get better and then relapses, they may return to the feelings of a previous stage at any time. The stages of grief which blend into each other are the following.

Initial shock

Even though parents and carers may suspect that their child has a serious or life-threatening illness, the confirmation of this will produce reactions of shock, denial, disbelief, numbness and panic. They may be too distressed to take in any of the explanations. They need the opportunity to ask questions and seek advice for a long time after the news is broken.

Confusion

This is a common reaction, probably because parents cannot understand why this is happening to their child. They may feel that their role as parent is in question and they cannot cope with what may happen in the future.

Fear

There may be an intense, almost physical, fear and a feeling of being trapped. This may result in what seems to be irrational behaviour to others.

Anger

There are feelings of unfairness that their child is seriously ill and may be dying. There may be reaction of 'Why is this happening to us?' Feelings of anger are very powerful and they may be directed at medical staff whom parents blame for their child's current condition. These outbursts should be treated with sensitivity and understanding – parents are often aware that they are not being reasonable, but they need to work through their emotions.

Guilt

Parents and carers often feel that their child's illness is their fault. They take personal responsibility for the situation, wishing that they had acted sooner or not done something. This is the 'If only' and 'What if?' stage of the grieving process. Because something has no rhyme or reason, parents try to explain it by blaming themselves.

Making decisions

Parents should be involved in every stage of their child's illness and be part of the decision-making process as much as possible, for example whether treatment should continue, what form it should take, where it should be given, such as physiotherapy at home or in hospital. Parents should also be asked what they believe their own and their child's needs are. The information given to families about their child's condition should be understood by them and given in language that they are familiar with; this will help them to make decisions for the child and for the family as a whole. They should not leave an appointment with a professional feeling that they have not been consulted, or had their views taken seriously.

- Family-centred care provides for the needs of the family as a unit. Parental involvement and participation in the care of their child is crucial.
- The cultural, religious and social circumstances of the family should be taken into account so that they are not expected to adopt behaviour that they are unaccustomed to.
- The physical and emotional needs of the parents are important. They should not be expected to perform technical tasks that they are uncomfortable with, such as using suction or changing dressings.
- Parents should be involved in developing care plans for the child at home, with the assistance and support of community nurses.

Professionals responding to parents

Qualified carers in the medical and allied professions should respond in the following ways.

- Be honest. Tell parents what is happening and give them time to ask questions and absorb information. Shutting them out by appearing to be too busy is destructive and prolongs their feelings of helplessness.
- Encourage parents to cry and show their feelings. It is important for them to find an emotional release. This applies to men and fathers too, who can find it difficult to express their intense sadness. Suppressing feelings may lead to psychological problems and later relationship difficulties.
- Allow parents to display their emotions. Feelings of sadness shown to parents by other carers can help them in their grieving process. It is important for parents to know that someone cares enough to share some of their feelings.

Good Practice

Childcare workers can be a valuable support for parents. They should be willing listeners and let the parents talk about their feelings and experiences. They should not avoid the subject or pretend that it has not happened.

Social implications

Parents at home with an ill child may feel the effects of isolation and loneliness because of difficulties in getting out of the home. They may also feel different from other families who are not having to cope with a seriously ill or disabled child. It is important for them to be able to meet new families and support groups involved in and experiencing similar difficulties.

There may be role changes within the family if a child needs long-term care. Both parents and siblings may need to rearrange their priorities and participate in the care of the ill child.

Relationship problems and marital difficulties are sometimes associated with caring for chronically ill children, because of the immense strain of caring for an ill child for 24 hours a day and 7 days a week.

Support from extended family is valuable if they are geographically close enough.

Financial implications

Parents who are caring for an ill child for a long period of time will probably have to make some financial readjustments. It could be that one parent has to stop working to provide full-time care at home for their ill child. This will mean that the household budget is drastically reduced. This, combined with increased costs to heat and light the home and even extra laundry, will make household bills larger. Transport costs to get to the hospital or assessment centre add to the financial burden. The family could experience the associated difficulties of poverty as a result.

Remember
Parents may need reassurance from professionals that how they feel is important and quite normal reactions to circumstances.

The Department of Social Security is the statutory body for authorising financial allowances and benefits paid by the Benefits Agency. Parents can claim certain state benefits, some of which are means tested (dependent upon the amount of household savings and income), and some of which are an entitlement regardless of savings or income. Parents should apply to the Benefits Agency who will have all the relevant information about which benefits the family may be entitled to claim. Benefits and allowances are constantly changing, the Citizens Advice Bureau and Welfare Rights organisations can give accurate and topical advice about which financial assistance a family is eligible to claim for.

Mobility may be difficult if the child finds walking impossible or difficult.

Case study

Rowena and Chris were very excited about the imminent birth of their first child who would be the first grandchild on both sides of the family. Baby Sam was born after a very difficult delivery when he was starved of oxygen and was diagnosed with severe cerebral palsy. The hospital staff were kind as they explained that Sam would be severely disabled and would need 24 hour care for the rest of his life. He was not expected to live for more than a few months. Rowena and Chris were devastated. They could not believe that their beautiful son, with his shock of blonde hair and peaceful expression, was going to die. Sam stayed in the hospital special care unit for 8 weeks before he was allowed to go home. He could not respond to sound or sights and found it difficult to cry. Rowena and Chris protected and cared for him for 24 hours a day, giving him their complete attention – going for hospital appointments, giving physiotherapy and oxygen, giving complicated doses of medicines and feeds. Sam's condition continued to deteriorate and he died in his sleep when he was 8 months old.

1 When and why do you think the grieving process started for this family?
2 Why was honesty from the health care team preferable?
3 What extra help was available from the support services?
4 What other support could be offered to the family?

Siblings

Brothers and sisters may feel the effects of having a very ill sibling in a variety of ways. Their experiences and reactions are not necessarily negative, a lot will depend upon their age and stage of development. Many siblings continue their special bond with their ill brother or sister. They are protective and supportive, and can help with general care and play suitable games together. Siblings can feel that their practical help is of real value, and so benefit from feelings of self-worth.

Other reactions may include other feelings.

Jealousy

The usual routine in the home may be abandoned as everything revolves around the needs of the ill child. A sibling may feel resentment and jealousy about all the attention that is given to their brother or sister. They may regress and develop attention-seeking behaviour as a reaction to the situation.

Neglect

Siblings may feel lonely, unloved and shut out as the attention of the family and the outside world is focused on the needs of the ill child. They may feel isolated because their previous activities have been postponed and they feel different to their friends.

Exploitation

Siblings may be required to take over some household tasks which were not previously asked of them. Parents may be tired if they have sleepless nights, and lack energy both as a result of their shock and grief and because of the physical and emotional resources required to provide 24-hour care for their sick child – caring for a seriously ill child is exhausting.

Guilt and fear

Feeling guilty that they are well and their sibling is very ill, and sometimes associated fear that they may 'catch' the illness. They may see their parents' sadness and be frightened by the adults' feelings.

Grief

Children, too, may react to the news, that their brother or sister is seriously ill or dying, by going through the grieving process. This can give the appearance of mood swings. Grief can be such an overpowering experience that the child may be affected in every area of growth and development. They may lose their appetite and energy, feeling too sad to play or to communicate. It is not unusual for grieving children to be self-absorbed and unable to concentrate, not wanting the company of their friends or relatives. It is essential to have an awareness of this when working with children who are experiencing grief.

> **Remember**
> Sibling reactions to traumatic events will depend a great deal on their age and stage of development.

Supporting siblings in their childcare establishment

Knowledge of the home circumstances will enable childcare workers to provide the correct balance of support and stimulation for the sibling(s) attending nursery or school. Carers should try to keep well informed of the situation and be aware of the child's level of knowledge to prevent them from disclosing incorrect or insensitive information. This awareness will enable them to:

- understand the child's feelings and behaviour
- be sensitive to the child's needs
- be able to provide and care for the child in the most appropriate way.

The following points draw attention to some aspects of the care which will help to support the child in all developmental areas.

- A key worker who has a strong bond with the child and will be able to provide continuity and consistency of care is vital in this situation.
- Observing the play and behaviour of the child will highlight any particular difficulties the child is experiencing.
- Encouraging the child to use play as a therapy will help them to work through their anxiety and express their feelings, for example resentment and sadness. Messy activities such as dough, sand, water and painting will enable children to release tension. Small world play and the home corner allow them to try to come to terms with the events in their home life.
- Making time to listen to the child and giving them the opportunity to speak to someone who will not judge them or be critical of them will allow them to express their feelings.
- Reassure them that they are special and very much loved by their family and carers. They may also need reassurance that this illness is not their fault and that they will not be affected by the same illness.

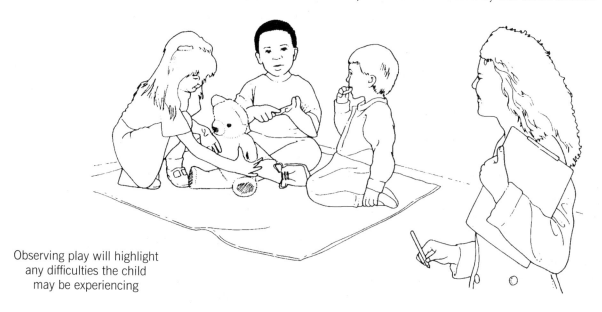

Observing play will highlight any difficulties the child may be experiencing

Dealing with a grieving child

The strength of feeling children have when they lose someone is directly linked to the strength of feeling they have for the person. The length of time the feelings last varies with the importance of the loss. Children may work through the stages of grief for a person within a year but it may take longer. The dates of special anniversaries associated with the lost person will generate memories.

People usually experience grief when they lose a person with whom they have an emotional bond. In any person's life the number of people with whom they have such a bond is quite limited. A child will probably only experience grief at the loss of a close carer or sibling.

Children are very vulnerable at times of loss. They need special consideration and care. However, it is probable that the adults who are closest to them are also suffering loss. This means that the child's needs may not always be given the highest priority. It is very common in white British culture, unlike, perhaps, Asian families, for children to be excluded during the period of mourning. They may not be informed of a death until later, they may not be allowed to attend a funeral even if they want to, or they may be sent away to stay with people who are not directly involved. This exclusion is probably the result of adults believing it is better not to upset the child, and also feeling that they do not have the emotional energy to cope with the child's grief as well as their own. Whatever the reasons, all available research shows that excluding a child at this time can create problems for the child. In the long term, their unexpressed and unresolved feelings can return and complicate their adult mental health. Children should be involved with the process of mourning and be allowed to say good-bye and to attend the funeral.

Adults who are not themselves involved in the grief of a child, for example childcare workers and teachers, can be of great help to a child. They can give the child uncomplicated attention and consideration. Despite this many adults find such involvement difficult. This may be because:

- they do not understand the process of grief or the appropriate way to respond
- some adults have unresolved grief. This could be because they were denied a period of mourning when they were young. Contact with a grieving child can therefore activate painful memories
- they have a fear of death which is very common, and unconsciously want to avoid any contact with it.

Avoidance of the subject will not help the child. It should be a part of all childcare workers' training to learn about the process of grief and examine their own feelings and attitudes.

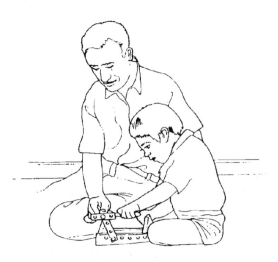

Uncomplicated attention from the child-care workers can help children to cope with grief

✅ *Progress check*

1 Why is it important for professionals to be careful about the way they tell parents about their child's illness?
2 What are the stages of grief which parents may experience?
3 Why do you think parents may feel guilty about the diagnosis?
4 How can parents be supported to make decisions on behalf of their child?
5 How can professionals help parents to cope with their situation?
6 What are the social implications for a family caring for a chronically ill child?
7 Why do some families experience financial difficulties as a result of a child's chronic illness?
8 Which feelings may siblings experience when their brother or sister is very ill and why?
9 How can siblings be supported to cope with the situation?
10 Why do some adults find it difficult to cope with a grieving child?

Case study

Anthony aged 7 years and Jessica aged 4 years were devoted to their grandparents, Arthur and Margaret, who lived 60 miles away from the family. Despite the distance, granny and granddad visited often, usually bringing small presents for the children. They went on holidays with the family and took the children for exciting trips to the fair, pantomimes and circus. The family also visited them at weekends, and the children sometimes stayed for a few days enjoying the undivided attention that they received, going for bike rides with granddad and devouring granny's tasty homemade cakes and biscuits. Margaret had a heart attack suddenly one Saturday. The children's mother, Lesley, went to comfort Arthur after explaining to the children that granny was very ill. She died early on Monday morning. Lesley left her father with her brother, to return home and collect the children. She met Anthony from school and gently told him that granny had died. He was distraught and wanted to see her. Jessica took the news more calmly and asked several questions about dying. Lesley answered as best she could despite her own intense grief. The children went to see their granny in the chapel of rest and kissed her good-bye. They thought she looked as though she was asleep. They stayed with their mother and grandfather and helped to arrange the funeral. Anthony read a children's prayer at the service and both children laid a red rose on the coffin. The family continued to talk about Margaret, and after the initial deep sadness they could laugh about their happy memories and be glad that they had had such a special grandmother.

1 How do you feel about the way that this family handled the grieving process for the children?

2   What are the benefits of including children in the period of mourning?
3   Write down any memories you have about the death of a loved adult when you were a child. Think about how your experiences may affect your ability to relate to a grieving child.

Activity

Research the different religious and cultural beliefs and customs about death and mourning which may relate to the families in your establishment.

Support for families

There are several support networks for families who are caring for a child with a long-term illness at home. They are mainly provided by the statutory agencies (the health service, social services and local education authorities) and are complemented by a range of voluntary agency provision. Ideally, the professional workers from each area should liaise with each other to provide the care which meets the individual needs of the child and family. In reality the level of support offered to families can depend on:

- where the family lives
- the nature of the illness
- the hospital caring for the child
- awareness of local health visitors and GPs.

National Health Service support

Hospital paediatric services

Doctors, nurses, physiotherapists, occupational therapists and dieticians provide:

- care for the child
- support and advice for their colleagues working in the community.

Some children will require regular periods of intensive treatment in hospital and may go home feeling very ill, especially after chemotherapy. Liaison between hospital, the primary health care team (PHCT) and parents is vital if good care is to be maintained.

Primary health care team

The services provided in the community include the Community Child Health Services. As well as the services of the GP and health visitor, home nursing may be provided by trained community paediatric nurses who can provide specialised care and support. Specialist therapists in the

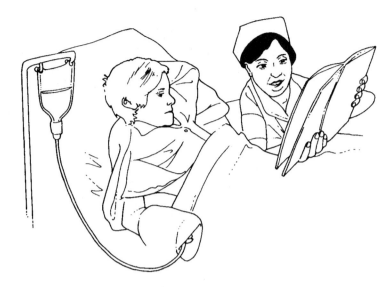

Hospital staff support and
care for ill children

community may be involved, depending on the individual circumstances, such as physiotherapy for a child with cystic fibrosis. Families with a supportive PHCT are the families who cope most successfully with a child with a serious illness.

More details of the PHCT and other health services are given in Chapter 5.

School health service

When the child returns to school, the school nurse and community paediatrician will be involved in monitoring the child's health and their ability to cope with full or part-time school.

Aids and equipment

Health and social services will arrange for the loan of vital pieces of equipment such as wheelchairs, ramps, bath aids etc.

Respite care

Some health authorities are able to arrange for parents to have a break from their 24-hour care. Comfortable and homely settings are preferable. Children's hospices and paediatric hospital wards may offer care if the child is terminally ill (see page 383).

Social Services support

Social workers

Families with a seriously ill child may require the assistance of a hospital based or community social worker. The social worker can help by offering support and advice about available resources, benefits, day care and respite care facilities and counselling.

Family centres, day nurseries and nursery centres

Family centres work to support the family by helping them to adjust to new circumstances and offering practical help in their childcare arrangements.

Day nurseries offer high quality care for the ill child enabling the family to spend time with their other children

Nursery centres are jointly organised with the local education authority (LEA).

Any of these facilities may be also available to the siblings of an ill child who may benefit from additional stimulation and contact with their peer group.

Family aides

These workers can visit the home on a daily basis to offer practical household help and child care.

Transport costs

Visits to hospital and travelling to day care settings can be expensive. Social services may be able to help the family by providing transport or covering the cost of taxis, trains or buses.

Financial advice

Social services departments can sometimes provide cash grants to families in need. They may be able to help the family untangle the complicated benefits system and provide assistance in competing applications for grants and benefits.

 Progress check

1 Which agencies offer support to families who are caring for a child with a chronic illness?
2 What does the level of support offered to families depend upon?
3 What is respite care?
4 How can social services childcare provision help the whole family?

Case study

Jawaid is 5 years old and had bacterial meningitis at the age of 3. His serious illness resulted in damage to his brain leaving him deaf and with severe learning difficulties. His epilepsy is controlled with drugs but he still has frequent seizures, usually at night which means that his parents and four brothers are often woken by his screams of fear. He cannot be comforted by voice and sounds, so his parents soothe him and gently massage him back to sleep. He attends a unit for hearing impaired children and is assisted there by a special needs support assistant. Family life has changed since he was a bright and lively 3-year-old.

1 Which statutory services could be used to benefit Jawaid and his family?
2 What are the effects on the family of coping with a child with special needs after such a sudden illness?

Effects of long-term illness on development

Childcare workers should consult with health staff about the possible effects of a particular condition so that they are well prepared and are able to offer appropriate care and activities to stimulate and interest the child. Consulting with parents and colleagues who have experience of the child and also reading topical literature will all help to provide an overview of the child and their condition. This research will be valuable in enabling the highest quality of provision to be offered in the childcare establishment and at home.

The effects of chronic illness will vary and depend on the nature and length of the illness. However, there are some factors which are common to many chronic illnesses.

Schooling

Childcare workers must work closely with parents and other carers to minimise the disruption caused by erratic school and nursery attendance. Written information about the particular child is valuable. Two-way communication about the child's progress at home and at school enables a thorough sharing of information.

- Frequent and recurrent illness will lead to poor school attendance.
- Associated difficulties in 'keeping up' with other children of the same age.
- All areas of development may be affected, for example play, communication skills such as reading and writing, and physical achievements will depend on the child's motor development and capability.

Emotional and social

- Development of strong peer group relationships may be difficult if attendance at school is disrupted. The child may lack confidence in making relationships.
- Some parents and carers may respond to chronic or life-threatening illness by over-protecting the child. This will affect self-esteem and prevent the child from learning from their own experience.
- Bullying of children who have chronic illness is more common as some children focus on the most vulnerable members of the group.

Childcare workers must be aware of this and be constantly vigilant for anti-social behaviour from other children and any signs of anxiety, distress or fear from the ill child.

■ Loss of independence or failure to develop independent living skills will reduce a child's self-esteem. This may be because adults find it easier to do a task for a child instead of allowing them the time to do it for themselves. Carers should allow the required amount of time and remain patient and relaxed if the child feels well and prefers to complete a task themselves.

Physical

Effects on physical skills will depend upon the nature of the illness and the parts of the body which are involved. Long-term illness and lack of exercise can result in muscle weakness and loss of previously acquired physical skills. Children will need gentle encouragement to increase their physical activity as they recover and regain their energy and strength.

Children with physical disabilities need physiotherapy to encourage mobility and movement and to help with posture and balance. They may need help with using the toilet and getting dressed and some children may need to be fed by their carer(s).

If children need to be lifted or carried, carers must be instructed about the most appropriate methods to use, to ensure both the safety of the child and their own well-being.

Equipment

Specialised equipment may be required, for example:
■ wheelchairs, crutches, braces, frames and callipers to enable the child to be mobile
■ aids for feeding.

Intellectual

Regression in all areas of development is to be expected when a child is ill. Drug treatments may cause difficulty in concentration and memory, problem solving and imagination may be impaired.

Language

Children need to be able to listen, to understand and to speak so that they can interact verbally. Any condition which affects any of these skills will affect their ability to communicate verbally.

Lack of stimulation and feeling too poorly to participate verbally in conversations will affect language development.

Good Practice

Supporting children with chronic illness in an educational setting can be achieved in various ways.

1 Allocating a key worker to the child who can maintain personal contact and involvement with the child and the family.
2 Involving parents in their child's care and working in partnership with them to achieve goals.
3 Knowing and meeting the child's individual needs:
   - physical needs, for example feeding, toileting or exercise should be met with sensitivity
   - enabling the child to access equipment and resources
   - encouraging relationships and independence skills
   - boosting self-esteem by offering praise and achievable tasks
   - offering a language-rich curriculum.
4 Keeping thorough records of the child's achievements:
   - observations
   - behaviour
   - peer group relationships.
5 Holding regular team meetings to discuss the child's progress and to plan future activities. These should be recorded.
6 Liaison with other professionals, as necessary, within the establishment and in other organisations.

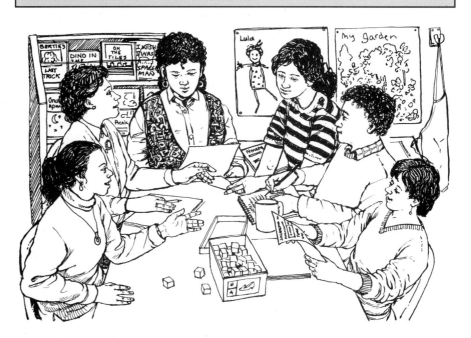

Regular team meetings provide the opportunity to discuss children's progress

Telling the child

Children should be told the truth about traumatic events that involve them personally or concern their family. If they are told simply, and in a way that they will understand, they can learn to accept changes. It is essential that adults are honest with children if they know what is going to happen. Children need the opportunity to ask questions and be able to trust that they will be answered honestly. They will then need help and support to adjust to the life-changing events. How they are told can affect the way they cope with the news.

Children under 4 years find it difficult to accept the permanence of change or understand that somebody who has died will not come back. Gentle reassurance from adults who understand that children do not have the same sense of proportion will enable them to come to terms with the situation.

Parents may delay telling children about divorce or death because they think that the child will not be able to cope or that the time is not right for disclosure. This is not helpful as children will feel shut out and may feel responsible for the event if they have been excluded from the process. They need reassurance that it is not their fault.

Good Practice

Childcare workers can help children to come to terms with traumatic events by:
- giving the child the opportunity to talk about how they feel, knowing that they will be listened to and not judged
- offering reassurance and support, physically and emotionally
- providing consistency of care and some stability will help the child to feel secure and more able to cope.

 Progress check

1 How can childcare workers prepare themselves for caring for a child with chronic illness?
2 How can recurrent absence from school affect development?
3 How can long-term illness affect emotional and social development?
4 How can a child best be supported in a childcare establishment?
5 Why is it important to always tell a child the truth?
6 How can childcare workers help children to come to terms with traumatic events?

Activity

Using the information contained in this chapter and in Chapters 13 and 14, make a table highlighting the possible effects on development of the following conditions:
- cystic fibrosis
- muscular dystrophy
- asthma

Use a format similar to this:

	Cystic fibrosis	Muscular dystrophy	Asthma
Physical			
Intellectual			
Language			
Emotional			
Social			

Terminal care

A terminal illness is an illness which cannot be actively treated with drugs or any other therapy. Relief of signs and symptoms is the aim of terminal care because the condition cannot be cured.

Some parents will know that their child is going to die because the treatment has not been successful or there is no cure for the condition. This knowledge will enable them to plan for the care of the child and decide where they want their child to die. In may be possible for doctors to give some indication of how long the child will live, but this is not always accurate. The death may be sudden or the child may live for a longer time than expected.

Each family can decide upon their own plan of care in liaison with the care team, they may prefer the child to be cared for in a hospice or in hospital but most children with terminal illness die at home. Although families may be apprehensive about their child dying at home, good support and a feeling of being in control in familiar surroundings will often create the best and most comfortable circumstances for all the family. Families are supported so that they can care for their child at home. The family can be in frequent contact with the home-care paediatric nurse who acts as the consultant to the family in providing care for their child. During the home visits home-care nurses also provide emotional support to the child's family.

Hospices for children

Some dying children are cared for in children's hospices which, as well as providing terminal care, also offer respite care for children whose families need some relief from the constant pressure of caring for a seriously ill child. There are very few hospice facilities for children nationally and they offer practical and emotional support for children and families. Staff consider the all round well-being of the child as the central focus of the care which is offered.

Some hospices provide community teams to go into homes to give family support and intensive physical care to the child. They also provide education for other professions such as the police, GPs, paediatricians and funeral directors in the practicalities and counselling skills needed for dealing with death in childhood.

Coping with the death of a child

The death of a child is always difficult to accept now. A hundred years ago it was not unusual, it was expected that some children would not survive to adulthood, and most families experienced infant death. The death of a child today, when there are so many ways of preventing death, seems to be a far greater tragedy. The loss of a child is devastating and the parents and family are left with a void in their lives.

Relating to parents

- Be prepared to face difficult situations. You may feel that you don't know what to say. This is because we are conditioned to try to make things better, and we realise that words can never take away the sadness when a child dies. A simple gesture like a touch of the hand may give more comfort than any words.
- Never say 'I know how you feel'. Unless you have experienced the death of a child it is impossible to know how it feels.
- Remember that the whole family is grieving and give a lot of attention to brothers and sisters. They will be finding it difficult to cope with the loss of their sibling and not know how to deal with their feelings.
- Offer support and practical help without imposing solutions. Parents may benefit from time on their own to deal with their feelings. Caring for the other children for a few hours to give them some space is a practical way to help.

Cultural awareness of grief and mourning

A knowledge of and a respect for different customs and beliefs is very important when working with children whose cultural and religious background is different from your own. The mourning period is the time when people show conventional signs of grief, such as wearing black or wearing white, weeping together, closing curtains. Different cultural practices for dealing with death and mourning should be accepted and respected. Without this knowledge a childcare worker might respond inappropriately by offering words of comfort that may even be offensive.

A child's perception of death

Children may have some experiences of death, the loss of a loved pet for instance. Loss and separation are also a part of many of their experiences. How they think about these things depends on how the adults close to them react and on the explanations they give. Death is often a subject which is not spoken about and the thought is pushed away. Adults should confront their feelings and think through ideas so that they are able to answer children's questions. Avoidance of the subject will not help the child.

The child's understanding will be limited by:
- previous experience

- language development
- grasp of the concept of time
- intellectual development.

Children who are dying often have very clear images, fears and concerns about death. Adults may say that a child does not know that they are dying, but many children do realise and must be given the opportunity to express their feelings, however difficult this may be for adults. Usually, when adults say that a child does not talk about death, it means that the child has not been given the chance to talk freely and honestly.

The young child, under 7, thinks that death is reversible, a state of sleep or separation, from which the person could return. Perhaps the main fear for the young child who is dying is thinking about separation and going into a darkness where there is no one familiar to give love and comfort.

Children will express their fears in very different ways:

- they may want close physical comfort and someone to listen and talk to them.
- they may also express their fears in anger.

Their anger can often be directed at the person closest to them emotionally, someone they love and trust. This can often be very hard for loving parents and carers, but it is an indication of the child's feelings of trust in them.

✔ Progress check

1 What is terminal care?
2 How can families be supported to care for a terminally ill child at home?
3 What sort of support can children's hospices offer?
4 How can carers relate to parents and offer support when the child has died?
5 Why should carers have an awareness of cultural variations in grief and mourning?
6 What does a child's perception of death depend on?
7 How may children express their fears?

Case study

When he was 4, Joe was diagnosed with acute lymphoblastic leukaemia. He was constantly in hospital having treatment for the condition which included chemotherapy to kill the abnormal cells. Although this was difficult at times, his hair fell out and he caught various infections, Joe went into remission and it seemed that the condition had been cured. Nine months later a routine blood test revealed that the leukaemia was back. Tests had already shown that his older sister Mary, aged 7, was a suitable match to be a bone marrow donor. Again, Joe had massive doses of chemotherapy to destroy all his bone marrow and Mary had a general anaesthetic to donate her healthy marrow for transfusion to Joe. The procedure went well and seemed to have worked, but Joe's body eventually rejected the bone marrow transplant and the leukaemia returned. His parents decided that Joe should not have to endure any more aggressive treatment so that he could enjoy the life he had left. The doctors said that he may survive for up to a year, so the family planned to do as much as possible together.

Soon after returning from a trip to EuroDisney Joe's condition began to deteriorate. He asked his father if he was going to die now but his father could not answer him. His parents struggled with their earlier decision to stop the treatment, but consoled themselves with the knowledge that Joe had had the time of his life in the past 6 months. They cared for him at home and the GP and community nurses provided treatment and support for Joe and his family. He died peacefully in his bedroom at 3 o'clock one morning while his parents held him.

1 Explain how the course of Joe's illness, treatment and death may have affected Mary.
2 What do you think about the parents' decision to discontinue Joe's treatment?
3 Why did Joe's father find it difficult to talk to him about death?
4 How could Joe have been helped to talk about his feelings?

Dealing with sudden infant death in a childcare establishment

Sudden infant death does not only occur at night when a child is sleeping in their bed or cot at home. It is no respecter of time or place. Unfortunately, some deaths have occurred whilst young children have been sleeping in their day nursery cot or whilst in the care of a nanny or child-minder. It is important for all childcarers to know:
■ what to do in the event of finding such a child
■ how to deal with the practical situation
■ how to respond to parents
■ the possible impact of their feelings.

If a child is pale and unresponsive when the childcare worker attempts to rouse him/her from a nap, check for breathing and pulse and if they are absent the staff team should do the following.
■ Give first aid immediately following the approved guidelines – Cardio-Pulmonary Resuscitation (CPR) by the first aider on duty.
■ Call an ambulance.
■ Contact parents and explain that the child is very ill and the ambulance has been called. Suggest that they go directly to the hospital.
■ Remove all the other children to a play area away from the ill child.
If you are a nanny or child-minder working on your own, start CPR and

carry the child to the phone continuing resuscitation while you wait for the ambulance to arrive.

Good Practice

Each childcare establishment should have a certified first-aider in duty at all times, and it is recommended that all carers complete a recognised first aid qualification.

The police will be involved and may need to take evidence from the home or nursery, such as the mattress, bedding and clothing. Statements will be taken from those people directly involved.

When anyone (a child or an adult) dies suddenly and unexpectedly, a post mortem has to be conducted to find the cause of death. The results of the post mortem are reported to the coroner who may hold an inquest to establish exactly who died and when, where and how death occurred.

Support for staff

Everyone involved in the death of a child will be severely traumatised by it. The staff of a nursery will be in a state of shock – as they work with healthy children, they do not expect to experience death in the setting and consequently feel that they have failed. Their family and friends may not understand the depth of their feelings of sadness and loss and urge them to pull themselves together. To avoid feeling isolated staff need to work through their grief together – they are the ones who understand each other. They can be helped in this by counselling organisations such as CRUSE and FSIDS.

 Progress check

1 Why may SIDS happen in a childcare establishment?
2 What should a childcare worker do if s/he finds an unconscious child?
3 How could staff support the parents and each other if this happened in a nursery?

Key terms

You need to know what these words and phrases mean. Go back through the chapter and find out.

chronic illness	**respite care**
family aides	**school health service**
family centres	**social worker**
hospice	**terminal care**
primary health care team	**terminal illness**

Glossary

aromatherapy Using natural oils from flowers, fruits and other parts of plants to improve physical and mental well-being.

active immunity The body develops immunity by producing antibodies.

amniocentesis The removal of a small sample of amniotic fluid from the uterus, via the abdominal wall.

analgesic Painkilling drug e.g. paracetamol.

antibiotic A drug which kills bacteria.

antibodies Proteins which protect the body against infection. They have a 'memory' and can recognise antigens (foreign substances) they have been in contact with before.

antiemetic A drug which treats sickness and nausea.

antifungal A drug which kills fungi.

antihistamine A drug which prevents itching.

antiparasitic A drug which kills parasites infesting the body.

antiseptic A chemical which prevents the growth of germs without necessarily killing them all.

ASC (Action for Sick Children) A voluntary organisation to promote the interests of children in hospital.

assessment The term used to describe what happens when a child is being examined to detect what the problem is i.e. when the diagnosis is being made.

axillary temperature Under the arm temperature.

bacteria A pathogenic micro-organism.

bronchodilator A drug which dilates the breathing passages.

child development centre A unit to provide specialised assessment, support and treatment for chronically ill or disabled children.

child guidance Specialised support for children and their families.

child health clinic Health visitor's and GP's clinics to monitor the health, development and progress of children under the age of 5 years.

child health surveillance A system of reviewing children's progress.

Children's Charter Published in 1996 to propose new standards for child health services in England.

chiropodist A professional specialising in care of the feet and treatment of foot conditions.

chorionic villus sampling The removal of a small sample of placental tissue via the cervix.

chromosome A unit of inheritance.

chronic illness A long-term disease or disorder.

cilia Fine hair-like projections which waft mucous, germs and dirt outside the body.

complementary medicine Treatment which provides a holistic approach i.e. cares for the whole child or person which can be used to complement traditional treatments.

complications Further illness or disability caused by the original illness.

congenital A condition that has developed during pregnancy and can sometimes be prevented.

congenital dislocation of the hip Misplacement of the hip joint.

contraception Preventing pregnancy.

corticosteroid A drug which reduces the inflammatory

response in some conditions.

day care surgery Children are admitted in the morning, a few hours before the surgery takes place, and as soon as they have recovered sufficiently they can be taken home.

dental caries Tooth decay.

developmental surveillance A continuous process which monitors a child's whole progress, not restricted to particular ages.

diarrhoea Loose, frequent motions.

disinfectant Chemicals which kill all micro-organisms.

distraction hearing test Routine test, of a baby's ability to locate sounds, performed between 6–9 months of age.

distraction techniques Play used when children are going through a particular procedure to take their attention away from their situation. It helps to relieve their anxiety.

distress syndrome During periods of separation children usually experience a similar sequence of behaviour distress, despair and detachment.

dominant inheritance One parent carries a dominant gene for a particular disorder so there is a 1:2 chance of this being passed on with each pregnancy.

drug Any substance which is used for its effects on the way the body works.

earache Pain in and around the ear.

eclampsia The onset of convulsions during pregnancy.

education social worker A profes-sional who is primarily concerned with school attendance.

educational psychologist A professional who is primarily concerned with the assessment of children's learning difficulties.

emergency admission Admission to hospital as the result of an accident or sudden, unexpected disease.

EMLA cream Ointment which is used to anaesthetise the skin on the injection site.

endocrine Ductless glands which pass their secretions directly into the bloodstream, for distribution around the body, to their 'target' organ.

family aides Workers who visit the home on a daily basis to offer practical household help and child care.

family centres Facilities to support the family by helping them to adjust to new circumstances and offering practical help in their childcare arrangements.

febrile convulsion A seizure caused by a raised temperature in childhood.

fleas Small insects which are able to bite through skin and suck blood.

folic acid A vitamin which is important in the formation of the brain and spinal cord.

fungi Simple, parasitic life-forms.

genetic counselling A service offered to couples with a family history of any inherited condition. They are informed of the potential risks to their future pregnancy and services are provided for prenatal testing.

genetics The study of inherited conditions which are passed from parent(s) to child.

Guthrie test A heel prick blood test performed on the 6th day to detect phenylketonuria and cystic fibrosis.

head lice Small insects living in hair close to the scalp.

health education The education of children, parents and carers about issues that affect health.

health promotion Encouraging positive and healthy lifestyles by promoting good health practices.

health visitor A professional specialising in preventive health, sometimes concentrating on the under-fives.

herd immunity The phrase used to describe the status of the whole population when enough people are immunised to prevent the spread of the disease.

hip tests Manoeuvres to check the stability of the hip joints.

holistic The holistic approach to child health means meeting the needs of the *whole child* and not concentrating on one part at a time.

homeopathy Treatments based on using natural substances to treat a wide range of conditions.

hormone A chemical substance which is made in one part of the body and carried in the bloodstream to act on tissues or organs in another part

hospice Dying children may be cared for in a children's hospice which, as well as providing terminal care, also offers respite care for children whose families need some relief from the constant pressure of caring for a seriously ill child.

hospital school A school for children of compulsory school age who are in hospital, usually run in partnership with the local education authority.

hygiene The study of health involving all aspects of keeping children well and healthy, including promoting cleanliness and safety and preventing the spread of infection.

immunisation The use of vaccines to protect people from disease.

immunity The ability of the body to resist infection.

inequalities in health Social status and the provision of health care affect people's health status.

inverse care law The amount of health care and advice available and accepted is inversely proportional to the level of need.

laxative A drug which softens faeces.

leucocytes White blood cells.

lumbar puncture A procedure used to provide a sample of cerebro-spinal fluid from the back in the lumbar region.

lymphoid tissue Cells which produce antibodies with a protective role in preventing and fighting infection.

malaise Tiredness and lethargy.

Maslow's hierarchy of needs A theory of needs which places all needs in an order of priority.

medication Treatment with drugs to reduce symptoms and/or cure the illness.

micro-organisms Very small cells.

mortality rates Statistics gathered yearly to assess the death rates for a range of conditions and age-groups.

mucous membrane The lining of all the external entrances to the body which secrete mucous to trap germs and other particles carried in the air.

nature and nurture The amount of potential given to a child is decided by heredity (nature) and the environment determines the extent to which that potential develops (nurture).

neonatal mortality Death in the first 28 days of life.

non-accidental injury Deliberate injury caused to a child.

occupational therapist A professional usually based in the local authority social services department who may visit homes to assess disability and recommend aids and equipment for families with a disabled child/ren.

osteopathy The practice of manipulation, correcting disorders of the body with massage, movement and exercise.

paediatric nurse A qualified children's nurse.

paediatric services Care for the child provided by doctors, nurses, physiotherapists, occupational therapists, dieticians and other specialised health staff.

passive immunity The body develops resistance to infection after antibodies, created in another organism, are introduced into them.

pathogen Disease causing micro-organism

perinatal At the time of birth

Personal Child Health Record Children's main surveillance and health record which is held by the parents.

physiotherapist A professional specialising in exercise and physical activity programmes to encourage gross motor skills and co-ordination, and to prevent the disabling effects of illness or accidents.

play specialist A qualified nursery nurse who has completed some extra training in hospital play.

pollution The result of contamination with harmful substances.

postnatal The period of 6 weeks after the birth.

post-procedural play Play which allows children to play out their experiences after the medical or surgical treatment.

practice nurse A qualified nurse employed by a GP who is responsible for performing practical treatments in the surgery or health centre.

pre-admission unit Children may be invited to a clinic a few days before their admission so that they can be examined before they come into hospital.

pre-conceptual Before pregnancy begins.

pre-eclampsia A condition that occurs only during pregnancy which is characterised by high blood pressure, swelling of the tissues (oedema), protein in the urine and excessive weight gain.

prenatal The period of pregnancy before birth.

pre-procedural play Play preparation used by play specialists and other professional hospital staff to help children to prepare for medical or surgical procedures e.g. a blood test, an operation, an X-ray.

primary health care team A team of health professionals based in the community to meet the health needs of the population.

primary prevention The first stage of disease prevention which involves attempts to reduce the number of children being affected by a disease or disorder.

pyrexia High temperature.

recessive inheritance If both parents carry a defective gene for a particular disorder there is a 1:4 chance of the disorder being passed on with each pregnancy.

rectal administration Drugs given by suppositories into the rectum.

reflexology A deep foot massage which stimulates the reflexes in the foot and hopes to return the body to a state of balance.

refractive errors A term used when the eye is not functioning as a perfect visual system.

regression Reverting to a slightly earlier developmental stage.

respite care A period caring for children who have a long-term illness or disability, to review their care and treatment and also to give their main carers a break.

roundworm Intestinal worms that are round when cut in cross-section and are pointed at both ends.

scabies External animal parasites affecting areas where the skin is thin.

school health service A team of professionals concerned with the health care of children at school.

screening The examination of apparently healthy children to find those who probably do have a condition from those who probably do not.

sebum A bactericidal substance (preventing the growth of bacteria) produced by the skin which prevents the drying of the skin.

secondary prevention The second stage of disease prevention, detecting early signs of illness so that the effects of the illness can be reduced.

sedative A drug which reduces anxiety.

sex-linked inheritance A condition passed from mothers to their sons on the X chromosome.

sign A symptom of illness which can be seen e.g. rash.

social disadvantage The situation of people who do not have the equal opportunity to achieve what other people in society regard as normal.

social worker A trained person who specialises in offering support and advice about available resources, benefits, day care and respite care facilities and counselling for children and families.

speech discrimination test A test involving the use of a set of small toys all with a single syllable name which will test the child's ability to hear different consonants like p, g, d, m, s, f, b.

sputum sample A specimen of the fluid coughed up from the respiratory tract.

squint The eyes do not work together properly, one eye seems to be looking in another direction.

stool specimen A sample of faeces.

sudden infant death syndrome Unexpected and unexplained death in infancy.

surveillance A programme of care to monitor children's health and prevent illness.

sweep test A hearing test on school entrants which involves the child in wearing a pair of earphones and listening for tones produced by an audiometer.

symptom Something experienced by the individual concerned e.g. pain or discomfort or general feelings of illness.

tapeworm Worms with flattened bodies which belong to a group of animals known as flatworms.

tepid sponging Attempts to reduce the temperature by bathing with lukewarm water.

terminal care The relief of signs and symptoms when the condition cannot be cured.

terminal illness An illness which cannot be actively treated with drugs or any other therapy and will lead to death.

tertiary prevention The third stage of disease prevention, aimed at reducing the effects of a particular disease or condition and minimising the suffering caused.

therapeutic play Play to encourage exercise and feelings of well-being which will help the child to cope with their illness.

threadworm Worms which live in the bowel and look like small, white threads in freshly passed stools.

ultrasound scan An echo-sounding device which uses high-frequency sound waves used to check fetal development in pregnancy.

virus Smallest pathogenic organism which cannot be seen under a traditional microscope.

vomiting Sickness resulting in the expulsion of the contents of the stomach.

Index